Heinz Häfner (Editor)

Risk and Protective Factors in Schizophrenia

Heinz Häfner (Editor)

assisted by
Wolfram an der Heiden · Franz Resch · Johannes Schröder

Risk
and Protective Factors
in Schizophrenia

Towards
a Conceptual Model
of the Disease Process

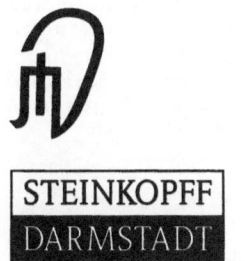

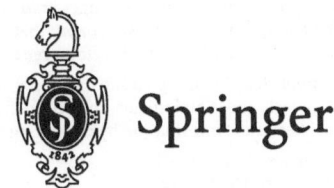

Editor
PROF. DR. DR. DRES. H. C. HEINZ HÄFNER
Schizophrenia Research Unit
Central Institute of Mental Health
J 5
68159 Mannheim, Germany
hhaefner@as200.zi-mannheim.de

assisted by
DR. WOLFRAM AN DER HEIDEN
Schizophrenia Research Unit
Central Institute of Mental Health
J 5
68159 Mannheim, Germany
adheiden@as200-zi-mannheim.de

PROF. DR. JOHANNES SCHRÖDER
Section of Geriatric Psychiatry
University of Heidelberg
Voßstraße 4
69115 Heidelberg, Germany
johannes_schroeder@med.uni-heidelberg.de

PROF. DR. FRANZ RESCH
Department of Child and Adolescent
Psychiatry
Psychiatric University Hospital
Blumenstraße 8
69115 Heidelberg, Germany
franz_resch@med.uni-heidelberg.de

ISBN 978-3-642-63282-2   ISBN 978-3-642-57516-7 (eBook)
DOI 10.1007/978-3-642-57516-7

Cataloging-in-Publication Data applied for
Bibliographic information published by Die Deutsche Bibliothek. Die Deutsche Bibliothek lists this publication in the Deutsche Nationalbibliografie; detailed bibliographic data is available in the Internet at http://dnb.ddb.de

http://www.steinkopff.springer.de

© Springer-Verlag Berlin Heidelberg 2002
Originally published by Steinkopff Verlag Darmstadt in 2002
Softcover reprint of the hardcover 1st edition 2002

The use of general descriptive names, registered names, trademarks, etc. in this publication does not imply, even in the absence of a specific statement, that such names are exempt from the relevant protective laws and regulations and therefore free for general use.

Product liability: The publishers cannot guarantee the accuracy of any information about the application of operative techniques and medications contained in this book. In every individual case the user must check such information by consulting the relevant literature.

Production: Heinz J. Schäfer
Cover Design: Erich Kirchner, Heidelberg
Typesetting: Typoservice, Griesheim

SPIN 10884113   80/7231 – 5 4 3 2 1 0 – Printed on acid-free paper

Contents

Indicators of Schizophrenia in Childhood and Adolescence

Psychopathological Predictors of Onset and Course of Schizophrenia

Perspectives of Neuroprotective Interventions

Psychoprotective Factors

Developments and Perspectives

Authors' addresses

Behl, Christian, Prof. Dr.
Institute of Physiological
Chemistry and
Pathobiochemistry
Duesbergweg 6
55099 Mainz, Germany
cbehl@mail.uni-mainz.de

Done, D. John, Dr.
Department of Psychology
University of Hertfordshire
Hatfield, Herts AL10 9AB, UK
d.j.done@herts.ac.uk

Ehrenreich, Hannelore,
Prof. Dr. Dr.
Max-Planck-Institute for
Experimental Medicine
Hermann-Rein Straße 3
37075 Göttingen, Germany
ehrenreich@em.mpg.de

Falkai, Peter, Prof. Dr.
Psychiatry and Psychotherapy
Neuro-Psychiatric Clinic
and Out-Patient Unit
The Saarland University
Hospital
66421 Homburg/Saar, Germany
pspfal@uniklinik-saarland.de

Gattaz, Wagner F., Prof. Dr.
Department of Psychiatry
Faculty of Medicine
University of São Paulo
P.O Box 3671
05403-010 São Paulo – SP –
Brazil
gattaz@usp.br

Gouzoulis-Mayfrank,
Euphrosyne, Dr.
Department of Psychiatry and
Psychotherapy
University Hospital
Pauwelsstraße 30
52074 Aachen, Germany
egouzoulis@ukaachen.de

Häfner, Heinz, Prof. Dr. Dr.
Dres. h. c.
Central Institute of Mental
Health
Schizophrenia Research Unit
J 5
68159 Mannheim, Germany
hhaefner@
as200.zi-mannheim.de

Harrison, Glynn, Prof. Dr.
Division of Psychiatry
University of Bristol
Cotham House, Cotham Hill
Bristol BS6 6JL, UK
g.harrison@bristol.ac.uk

Jones, Peter B., Prof. Dr.
Department of Psychiatry
University of Cambridge
Box 189 Addenbrooke's Hospital
Cambridge CB2 2QQ, UK
pbj21@cam.ac.uk

Klingberg, Stefan, Dr.
Department of Psychiatry and
Psychotherapy
University of Tübingen
Osianderstraße 24
72076 Tübingen, Germany
stefan.klingberg@med.uni-
tuebingen.de

Klosterkötter, Joachim, Prof. Dr.
Department of Psychiatry and
Psychotherapy
University of Köln
Joseph-Stelzmann-Straße 9
50924 Köln, Germany
sekretariat.psychiatrie@medizin.
uni-koeln.de

Kulkarni, Jayashri, Prof. Dr.
Alfred Psychiatry Research
Centre
Old Baker Building
Alfred Hospital
Commercial Rd
Prahran, Vic 3181, Australia
jayashri.kulkarni@med.monash.
edu.au

Maier, Wolfgang, Prof. Dr.
Clinic of Psychiatry and
Psychotherapy
University of Bonn
Sigmund-Freud-Straße 25
53105 Bonn, Germany
w.maier@uni-bonn.de

Maurer, Kurt, Dr.
Central Institute of Mental
Health
Schizophrenia Research Unit
J 5
68159 Mannheim
maurer@as200-zi-mannheim.de

Mortensen, Preben Bo, Prof. Dr.
National Center for Register-
based Research
University of Aarhus
Taasingegade 1
8000 Aarhus C, Denmark
pbm@ncrr.au.dk

Parnas, Josef, Prof. Dr. Dr.
Cognitive Research Unit
University Department of
Psychiatry
Hvidovre Hospital
Brøndbyøstervej 160
2650 Hvidovre, Denmark
parnas@hh.hosp.dk

Resch, Franz, Prof. Dr.
Department of Child and
Adolescent Psychiatry
Psychiatric University Hospital
Blumenstraße 8
69115 Heidelberg, Germany
franz_resch@
med.uni-heidelberg.de

Schröder, Johannes, Prof. Dr.
Section of Geriatric Psychiatry
University of Heidelberg
Voßstraße 4
69115 Heidelberg, Germany
johannes_schroeder@med.uni-
heidelberg.de

Schultze-Lutter, Frauke, Dr.
Department of Psychiatry and
Psychotherapy
University of Köln
Josef-Stelzmann-Straße 9
50924 Köln, Germany
frauke.schultze-lutter@web.de

Tarrier, Nicolas, Prof. Dr.
Academic Division of Clinical
Psychology
School of Psychiatry and
Behavioural Sciences
University of Manchester
Wythenshawe Hospital
Manchester, M23 9LT, UK
ntarrier@fs1.with.man.ac.uk

Tienari, Pekka, Prof. Dr.,
Department of Psychiatry
University of Oulu
PL 5000
90014 Oulun yliopisto, Finland
pekka.tienari@oulu.fi

van Os, Jim, Prof. Dr.
Department of Psychiatry and
Neuropsychology
Maastricht University
P. O. Box 616 (PAR45)
6200 MD Maastricht, The
Netherlands
j.vanos@sp.unimaas.nl

Verdoux, Hélène, Prof. Dr.
University Department of
Psychiatry
Hôpital Charles Perrens
121 rue de la Béchade
33076 Bordeaux Cedex, France
helene.verdoux@
ipso.u-bordeaux2.fr

Weiser, Mark, Dr.
Psychiatric Outpatient Clinic
Sheba Medical Center
Tel Hashomer 52621, Israel
mweiser@netvision.net.il

Introduction

H. HÄFNER
Schizophrenia Research Unit, Central Institute of Mental Health, Mannheim, Germany

The present volume contains the lectures and invited discussions of the symposium on "Risk and protective factors in schizophrenia – towards a conceptual model of the disease process", which was held at the International Science Forum of the University of Heidelberg from October 25 to 27, 2001. They are supplemented by a "Summary and outlook", in which Peter Jones gives a brief overview of the results and perspectives featured in the presentations and discussions. The contributions and discussions reflect the open-minded and creative atmosphere at the meeting.

The systematically structured program of the symposium continued the tradition of the Search for the Causes of Schizophrenia symposia, which were started in 1986 on the occasion of the 600th anniversary of the University of Heidelberg and which are co-organized with Prof. Wagner Farid Gattaz/Sao Paulo. The aim of these symposia and their proceedings volumes [6, 8–10] has been to reflect the state of the art in schizophrenia research at their time, and they have successfully done so. In contrast, the present symposium pursued a more limited objective and was of a different type. It brought together, around a large table at the International Science Forum in Heidelberg, 22 invited speakers and discussants and an equal number of young scientists working in the research fields in question, who were thus given an opportunity to listen and to participate. The invited speakers and discussants are all active and leading figures in the fields of schizophrenia research represented by the topics of their presentations. In addition, these participants were chosen because of their willingness to contribute to a discussion not limited to their own disciplines and research interests.

The members of the Program Committee of the symposium came from the Schizophrenia Research Unit of the Central Institute of Mental Health, Mannheim (H. Häfner and W. an der Heiden), from the Child and Adolescent Psychiatric Department (F. Resch) and the Psychogeriatric Section (J. Schröder) of the Psychiatric Department of the University of Heidelberg. All these members also contributed from their own research fields.

The cornerstone of the meeting was an intensive, comparative discussion of research results with the aim of arriving at a synthesis. This idea proved highly successful. It enabled an extraordinarily rich and fruitful exchange of substantial arguments, overarching views and lines of thought. Unfortunately, it will be reflected in the present volume only in the invited discussions and Peter Jones' concluding remarks. It has not been possible to reproduce all the discussions that ensued at the meeting among the participants gathered around the large table and to which almost half of the conference time was dedicated. But it is to be presumed that no participant left the meeting uninspired by the intensive discussion and the insights that the contributions produced. Hence, seminal effects may well ensue on the participants' heuristics and future research work.

One reason for organizing this meeting was that funding by the German Research Association (DFG) of the core project of the ABC Schizophrenia Study, which commenced on January 1, 1987, is now about to terminate (on Sept. 30, 2002). We feel deeply grateful for this long-term, generous support. Together with the studies following it, now underway and financed by the German Research Association and the Federal Ministry for Education and Research, the ABC Schizophrenia Study is probably one of the largest and most interesting projects in the field of schizophrenia research.

But there were also other reasons for holding this symposium. The topics included in the program go far beyond the results of the ABC Study. The contributions are mainly based on new findings on various levels of schizophrenia research. In many cases these findings stood on their own, and it was not clear how they were related to other findings. To illustrate this, I will briefly introduce some recent results that were included in the program.

According to epidemiological family studies, 20% to 30% of the first-degree relatives of persons with schizophrenia show minor neuropsychological anomalies and mild psychopathology. In genetic studies a growing number of susceptibility gene loci have been identified and replicated. Some of these genes are presumed to be widespread in the general population, but also to constitute a considerable risk for schizophrenia only in combination with other genes (cf. Maier et al., this volume).

The epidemiological adoption study conducted in Finland (Tienari et al., this volume) though seems to indicate that a favorable family setting in infancy and childhood can have a protective effect against the risk of schizophrenia in persons with a genetic predisposition to the illness.

Another major risk factor is constituted by pre- and perinatal complications and inflammatory diseases of the brain and the meninx (cf. Gattaz et al., this volume) in infancy. The role of psychological risk factors, maternal depression during pregnancy, after birth and in early infancy is being discussed without conclusive evidence having surfaced yet (Verdoux & Sutter, this volume).

The general-practice and population studies conducted by Verdoux et al. [20] and van Os et al. [19] have demonstrated that psychotic symptoms occur five to fifteen times more frequently in the general population than in people suffering from schizophrenia. They also constitute significant risk factors preceding the onset of schizophrenia (cf. van Os et al., this volume). It seems that Kraepelin's categorical disease entity has lost its validity as a discriminating diagnostic concept and as a representation of a homogeneous etiology.

In several large-scale prospective studies of population birth cohorts, especially those analyzed by Peter Jones, John Done and Jim van Os in Great Britain and Northern Finland [3, 4, 14, 15, 18] and by Poulton et al. [17] in New Zealand, early precursors of the disorder have been identified. Preceding the antecedents that emerge in adolescence, there are minor delays in developmental milestones (walking and speech) in early childhood, which are followed by mild cognitive deficits, emotional and behavioral anomalies and mild impairment in social functioning [1, 16, Weiser, this volume] as well as by some self-reported psychotic symptoms at age 11 in 42% of cases with a diagnosis of a schizophreniform disorder at age 26 [17].

Illness onset, in women several years later than in men, is followed by the most active stage in the disease process showing great variation in its pace of symptom development and decline in functioning [11]. After this initial stage persons affected, on average, show a plateau of neuropsychological deficits and negative symptoms [5, 7, 11].

The individual illness courses are very heterogeneous. Some 20% show full recovery after the first episode, and a small proportion suffers very gradual decline in cognitive abilities. As recently reported by Harvey et al. [12, 13] some suffer striking late-life decline in cognitive functions without signs of a dementia of Alzheimer's type.

With the help of new neuropathological and brain-imaging techniques, on which Falkai et al. (this volume) and Schröder et al. (this volume) will report, we have gained insight into what happens with brain morphology and functioning in these presumably neurodegenerative processes. Minor morphological brain anomalies are already there in the first illness episode. A few controlled multilevel studies, conducted e.g. by DeLisi et al. [2], have found mild progression in these anomalies, so far over 5 years of illness, in small groups of patients. Functional studies have provided information on the localization of single symptoms and on disconnectivities between cerebral regions as possible correlates of cognitive and other types of dysfunctioning. Although with the insights into the dysfunctioning of the brain we have made a great leap towards understanding the underlying pathophysiological processes, it has not yet been possible to clarify the etiology of the disorder. What actually happens in the morphology and functioning of the brain at the slowly or rapidly evolving early illness stage is one of the core questions of modern schizophrenia research.

The antipsychotic effect of estrogens and the use of this hormone as a substitute for a neuroleptic therapy (Kulkarni, this volume) are nourishing the hope of expanding our therapeutic and possibly also the preventive arsenal of the psychosis. The new research field of neuroprotection in which estrogens and erythropoietin play a central role might some day provide a key to early treatment or prevention that is capable of more than just acting upon a rather late and conspicuous component of the disorder: the psychotic symptoms. The protective effect of being raised in a favorable family environment on high-risk individuals was mentioned above.

This brief and selective overview of the topics included in the program illustrates the great variety of research findings and perspectives currently pursued. It also reflects a major flaw of today's scientific research in many fields: while rapid progress is being made in single disciplines and methods, a comprehensive view of the whole refuses to emerge, in our case, of the complex illness called schizophrenia. This is exactly the task that we gave ourselves with this symposium and the reason why this particular type of meeting and of publishing its proceedings was chosen, namely, to enable an intensive exchange of results and ideas in order to arrive at a new view of the disorder.

I am greatly indebted to my colleagues Wolfram an der Heiden, Franz Resch and Johannes Schröder for their cooperation in planning and organizing the symposium as well as to the sponsors of the symposium: the Deutsche Forschungsgemeinschaft also for financing the ABC Schizophrenia Study, the University of Heidelberg Foundation, Astra-Zeneca and Novartis Pharma GmbH. I am grateful to Eli-Lilly Germany in particular, Astra Zeneca and Novartis Pharma GmbH for sponsoring the publication of the proceedings. I also wish to thank my secretaries Angelika Heimann and Auli Komulainen-Tremmel for their dependable, excellent support.

References

1. Davidson M, Reichenberg A, Rabinowitz J, Weiser M, Kaplan Z, Mark M (1999) Cognitive and behavioral markers for schizophrenia in a population of apparently healthy male adolescents. Am J Psychiatry 156: 1328–1335
2. DeLisi LE, Sakuma M, Tew W, Kushner M, Hoff AL, Grimson R (1997) Schizophrenia as a chronic active brain process: a study of progressive brain structural change subsequent to the onset of schizophrenia. Psychiatry Res 74: 129–140
3. Done DJ, Sacker A, Crow TJ (1994) Childhood antecedents of schizophrenia and affective illness: intellectual performance at ages 7 and 11. Schizophrenia Res 11: 96–97
4. Done D, Crow TJ, Johnstone EC, Sacker A (1994) Childhood antecedents of schizophrenia and affective illness: social adjustment at ages 7 and 11. Br Med J 309: 699–703
5. Fenton WS, McGlashan TH (1991) Natural history of schizophrenia subtypes. II. Positive and negative symptoms and long-term course. Arch Gen Psychiatry 48: 978–986
6. Gattaz WF, Häfner H (eds) (1999) Search for the causes of schizophrenia, vol. IV: Balance of the century. Steinkopff-Verlag, Darmstadt and Springer-Verlag, Berlin Heidelberg New York
7. Goldberg TE, Hyde TM, Kleinman JE, Weinberger DR (1993) Course of schizophrenia: neuropsychological evidence for a static encephalopathy. Schizophr Bull 19: 797–804
8. Häfner H, Gattaz WF (eds) (1991) Search for the causes of schizophrenia, vol. II. Springer-Verlag, Berlin Heidelberg New York
9. Häfner H, Gattaz WF (eds) (1995) Search for the causes of schizophrenia, vol. III. Springer-Verlag, Berlin Heidelberg New York
10. Häfner H, Gattaz WF, Janzarik W (eds) (1987) Search for the causes of schizophrenia. Springer-Verlag, Berlin Heidelberg New York
11. Häfner H, Maurer K, Löffler W, an der Heiden W, Könnecke R, Hambrecht M (1999) Onset and prodromal phase as determinants of the course. In: Gattaz WF, Häfner H (eds) Search for the causes of schizophrenia, vol. IV: Balance of the century. Steinkopff Verlag, Darmstadt, Springer, Berlin, pp 1–24
12. Harvey PD, Howanitz E, Parrella M, White L, Davidson M (1998) Symptoms, cognitive functioning, and adaptive skills in geriatric patients with lifelong schizophrenia: a comparison across treatment sites. Am J Psychiatry 155: 1980–1986
13. Harvey PD, Parrella M, White L, Mohs RC, Davidson M, Davis KL (1999) Convergence of cognitive and adaptive decline in late-life schizophrenia. Schizophrenia Res 35: 77–84
14. Jones PB, Done DJ (1997) From birth to onset: a developmental perspective of schizophrenia in two national birth cohorts. In: Keshavan MS, Murray RM (eds) Neurodevelopmental and adult psychopathology. Cambridge University Press, Cambridge, pp 119–136

15. Jones PB, Rantakallio P, Hartikainen AL, Isohanni H, Sipilä P (1998) Schizophrenia as a long-term outcome of pregnancy, delivery and perinatal complications: a 28-year follow-up of the 1966 North Finland general population birth cohort. Am J Psychiatry 155: 355–364
16. Malmberg A, Lewis G, David A, Allebeck P (1998) Premorbid adjustment and personality in people with schizophrenia. Br J Psychiatry 172: 308–313
17. Poulton R, Caspi A, Moffitt TE, Cannon M, Murray R, Harrington H (2000) Children's self-reported psychotic symptoms and adult schizophreniform disorder: a 15-year longitudinal study (In Process Citation). Arch Gen Psychiatry 57: 1053–1058
18. Van Os J, Jones PB, Lewis G, Wadsworth M, Murray RM (1997) Developmental precursors of affective illness in a general population birth cohort. Arch Gen Psychiatry 54: 625–631
19. Van Os J, Verdoux H, Maurice-Tison S, Gay B, Liraud F, Salamon R, Bourgeois M (1999) Self-reported psychosis-like symptoms and the continuum of psychosis. Soc Psychiatry Psychiatr Epidemiol 34: 459–463
20. Verdoux H, Maurice-Tison S, Gay B, Van Os J, Salamon R, Bourgeois ML (1998) A survey of delusional ideation in primary-care patients. Psychol Med 28: 127–134

■ Genetic and Population-related Risk Factors

Genetics of schizophrenia and related disorders

W. Maier, M. Rietschel, M. Linz, P. Falkai
Department of Psychiatry, University of Bonn, Germany

Schizophrenia, like all other common diseases, aggregates in families. The patterns of familial transmission are irregular and do not fit a Mendelian pattern. Simultaneously, twin and partly also adoption studies revealed for all common diseases a strong genetic influence without ruling out nongenetic environmental factors. It can be derived from incomplete concordance rates among monozygotic twins that nongenetic factors also contribute to all common disorders. The impact of nongenetic determinants is thought to be comparable by magnitude to genetic factors in most common diseases; twin studies – as far as they are available – support this assumption. The term "complex diseases" indicate a presence of genetic determination in the absence of Mendelian, monogenic transmission and of nongenetic environmental factors.

In previous decades, the search for risk factors in common diseases has focussed on nongenetic environmental factors. For example, in schizophrenia obstetric complications, season of birth, upbringing in cities, lowered intelligence and CNS infections in childhood were found to contribute to the emergence of schizophrenia without defining altogether most of the mass of risk [57]. The strongest predictor for schizophrenia, however, is the relationship to an affected subject (with relative risks of 7.0–9.3 among 1st degree relatives [37]). Twin studies of this syndrome suggested that familial aggregation is nearly exclusively due to genetic factors [35]. These postulated genetic factors should correspond to sequence variations in the genome (DNA).

The multiplicity of contributing genes in concert with environmental factors are postulated as being necessary to understand the complex genetic basis of common diseases. These assumed contributing specific genetic variants promise to define valid and robust risk factors which are stable and premorbidly observable. Because of the recent technological and conceptual developments in molecular genetics, the search for genetic risk factors on the DNA level became especially promising for all common disorders and for schizophrenia in particular. Elucidation of at least parts of the genetically influenced etiological puzzle offers the prospect to derive more powerful diagnostic and therapeutic tools. Additionally, the identification of specific influential genetic mutations can help to develop new therapeutic drugs with innovative mechanisms of action.

Therefore, enormous research efforts were and are invested in each of the common diseases to shed light on at least some of the disease genes. The progress of the human genome project has greatly promoted the efforts, investments and activities in clinical genetics. For each of the common diseases, the search for specific DNA variants influencing the genetic risk has lasted now for more than 10 years. However, the genetics of the common diseases still remains widely obscure; the research achievements have more or less reached a very similar state of knowledge for each of these diseases.

This paper reviews the present status of the search for specific genes contributing to schizophrenia, and new research strategies in this field. We will also try to use the progress of knowledge to refine our concepts of the origin of psychoses. Although other psychoses also cluster in families of schizophrenic patients, molecular-genetic research has nearly exclusively been applied to schizophrenia [26]. Therefore, this present state of knowledge report focusses also on schizophrenia.

▓ Present state of knowledge on specific contributing genes and their localization

Principally, two search strategies for disease-gene identification are possible: linkage and association/linkage disequilibrium studies. Advantages and disadvantages of both methods have recently been reviewed extensively [2]. Both methods are complementary and not competitive approaches in genetics of complex diseases; each of these techniques has a specific position in the search for disease genes. Classically, linkage stands for a systematic, hypothesis-free and genome-wide approach, while association studies stand for a candidate-oriented approach which is particularly able to pick up the "low-hanging fruits" emerging from our current knowledge of the etiology and pathophysiology of the disease under study.

Association studies with candidate genes

Association studies explore whether a specific genetic variant (allele) occurs more often among affected versus nonaffected probands. These studies are most easily to perform as no families have to be collected and to be investigated. The association strategy is particularly successful if the pathophysiology of the disease is well known and a comprehensive set of candidate genes coding for pathophysiologically relevant proteins can be derived. Association only indicates that either the genetic variant under study or a genetic variant in linkage disequilibrium contributes to the disease risk; linkage disequilibrium in the mean holds up across 3000 base pairs, i.e., a region which might cover multiple genes. Thus, genetic association alone is not able to identify disease genes or their variants.

Despite the lack of comprehensive knowledge on the etiology and pathophysiological basis of schizophrenia, multiple genes involved with common polymorphisms are known and were tested for association with schizophrenia. Numerous association studies were published, most of them with negative results. Association to some candidate gene variants reported partly replicable results with at least some of the replication tests being in line with the original positive finding. There is not a single genetic variant with only positive association results in multiple independent studies (like it is the case for ApoE4 in late-onset Alzheimer's disease). As a high false-positive rate in association studies is to be expected (given the statistical rationale), multiple replications are needed for positive findings. In addition, metaanalyses are more conclusive in this respect as they offer a quantitative trade-off between positive and negative findings. The following genetic variants were tested for association to schizophrenia with at least some positive results (see also Fig. 1, left column):

▨ The serotonin-2A receptor (5-HT-2A) gene carries an exonic polymorphism T102C. The C-allele is more common among patients suffering from schizophrenia compared to controls according to some but only a minority of association tests. Inconsistent results motivated a metaanalysis combining 15 studies published until 1997. A very modest but significant elevation of relative risk (1.18) was obtained without evidence of heterogeneity [63].

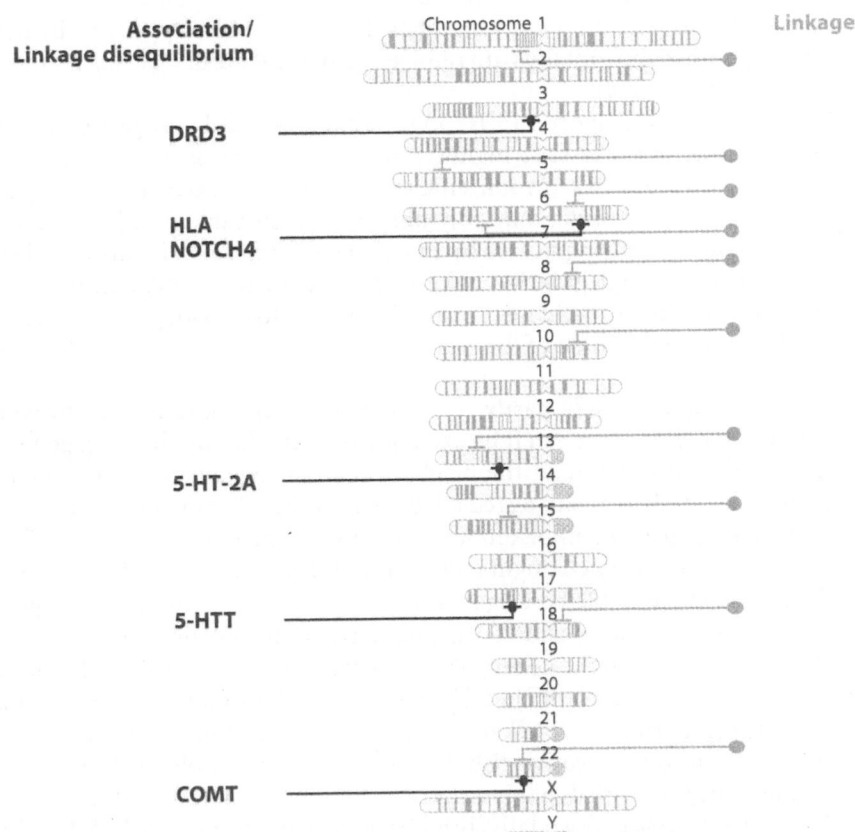

Fig. 1. Association/linkage disequilibrium and linkage findings in schizophrenia.

■ The dopamine-3 receptor (DRD3) gene reveals a biallelic exonic (Ba II) and four other polymorphisms [23]. Both forms of homozygotes of the Ba II polymorphisms were found to be more common among patients with schizophrenia versus controls according to some but not all association studies; in contrast, the frequencies of single alleles of this specific polymorphism were not different between groups. Again, a metaanalysis combining 30 studies found a weakly but significantly increased disease risk (1.28) for homozygosity at the Ba II polymorphism [64]. The interpretation of this finding could be based on highly significant associations of haplotypes of three D3 receptor gene polymorphisms to schizophrenia (what was reported by one study recently [23]) or refer to the presumed general principle of an advantage of heterozygosity which provides more adaptive flexibility.

■ The dopamine-degrading enzyme COMT exists in two different genetic variants: a low- and a high-activity variant as a consequence of an amino acid substitution Val$^{108/158}$Met. Several association studies report weak associations of schizophrenia to the low-activity genetic variant although there is the same number of negative reports or even one report with the reverse relationship [12]. It is difficult to decide if this COMT gene is really influencing the etiology of the disease or if it only modifies the disease phenotype (e.g., by reducing dopamine prefrontally with reduced achievements of working memory as a consequence) [20].

■ The serotonin transporter (5-HTT) gene shows several polymorphisms. One intronic (i.e., unexpressed), highly variable polymorphism (VNTR) was found to be associated with schizophrenia in our German-Israeli family sample but not so alleles of the functional polymorphism of the same gene [21]. This finding was surprisingly replicated by an independent German family sample with an excessively high relative risk (6.5) [24]. Further replication tests are required in order to validate the association and to provide more precise estimates of the magnitude of the relative risk.

Altogether, some of these partly replicated association findings might be true positives. In neither case can it be excluded that the risk-modulating gene variant is located somewhere in the neighborhood of the gene with the polymorphism under study, i.e., the tested allele and the "true" influential genetic variant are in linkage disequilibrium which extends in general across thousands of base pairs (a region which might include multiple genes). Thus, the true relative risk and the attributable risk figures remain obscure. Therefore, these genetic variants cannot yet be considered as predictive or diagnostic tools.

In any case, most of the genetic variance contributing to the manifestation of the disease remains unexplained by these association findings. The estimated variant-specific risks are small and remain small in combinations (particularly in comparison to the relative risk defined by having a biological relative with schizophrenia). The attributable risks (e.g., for the associated 5-HT-2A variants) might be higher due to the relatively high frequency of the associated allele in the general population; however, this observation is only valid if the associated allele is directly influencing the risk and not another allele in linkage disequilibrium.

Consequently, the genetic variants identified by the candidate-gene association approach cannot define the whole genetic risk for schizophrenia. Thus, we
need approaches in the search of disease genes beyond the candidate genes on
the basis of our present pathophysiological understanding. Principally, all genes
expressed in the brain are putative candidates. A hypothesis-free, genome-wide
search is therefore indicated. Under previous and current technical conditions,
genome-wide linkage studies offer appropriate opportunity.

Hypothesis-free linkage studies

Linkage explores the cosegregation between a marker gene and the disease gene
in families; like association studies, linkage provides only positional information. Linkage might lead to the disease gene; however, identification of disease
genes requires neurobiological evidence. Unit of analysis are informative families with at least two affected subjects (either pairs of affected siblings or extended
multiplex families with multiple generations).

Linkage studies starting without an a priori hypothesis were enormously
effective in discovering disease genes for Mendelian, monogenic diseases.
Although linkage studies propose only candidate regions on the genome (positional cloning), including the disease gene, continuous application of this strategy helps to identify the disease gene in monogenic diseases. The genes for most
of these monogenic diseases have been cloned in the meantime; the genetic basis
for the remaining (monogenic) diseases will be discovered by this strategy with
certainty.

Similarly, genome-wide linkage analyses can be considered as the most promising starting point for the search of disease genes in complex disorders. However, the crucial step in exploring linkage in monogenic diseases does not work
here as well: The recombination between marker genes and the disease gene is
less informative in the case of multiple genes. Instead, sharing of alleles between
affected siblings is a major rationale for establishing linkage in complex diseases.
Thus, in contrast to monogenic diseases, pairs of affected siblings present the
most informative family sample for complex diseases.

Successful linkage studies provided the gateway for the detection of disease
genes already in some complex diseases. Two examples:

■ ApoE4 influencing the risk of late-onset Alzheimer's disease was detected after
  a report of a weak linkage on chromosome 19, and stimulated association
  studies to candidate gene variants in the linked region [39, 40].
■ Haplotypes in the until recently unknown calpain-10 gene were demonstrated
  to influence the risk for diabetes mellitus type II after linkage studies detected
  a candidate region on chromosome 2p; a subsequent combined linkage-asso-
  ciation approach narrowed the region down to a new gene which was called
  calpain-10 gene [22].

Multiple, genome-wide linkage scans were carried out in schizophrenia (10 published) using an affected sibpair approach in outbred populations (e.g. [7, 10, 25,
30, 48, 53, 54, 65]). In addition, several linkage analyses in highly loaded com-

plex pedigrees, mostly with assumed homogeneous genetic background (inbred), were also successfully performed (e.g., [8]). In all studies the identified candidate regions were always broad and the linkage signals were weak (although of borderline significance). This pattern is observable in all common diseases and reflects the oligo-/polygenic nature and the nongenetic influences. Consequently, it is difficult to distinguish between "false" and "true" positives. Replicability of an initial positive linkage finding is, therefore, the major criterion for the validity of a linkage finding in complex diseases. Unfortunately, replication of a "true" finding requires larger sample sizes in complex diseases compared to the original finding [55].

The identified regions with suggestive and probable linkage with schizophrenia across these analyses reveal no consistent pattern with regard to replicability. Not a single linked region could be identified across all or most of the analyses. The main reason for those inconsistencies are:

■ *Sample sizes:* Detection of genes with small effect size requires unrealistically high numbers of informative families in order to obtain a high statistical power (> 50%). Thus, when linkage is not initially replicated, the positive result does not need to be discarded as long as the power to detect linkage under realistic sample size conditions is 5 – 10% (assuming modest effect sizes per gene) [55].

■ *Population heterogeneity:* Given multiple contributing genes, some of these genes might only operate in specific clinical subsyndromes or in different populations. Population dependence has been particularly observed for linkage to 15q11-13, a region including the gene for the nicotinergic acetylcholine receptor subunit 7α. Linkage to this region turned out to be replicable in African or Afro-American populations but not in European-descent populations [25, 43].

Thus, which of the identified candidate regions are worthwhile to follow-up? Two strategies might help to decide this question:

■ *Metaanalyses across different linkage studies:* Due to a substantial increase in sample size there is a better chance to find true positives. Only a single meta-analysis covering all of the relevant candidate regions is published and combines eight samples from different countries which were collected and analyzed under comparable condition [31]. The most comprehensive available affected sibpair samples are included. Four linkage findings on chromosomes 6p, 6q, 8p and 13p received support by metaanalyses.

■ *Replications:* Given the limited number of genome scans (see above) a single replication of a suggestive linkage finding in a limited number of replication tests is far beyond being a random event (given that p = 0.0001 for suggestive linkage [28]). Thus, it is impossible to calculate exactly the probability that the observed partial overlap between the published 10 genome-wide linkage studies just occurred by chance given the very restrictive p-value for suggestive linkage.

Using the criterion of "being replicated at least in one independent linkage analysis", a more diverse pattern is emerging. These findings were recently reviewed extensively by Riley and McGuffin [42]. The most convincing candidate areas are summarized in Fig. 1, right column.

The comparison between the chromosomal localizations of linkage and of association findings, however, reveals much diversity (Fig. 1). What are the reasons for the lack of consistency between association and linkage studies? Both strategies have different sensitivities for stronger gene effects with genetic association studies having a higher power to detect smaller genetic effects. Thus, it does not come as a surprise that the observed associations are not always placed in linked candidate areas. The susceptibility genes in linkage candidate regions with impact on the disease risk have still to be detected.

▓ Consequences of the present status of research in association and linkage studies

Linkage and association studies demonstrate that schizophrenia reveals a multilocus etiology in a genetic perspective. Thus, although we still do not know with certainty any single contributing gene, a poly- or oligogenic etiology can be assumed. Given twin and epidemiological studies (e.g., [37]), nongenetic environmental conditions are also influential. It is unresolved if the genetic and nongenetic determinants are interacting or if they are operating additively [37].

Monogenic subtypes of schizophrenia?

Contribution of multiple genes to the disease risk is compatible with two models of heterogeneity:
- ▓ Each of the disease gene variants causes schizophrenia in a subset of cases; other contributing genes are relevant preferentially in other subtypes. This means, one or several etiological subtypes are monogenic diseases or are at least driven by a major gene; each of these causal genetic variants should be rare, given the prevalence of schizophrenia (or its subtypes).
- ▓ Neither of the individual contributing genes causes schizophrenia; only in concert with other susceptibility gene variants might the disease be a consequence under unfavorable environmental conditions. In this context, each of the susceptibility genes influences the risk without causing it (susceptibility or vulnerability gene). The effect size of each of the contributing variants is small. Genetic variants exerting only small effects are mostly common.

It is most likely that the first possibility is either irrelevant or only relevant for a minority of cases. Previously, periodic catatonia was assumed to be a monogenic condition by Beckmann et al. [4]. However, a genome scan in this subgroup by the same group did not support this hypothesis [51]. Classical former genetic investigations clearly demonstrated that monogenic determination is unlikely among the vast majority of cases [34]. Thus, the second possibility is very likely to define an appropriate model for most of the cases (see also Fig. 2). In this

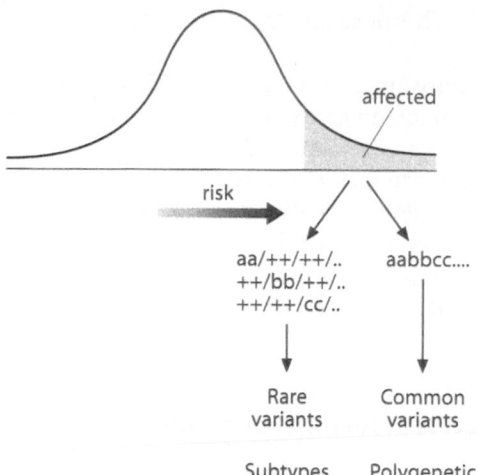

Rare
variants

Common
variants

Subtypes   Polygenetic
with main genes

Fig. 2. Multiple disease gene loci: alternative explanations [9].

model so-called sporadic cases (i.e., without a biological relative with the same disease) might also carry genetic variants associated with elevated risk.

Assuming that multiple genes are operating, can we also draw conclusions on the interplay between the different genes and nongenetic forces? Family studies reporting on the risk of relatives as a function of the degree of relationship to the index case with schizophrenia are informative in this respect: In schizophrenia a steep decline of risk is observed between relatives of 1st and 2nd degree, whereas the change between 2nd and 3rd degree is only small [33]. This constellation argues for superadditive (i.e., multiplicative) interaction between different susceptibility gene variants [44].

Sequelae of oligo-/polygenic etiology

Although linkage studies were not yet able to identify specific contributing genes, we may use the polygeneity for explaining epidemiological features of schizophrenia.

1. *Why are not only schizophrenia and related psychotic disorders more common among relatives of probands with schizophrenia than in the general population, but also less impeding phenotypes revealing schizophrenia-like features?*

This quantitative phenotypic variation can easily be explained assuming a polygenic/multifactorial transmission. Each individual genetic variant contributing to schizophrenia reveals only a small phenotypic effect by itself. Only in concert with other risk-modulating variants may schizophrenia emerge as a consequence (e.g., if a minimal number of susceptibility gene variants or a threshold of combined effects is reached). The combination of fewer or less powerful susceptibility gene variants presents as schizophrenia-related phenotypes, e.g., as schizotypal personality, schizoid behavior, specific schizophrenia-related neurophysiological, -chemical, -morphometric or –psychological traits (e.g., [13]). An aggregation of these genetic constellations is to be expected among close biological relatives of an index case with schizophrenia who may carry multiple susceptibility gene variants but do not reach the disease-specific threshold. Even clinically unaffected relatives of probands with schizophrenia reveal a higher mean number of susceptibility gene variants than expected by chance under this model. The aggregation of schizophrenia-related phenotypic traits among family members is in agreement with this model. Figures 3a and 3b illustrate these consequences by results of the Bonn Family Study (e.g., [6]): Unaffected relatives of patients with schizophrenia reveal quantitative deficiencies compared to unaffected general population controls both on a behavioral level (working memory by Subject Ordered Pointing Task) and in brain function (NAA/Cho coeffi-

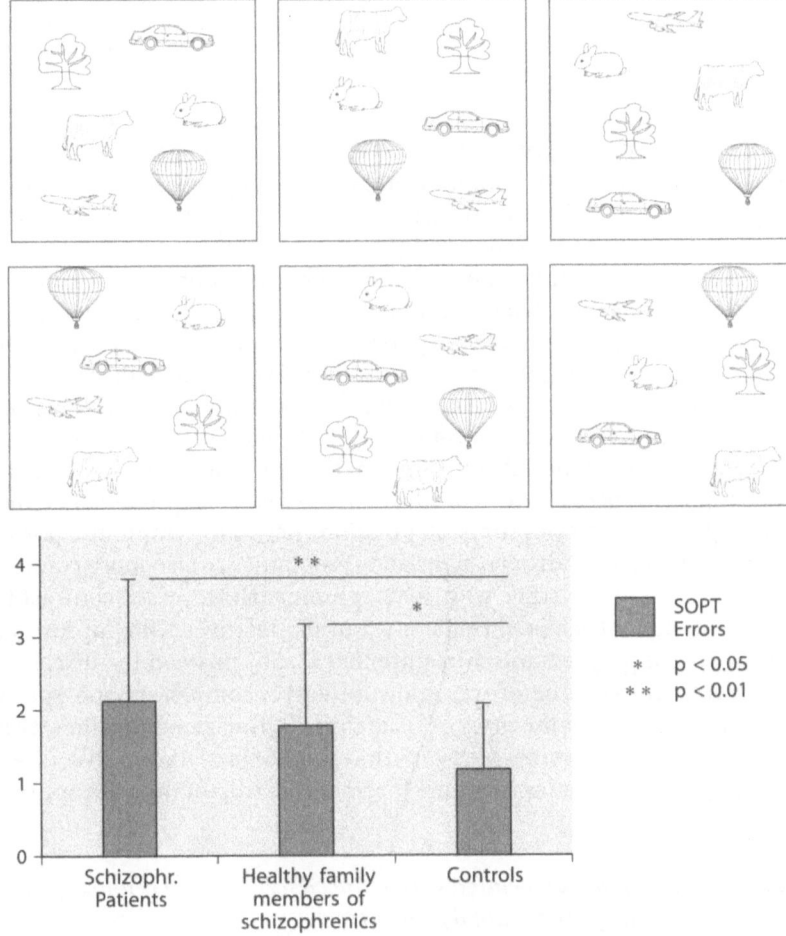

Fig. 3. a Neuropsychological impairment in the Subject Ordered Pointing Task (SOPT) in schizophrenic patients and their healthy family members in comparison with a healthy control group (Bonn Family Study).

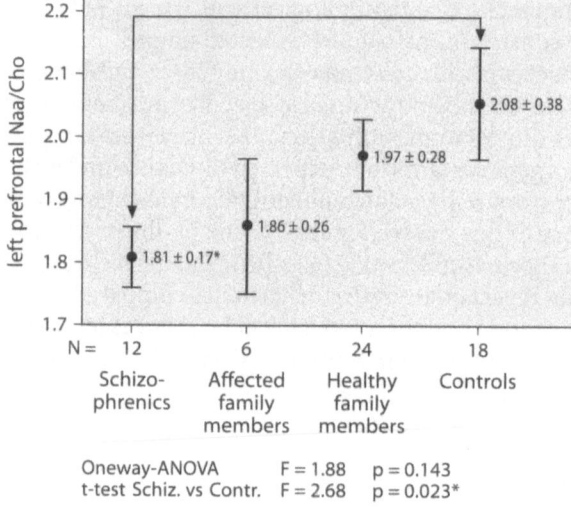

Fig. 3. b Quotient of N-acetylaspartate (NAA) and choline (Cho) in schizophrenic patients, in their affected and in their healthy family members in comparison with a healthy control group (Bonn Family Study).

cient indicating integrity of neurons in the forebrain detected by magnetic resonance spectroscopy). Both indicators are strongly correlated ($r = 0.5$).

On the basis of a polygenic model of schizophrenia, intrafamilial phenotypic heterogeneity is to be expected [38]. Starting with an affected index case with multiple susceptibility gene variants, different numbers and combinations of susceptibility gene variants among relatives will occur. Given that different susceptibility genes influence different aspects of behavior, intrafamilial phenotypic heterogeneity among nonpsychotic relatives will be the result.

In this context the apparently heterogeneous phenotypes clustering in families of patients with schizophrenia can also be viewed from the perspective of the staging model proposed by Häfner [18]: The symptom cluster diagnosed as schizophrenia occurs after a prodromal stage with symptoms occurring in a fixed order (unspecific symptoms, depression, negative symptoms, positive symptoms). All those prodromal signs and symptoms are also more common in family members of probands with schizophrenia. However, in contrast to subjects with subsequent schizophrenia, most of the relatives with "prodromal" symptoms do not progress to schizophrenia [32, 56]. Instead the disease process of schizophrenia stops before reaching the level of complete phenotype expression. It is most likely that the mass of risk (contributing genes together with environmental factors) produce an elevated but submaximal mass of risk (see Fig. 4); the etiological constellations cause a "premature" stop of the schizophrenic disease process.

2. Schizophrenia is associated with reduced fertility and is under genetic control. Why is schizophrenia not dying out?

Indeed, the pathogenic alleles of monogenic diseases with reduced fertility will decrease by frequency over generations. The alleles contributing to schizophre-

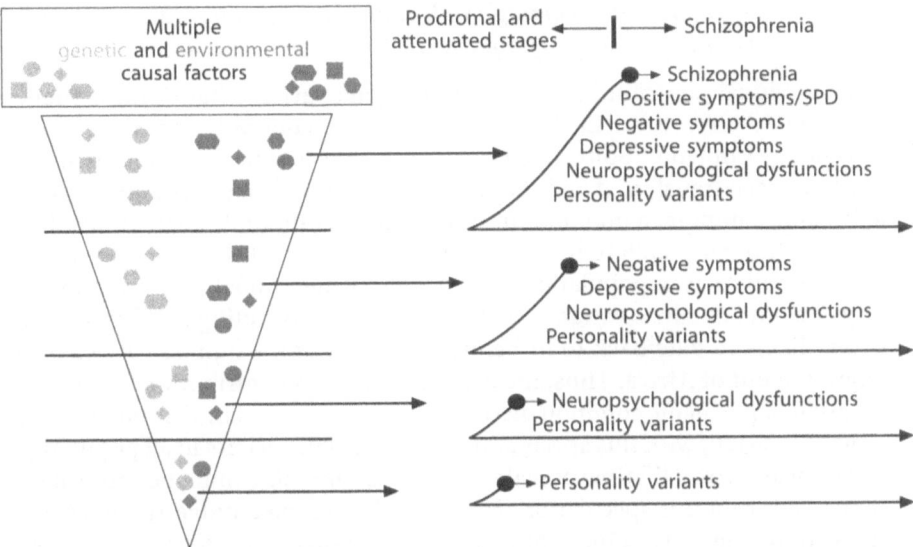

Fig. 4. Hierarchical model of schizophrenia.

nia, however, are not under selective pressure under most realistic assumptions: Multiple deleterious allelic variants are needed to induce schizophrenia, while a lower number of contributing gene variants only induces less deviant phenotypes. Only schizophrenia, but not the less impaired related traits, causes a reduction of mean fertility via disability before or during the lifespan with maximal reproduction rates and reduces the probability of mating and of having children (see Fig. 5).

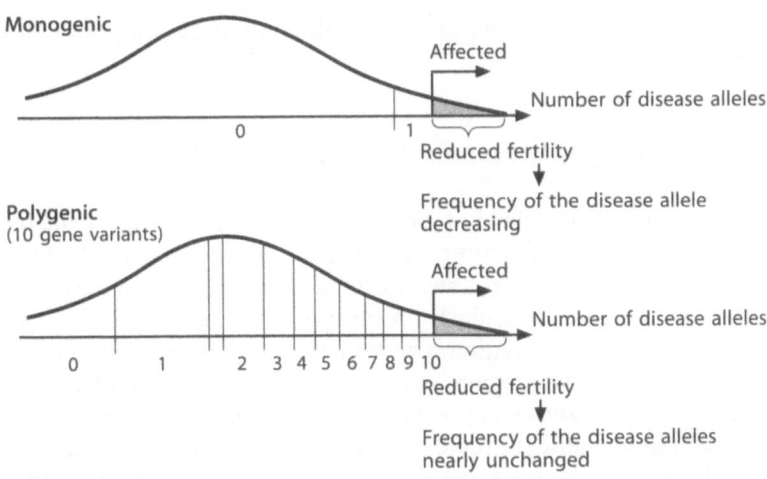

Fig. 5. Distribution of disease alleles/person in the population: consequence for the fertility in case of early onsetting, impairing disorders.

3. *Why is schizophrenia occurring in all countries with very different cultural conditions with comparable frequency?*

The individual contributing susceptibility gene variants have only a modest effect and, therefore, are likely to be common. Polymorphic variations at gene loci emerge from mutations which occurred for the first time previous in history and have been transferred and preserved over subsequent generations. In order to become common, a mutation must expand over multiple generations. However, the human population is very young, emerging 50,000-100,000 years ago from a small African population (2000 to 5000 generations). The mutation history of common allelic variants, including those contributing to schizophrenia, is very likely to date back to or before the origin of the human species or the migration out of Africa. Thus, the genetic mutations contributing to the manifestation of polygenic common diseases are to be expected in all human populations. Consistent with this speculation, schizophrenia occurs in all populations.

The nearly equal lifetime prevalence of schizophrenia cannot be compellingly concluded from this speculation. However, the assumed universal presence of susceptibility gene variants proposes a limited range of the variation of prevalence rates across various human populations.

4. *Why do affective disorders and schizophrenia overlap in families?*

There is considerable overlap between multiple candidate regions found by linkage analyses between schizophrenia and affective disorder. The extent of overlap is higher than expected by chance [5, 16]. This constellation motivated the suggestion of sharing of susceptibility genes between both disorders. Currently, this speculation cannot be proven. Only identification of identical vulnerability genes for both disorders can conclusively support this hypothesis. However, for neither of the two disorders have specific susceptibility genes been up to now identified. Curiously, this speculation is in agreement with clinical and genetic epidemiological evidence of shared vulnerability between both disorders [17, 33, 62].

■ Narrowing down candidate regions found by linkage analysis

The successful strategy in monogenic diseases for disease-gene identification is positional cloning: An initial linkage study identifies a candidate region which is subsequently narrowed down by expansion of the sample size. As mentioned, this procedure is particularly promising if the linkage signals are very sharp, and the initial candidate region is very small. In complex diseases linkage signals are weak, the candidate region is broad (~ 20 cM), and even extension of sample size (e.g., in metaanalyses, e.g., [31]) does not increase the significant linkage signals by amplitude, and are unable to narrow down the candidate region. This constellation is to be expected if the effects of individual susceptibility genes are small, are varying by magnitude across populations (because of the dependence on differential genetic population backgrounds), are modulated by environ-

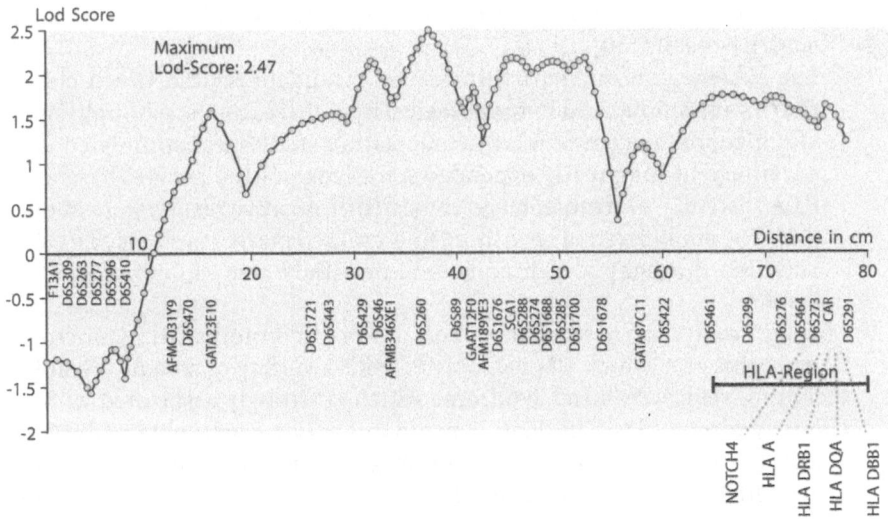

Fig. 6. Linkage on chromosome 6p: sibpair multipoint analysis with 35 microsatellite markers [47].

mental conditions, and, even more, if there are several etiological subtypes with different genetic underpinning.

As an example we present the linkage results on the chromosome 6p hot spot (Fig. 6) emerging from our genome scan [47]. The linkage figure reveals significantly but only modestly elevated linkage signals and a broad candidate region.

Thus, alternative strategies have to be considered. Most promising is narrowing down of candidate regions by association/linkage disequilibrium strategy using markers selected to cover the whole candidate region, i.e., densely located markers; the distance between markers should be smaller then the span of linkage disequilibrium in this area. The advantage of this strategy is that the spatial resolution of association/linkage disequilibrium analyses is substantially smaller compared to candidate regions identified by linkage analysis in complex diseases; the extension of linkage disequilibrium (detected by genetic association studies) is by a factor of about 10 smaller than the linked candidate areas (in the mean ~ 20 cM, corresponding to about 20,000 kilobases). Thus, the candidate region can be narrowed down by refining the marker system around associated markers step by step.

The most promising candidate areas for schizophrenia are currently under intensive examination using the same fine-mapping strategy and the progress in the growing availability of dense and/or informative marker systems. Two examples:
■ Linkage to chromosome 6p stimulated a series of association/linkage disequilibrium studies with candidate genes located in this region:
    – Promising first results for an association with the NOTCH4 gene were reported [60]. Because of the putative involvement of this gene in brain maturation and apoptosis, and its structural similarity to growth factor

genes, multiple replication tests were motivated, unfortunately with mainly negative results [50].
- The HLA region overlaps with the 6p candidate region. Given classical association studies and immunological hypotheses on the pathophysiology of schizophrenia, a new wave of association studies was stimulated taking advantage of the greatly expanded knowledge of the genetic basis of the HLA system. Unfortunately, no consistently positive results were obtained [49]. The application of new, more fine-grained marker systems (e.g., SNPs) and high-throughput techniques will hopefully come to more promising results.
- Linkage studies to chromosome 22q11.2 were first motivated by microdeletions in this area which were associated with a variety of somatic symptoms including velocardiofacial syndrome which is strongly associated with psychotic syndromes [3]; candidate genes in this region can be obtained from the analysis of the structure of deletions; in addition, the analysis of candidate genes with functional variants (COMT) located in this region provided promising results [12].

New strategies to identify candidate genes

New marker systems/genome-wide association studies

For some little time, a marker system is in development which meets the requirements for a high-density map to be applied in large case-control samples: the single nucleotide polymorphisms (SNPs) [61]. These polymorphisms are defined by just a single nucleotide exchange either in coding (possibly with functional consequences) or in noncoding regions. These markers are the main source of genetic variation in and between the populations. The estimated number across the human genome is up to 3 million SNPs (i.e., 1 SNP per 1000 base pairs) [52]. Up to now, about half of them have been identified due to the progress of the human genome project and the international SNP consortium. The allele frequency in the population is stable (due to low mutation rate and old age). Thousands of SNPs can be compared by frequency in parallel between thousands of patients and controls in automatized high-throughput technology (mass spectroscopy).

These technical developments offer new opportunities for positional cloning strategies using an association/linkage disequilibrium approach. For many years case-control studies have been hampered by lack of control of population-genetic comparability between samples. Recently, molecular-genetic control using anonymous markers became possible [41, 45]. Thus, the very efficient DNA-pooling strategy using high-throughput techniques is feasible [46]. These new technical opportunities offer a very efficient and dense marker system for association/linkage disequilibrium for
- Narrowing down of candidate regions found by linkage analysis applying a dense SNP map in an association/linkage disequilibrium analysis,

■ Genome-wide association/linkage disequilibrium analysis using a genome-wide SNP-marker map in case-control studies for hypothesis-free search for susceptibility genes with small effect sizes [27].

New strategies for phenotype characterization: endophenotypes

The simpler the genotype-phenotype relationship is, the more straightforward and the quicker contributing genes can be sought and identified. The search for susceptibility genes is impaired by the complexity of the genotype-phenotype relationship. Reduction of the complexity might be achieved by reducing the heterogeneity of the clinical phenotype: The clinical phenotype is associated with multiple neurochemical, physiological and psychological traits which are neurobiologically more deeply rooted than symptoms; as these traits are no obligatory but only facultative associates of schizophrenia it might be speculated that each of them reveals a simpler genotype-phenotype relationship than the more complex, comprehensive disease phenotype. Those neurobiological traits might substitute polygenetically determined clinical phenotypes in linkage and association studies, particularly if the following requirements are fulfilled:
■ Association with the disease
■ Clustering in families of affected persons (also among clinically unaffected relatives)
■ Stability over time and low impact of treatment
■ Genetic determination to be demonstrated by twin studies
■ Optimally:
  - Cosegregation with the disease in families
  - Presence already before manifestation of the disease
  - Evidence for a more Mendelian-like genetics.
Those traits are called "endophenotypes" [29].

This observation proposes that multiple pathways may result in schizophrenia. These diverse pathways might be under the influence of different susceptibility genes and/or environmental factors. Appropriate neurobiological associates of schizophrenia might help to decompose this genetic and etiological complexity into more simple components.

Neurobiological and genetic research in schizophrenia has proposed multiple hypothetical "endophenotypes" which fulfill most of the mentioned criteria. Some of them have already been successfully used in linkage and association studies, e.g.:
■ Lack of inhibition paradigms indicated by P50 potential [15]
■ Smooth pursuit eye movement [1]
■ Wisconsin card sorting test [12, 14].

As a disadvantage, all these three measures are not stable, and influenced by medication, nutrition or substance use (e.g., nicotine). Consequently, these three traits are no perfect "endophenotypes". We are, therefore, aiming at neurodevelopmental phenotypes which are present already before the manifestation of the disease, and stable across lifetime. One example is the pattern of gyrification [58]. This feature perfectly fits all requested criteria (publication in preparation).

Altogether, it is not yet proven that the endophenotype approach is more successful than the "disease"-phenotype approach. This strategy is still a kind of trial-and-error experiment.

▦ Functional genomics and new candidate genes

Our current knowledge on the molecular etiology and pathophysiology of schizophrenia is limited; new progress in the a priori selection of appropriate candidate genes being involved in the manifestation of schizophrenia requires the detection of new molecular pathways related to schizophrenia. Recent technical developments offer new opportunities in this respect.

The parallel investigation of the expression of thousands of genes in mRNA tissue became recently feasible [59]. Those microarray chips were first proposed in 1985 and are now widely available: Expression profiles can be compared between pathological and control tissue [11]. These techniques are able to map biochemical pathways on the mRNA level and to compare them between affected persons and controls. Changes in pathways might point at the impact of susceptibility genes, and help to identify new candidate genes. The prefrontal brain and hippocampus are the target brain areas of schizophrenia. It can be assumed that the susceptibility genes contribute to schizophrenia by changing the expression profile of relevant gene products either directly (e.g., through variation in promoter regions) or indirectly by changing the other related gene products (e.g., variations in transcription factors impact on expression of multiple gene products). Given the large magnitude of brain-related genes (10,000 or more), a focus on pathophysiological gene families is appropriate.

In particular, gene families, involved in brain maturation and in brain plasticity, were explored by these technical tools in schizophrenia. Genes coding for presynaptic proteins and for myelinization were found to be differentially expressed [19, 36]. New candidate gene-based association studies are stimulated by the results; of particular interest are candidate genes located in candidate regions on the genome identified by linkage studies.

Genetic causes of diseases are thought to refer to specific sequence variants in the DNA. However, as a complication the detection of genetic causes of schizophrenia by detection of influential mutations in the DNA sequence might be blurred by the possibility that inheritance across generations is not necessarily bound to DNA-sequence variation. Epigenetics is the study of heritable changes in gene expression that occurs without changes in the DNA sequence [66]. The main known epigenetic mechanism is inactivation of genes via methylation or acetylation which play a major role in two neuropsychiatric syndromes (fragile X-syndrome and Rett's syndrome). Although these epigenetic mechanisms are under genetic control in these two syndromes, environmental and other non-genetic influences might also be relevant. Another epigenetic mechanism is imprinting (i.e., differential effects on the phenotype depending on the parental origin of a disease allele). Epigenetic transmission might induce irregular patterns of familial aggregations of the disorder which do not correspond to sequence variations in the DNA. However, differential expression patterns of genes might distinguish diseases and disease stages. Thus, gene expression analyses receive growing importance to unravel the genetic basis of schizophrenia.

▓ Conclusion

Progress in psychiatric genetics as well as in genetics of other complex diseases is slower than expected on the basis of the successes in mapping genes of monogenic diseases. The main progress in recent years has been positional cloning of susceptibility genes to multiple candidate regions with some consistency across various linkage studies. Unexpectedly, the systematic search for vulnerability genes turned out to be very awkward and nearly impossible using classical techniques. New molecular-genetic developments offering an efficient strategy to disease-gene identification became available only recently. New approaches to define a less complex phenotype might also turn out to be useful. Thus, despite the previous obstacles in the search of risk-modulating genes for schizophrenia there are good reasons for rapid progress in the identification of vulnerability genes for schizophrenia.

▓ References

1. Arolt V, Lencer R, Purmann S, Schurmann M, Muller-Myhsok B, Krecker K, Schwinger E (1999) Testing for linkage of eye tracking dysfunction and schizophrenia to markers on chromosomes 6, 8, 9, 20, and 22 in families multiply affected with schizophrenia. Am J Med Genet 88: 603–606
2. Baron M (2001) The search for complex disease genes: fault by linkage or fault by association? Mol Psychiatry 6: 143–149
3. Bassett AS, Chow EW (1999) 22q11 deletion syndrome: a genetic subtype of schizophrenia. Biol Psychiatry 46: 882–891
4. Beckmann H, Franzek E, Stöber G (1996) Genetic heterogeneity in catatonic schizophrenia: a family study. Am J Med Genet 67:289–300
5. Berrettini, WH (2001) Susceptibility loci. Am J Psychiatry 158: 865
6. Block W, Bayer TA, Tepest R, Träber F, Rietschel M, Müller DJ, Schulze TG, Honer, WG, Maier W, Schild HH, Falkai P (2000) Decreased frontal lobe ratio of N-acetyl aspartate to choline in familial schizophrenia: a proton magnetic resonance spectroscopy study. Neurosci Lett 289: 147–151
7. Blouin JL, Dombroski BA, Nath SK, Lasseter VK, Wolyniec PS, Nestadt G, Thornquist M, Ullrich G, McGrath J, Kasch L et al. (1998) Schizophrenia susceptibility loci on chromosomes 13q32 and 8p21. Nat Genet 20: 70–73
8. Brzustowicz LM, Hodgkinson KA, Chow EW, Honer WG, Bassett AS (2000) Location of a major susceptibility locus for familial schizophrenia on chromosome 1q21-q22. Science 288: 678–682
9. Chakravarti A (1999) Population genetics – making sense out of sequence. Nat Genet 21 (Suppl): 56–60
10. Cloninger CR, Kaufmann CA, Faraone SV, Malaspina D, Svrakic DM, Harkavy-Friedman J, Suarez BK, Matise TC, Shore D, Lee H et al. (1998) Genome-wide search for schizophrenia susceptibility loci: the NIMH Genetics Initiative and Millennium Consortium. Am J Med Genet 81: 275–281

11. Duggan DJ, Bittner M, Chgen Y, Meltzer P, Trent JM (1999) Expression profiling using cDNA microarrays. Nat Genet (Suppl) 21: 10–14
12. Egan MF, Goldberg TE, Kolachana BS, Callicott JH, Mazzanti CM, Straub RE, Goldman D, Weinberger DR (2001) Effect of COMT Val 108/158 Met genotype on frontal lobe function and risk for schizophrenia. Proc Natl Acad Sci U S A 98: 6917–6922
13. Erlenmeyer-Kimling L (2000) Neurobehavioral deficits in offspring of schizophrenic parents: liability indicators and predictors of illness. Am J Med Genet 97: 65–71
14. Franke P, Maier W, Hain C, Klingler T (1992) Wisconsin Card Sorting Test: an indicator of vulnerability to schizophrenia? Schizophr Res 6: 243–249
15. Freedman R, Coon H, Myles-Worsley M, Orr-Urtreger A, Olincy A, Davis A, Polymeropoulos M, Holik J, Hopkins J, Hoff M et al. (1997) Linkage of a neurophysiological deficit in schizophrenia to a chromosome 15 locus. Proc Natl Acad Sci U S A 94: 587–592
16. Gershon ES (2000) Bipolar illness and schizophrenia as oligogenic diseases: implications for the future. Biol Psychiatry 47: 240–244
17. Gershon ES, DeLisi LE, Hamovit J, Nurnberger JI Jr, Maxwell ME, Schreiber J, Dauphinais D, Dingman CW 2nd, Guroff JJ (1988) A controlled family study of chronic psychoses. Schizophrenia and schizoaffective disorder. Arch Gen Psychiatry 45: 328–336
18. Häfner H (2000) Onset and early course as determinants of the further course of schizophrenia. Acta Psychiatr Scand Suppl 407: 44–48
19. Hakak Y, Walker JR, Li C, Wong WH, Davis KL, Buxbaum JD, Haroutunian V, Fienberg AA (2001) Genome-wide expression analysis reveals dysregulation of myelination-related genes in chronic schizophrenia. Proc Natl Acad Sci U S A 98: 4746–4751
20. Herken H, Erdal ME (2001) Catechol-O-methyltransferase gene polymorphism in schizophrenia: evidence for association between symptomatology and prognosis. Psychiatr Genet 11: 105–109
21. Hernandez I, Sokolov BP (1997) Abnormal expression of serotonin transporter mRNA in the frontal and temporal cortex of schizophrenics. Mol Psychiatry 2: 57–64
22. Horikawa Y, Oda N, Cox NJ, Li X, Orho-Melander M, Hara M, Hinokio Y, Lindner TH, Mashima H, Schwarz PE et al. (2000) Genetic variation in the gene encoding calpain-10 is associated with type 2 diabetes mellitus. Nat Genet 26: 163–175
23. Ishiguro H, Okuyama Y, Toru M, Arinami T (2000) Mutation and association analysis of the 5' region of the dopamine D3 receptor gene in schizophrenia patients: identification of the Ala38Thr polymorphism and suggested association between DRD3 haplotypes and schizophrenia. Mol Psychiatry 5: 433–438
24. Kaiser R, Tremblay PB, Schmider J, Henneken M, Dettling M, Müller-Oerlinghausen B, Uebelhack R, Roots I, Brockmoller J (2001) Serotonin transporter polymorphisms: no association with response to antipsychotic treatment, but associations with the schizoparanoid and residual subtypes of schizophrenia. Mol Psychiatry 6: 179–185
25. Kaufmann CA, Suarez B, Malaspina D, Pepple J, Svrakic D, Markel PD, Meyer J, Zambuto CT, Schmitt K, Matise TC et al. (1998) NIMH Genetics Initiative Millenium Schizophrenia Consortium: linkage analysis of African-American pedigrees. Am J Med Genet 81: 282–289
26. Kendler KS, McGuire M, Gruenberg AM, Spellman M, O'Hare A, Walsh D (1993) The Roscommon Family Study. II. The risk of nonschizophrenic nonaffective psychoses in relatives. Arch Gen Psychiatry 50: 645–652
27. Kruglyak L (1999) Prospects for whole-genome linkage disequilibrium mapping of common disease genes. Nat Genet 22: 139–144
28. Lander E, Kruglyak L (1995) Genetic dissection of complex traits: guidelines for interpreting and reporting linkage results. Nat Genet 11: 241–247
29. Leboyer M, Bellivier F, Nosten-Bertrand M, Jouvent R, Pauls D, Mallet J (1998) Psychiatric genetics: search for phenotypes. Trends Neurosci 21: 102–105
30. Levinson DF, Mahtani MM, Nancarrow DJ, Brown DM, Kruglyak L, Kirby A, Hayward NK, Crowe RR, Andreasen NC, Black DW et al. (1998) Genome scan of schizophrenia. Am J Psychiatry 155: 741–750
31. Levinson DF, Holmans P, Straub RE, Owen MJ, Wildenauer DB, Gejman PV, Pulver AE, Laurent C, Kendler KS, Walsh D et al. (2000) Multicenter linkage study of schizophrenia candidate regions on chromosomes 5q, 6q, 10p, and 13q: schizophrenia linkage collaborative group III. Am J Hum Genet 67: 652–663

32. Maier W, Lichtermann D, Minges J, Hallmayer J, Heun R, Benkert O, Levinson DF (1993) Continuity and discontinuity of affective disorders and schizophrenia. Results of a controlled family study. Arch Gen Psychiatry 50: 871–883
33. Maier W, Lichtermann D, Franke P, Heun R, Falkai P, Rietschel M (2002) The dichotomy of schizophrenia and affective disorders in extended pedigrees. Schizophr Res (in press)
34. McGue M, Gottesman II (1991) The genetic epidemiology of schizophrenia and the design of linkage studies. Eur Arch Psychiatry Clin Neurosci 240: 174–181
35. McGuffin P, Asherson P, Owen M, Farmer A (1994) The strength of the genetic effect. Is there room for an environmental influence in the aetiology of schizophrenia? Br J Psychiatry 164: 593–599
36. Mirnics K, Middleton FA, Marquez A, Lewis DA, Levitt P (2000) Molecular characterization of schizophrenia viewed by microarray analysis of gene expression in prefrontal cortex. Neuron 28: 33–67
37. Mortensen PB, Pedersen CB, Westergaard T, Wohlfahrt J, Ewald H, Mors O, Andersen PK, Melbye M (1999) Effects of family history and place and season of birth on the risk of schizophrenia. N Engl J Med 340: 603–608
38. Peltonen L, McKusick VA (2001) Genomics and medicine. Dissecting human disease in the postgenomic era. Science 291: 1224–1229
39. Pericak-Vance MA, Bebout JL, Gaskell PC Jr, Yamaoka LH, Hung WY, Alberts MJ, Walker AP, Bartlett RJ, Haynes CA, Welsh KA et al. (1991) Linkage studies in familial Alzheimer disease: evidence for chromosome 19 linkage. Am J Hum Genet 48: 1034–1050
40. Poirier J, Davignon J, Bouthillier D, Kogan S, Bertrand P, Gauthier S (1993) Apolipoprotein E polymorphism and Alzheimer's disease. Lancet 342: 697–699
41. Pritchard JK, Rosenberg NA (1999) Use of unlinked genetic markers to detect population stratification in association studies. Am J Hum Genet 65: 220–228
42. Riley BP, McGuffin P (2000) Linkage and associated studies of schizophrenia. Am J Med Genet 97: 23–44
43. Riley BP, Makoff A, Mogudi-Carter M, Jenkins T, Williamson R, Collier D, Murray R (2000) Haplotype transmission disequilibrium and evidence for linkage of the CHRNA7 gene region to schizophrenia in Southern African Bantu families. Am J Med Genet 96: 196–201
44. Risch N (1990) Linkage strategies for genetically complex traits. I. Multilocus models. Am J Hum Genet 46: 222–228
45. Risch N (2000) Searching for genetic determinants in the new millennium. Nature 405: 847–856
46. Risch N, Teng J (1998) The relative poser of family-based and case-control designs for association studies of complex human diseases. I. DNA pooling. Genome Res 8: 1273–1288
47. Schwab SG, Albus M, Hallmayer J, Hönig S, Borrmann M, Lichtermann D, Ebstein RP, Ackenheil M, Lerer B, Risch N et al. (1995) Evaluation of a susceptibility gene for schizophrenia on chromosome 6p by multipoint affected sib-pair linkage analysis. Nat Genet 11: 325–327
48. Schwab SG, Hallmayer J, Albus M, Lerer B, Eckstein GN, Borrmann M, Segman RH, Hanses C, Freymann J, Yakir A et al. (2000) A genome-wide autosomal screen for schizophrenia susceptibility loci in 71 families with affected siblings: support for loci on chromosome 10p and 6. Mol Psychiatry 5: 638–649
49. Schwab SG, Hallmayer J, Freimann J, Lerer B, Albus M, Borrmann-Hassenbach M, Segman RH, Trixler M, Rietschel M, Maier W, Wildenauer DB (2001) Investigation of linkage and association/linkage disequilibrium of HLA A-, DQA1-, DQB1-, and DRB1-alleles in 69 sib-pair- and 89 trio-families with schizophrenia. Am J Med Genet 114: 315–320
50. Sklar P, Schwab SG, Williams NM, Daly M, Schaffner S, Maier W, Albus M, Trixler M, Eichhammer P, Lerer B et al. (2001) Association analysis of NOTCH4 loci in schizophrenia using family and population-based controls. Nat Genet 28: 126–128
51. Stöber G, Saar K, Ruschendorf F, Meyer J, Nurnberg G, Jatzke S, Franzek E, Reis A, Lesch KP, Wienker TF, Beckmann H (2000) Splitting schizophrenia: periodic catatonia-susceptibility locus on chromosome 15q15. Am J Hum Genet 67: 1201–1207
52. Stoneking M (2001) Single nucleotide polymorphisms. Nature 409: 821–822

53. Straub RE, MacLean CJ, O'Neill FA, Burke J, Murphy B, Duke F, Shinkwin R, Webb BT, Zhang J, Walsh D et al. (1995) A potential vulnerability locus for schizophrenia on chromosome 6p24-22: evidence for genetic heterogeneity. Nat Genet 11: 287–293

54. Straub RE, MacLean CJ, Martin RB, Ma Y, Myakishev MV, Harris-Kerr C, Webb BT, O'Neill FA, Walsh D, Kendler KS (1998) A schizophrenia locus may be located in region 10p15-p11. Am J Med Genet 81: 296–301

55. Suarez BK, Hampe CL, van Eerdewegh P (1994) Problems of replicating linkage claims in psychiatry. In: Gershon ES, Cloninger C (eds) Genetic Approaches to Mental Disorders. American Psychiatric Association, Washington, pp 23–46

56. Tsuang M (1991) Morbidity risks of schizophrenia and affective disorders among first-degree relatives of patients with schizoaffective disorders. Br J Psychiatry 158: 165–170

57. Tsuang M (2000) Schizophrenia: genes and environment. Biol Psychiatry 47: 210–220

58. Vogeley K, Tepest R, Pfeiffer U, Schneider-Axmann T, Maier W, Honer WG, Falkai P (2001) Right frontal hypergyria differentiation in affected and unaffected siblings from families multiply affected with schizophrenia: a morphometric MRI study. Am J Psychiatry 158: 494–496

59. Watson SJ, Akil H (1999) Gene chips and arrays revealed: a primer on their power and their uses. Biol Psychiatry 45: 533–543

60. Wei J, Hemmings GP (2000) The NOTCH4 locus is associated with susceptibility to schizophrenia. Nat Genet 25: 376–377

61. Weiss KM, Terwilliger J (2000) How many diseases does it take to map a gene with SNPs? Nat Genet 26: 151–156

62. Wildenauer DB, Schwab SG, Maier W, Detera-Wadleigh SD (1999) Do schizophrenia and affective disorder share susceptibility genes? Schizophr Res 39: 107–111

63. Williams J, McGuffin P, Nothen M, Owen MJ (1997) Meta-analysis of association between the 5-HT2a receptor T102C polymorphism and schizophrenia. EMASS Collaborative Group. European Multicentre Association Study of Schizophrenia. Lancet 349: 1221

64. Williams J, Spurlock G, Holmans P, Mant R, Murphy K, Jones L, Cardno A, Asherson P, Blackwood D, Muir W et al. (1998) A meta-analysis and transmission disequilibrium study of association between the dopamine D3 receptor gene and schizophrenia. Mol Psychiatry 3: 141–149

65. Williams NM, Rees MI, Holmans P, Norton N, Cardno AG, Jones LA, Murphy KC, Sanders RD, McCarthy G, Gray MY et al. (1999) A two-stage genome scan for schizophrenia susceptibility genes in 196 affected sibling pairs. Hum Mol Genet 8: 1729–1739

66. Wolffe AP, Matzke MA (1999) Epigenetics: regulation through repression. Science 286: 481–486

Genotype-environment interaction in the Finnish adoptive family study – Interplay between genes and environment?

P. Tienari, L. C. Wynne,* A. Sorri, I. Lahti, K. Läksy, J. Moring, M. Naarala, P. Nieminen, K.-E. Wahlberg, J. Miettunen
The Department of Psychiatry, the University of Oulu, Finland
*Department of Psychiatry, the University of Rochester, NY, USA

▓ Introduction

Nature and nurture are not separate. Instead of studying them apart from each other, it is important to investigate the interplay between genes and environment and how they influence one another. To an important degree, genetic effects on behavior come about because they either influence the extent to which the individual is likely to be exposed to individual differences in environmental risk or they affect how susceptible the individual is to environmental adversities [17]. The disorders of greatest medical, research, and policy concern today, particularly in psychiatry, are likely to be complex. Such disorders may have not a single cause but a causal chain, or multiple such chains. These chains may involve genetic, biological, environmental and social risk factors. The effect of a single risk factor can only be fully understood in the context of all the others [7].

Vulnerability (predisposition, diathesis) to schizophrenia can be defined as the individual's characteristic threshold beyond which stressful events produce decompensation manifest in the clinically diagnosable symptom picture. The genetic components of vulnerability are inevitably shaped from conception onward throughout development as the result of transactions of the individual with the psychosocial and physical environment. Transactions seen in a developmental context imply the concept of *epigenesis* [30]. Rosenthal [14] calls this "reciprocal escalation", meaning that the inborn diathesis (vulnerability) and stressors heighten each other in an intensifying process until the schizophrenic break occurs. Rutter, Dunn and Plomin et al. [18] have in their review integrated this complicated issue of nature and nurture: The general principles include individual differences in reactivity to the environment, two-way interplay between intra-individual biology and environmental influences, and the need to consider broader social contextual features.

Ottman [9] described from an epidemiological point of view some theoretical alternatives. 1) The genetic susceptibility does not cause disease directly, but acts by increasing the level of expression of the risk factor. In this case, the genetic basis of disease is equivalent to the genetic basis of the risk factor, but the risk factor may have other, non-genetic causes. 2) The risk factor has a direct effect on disease susceptibility, and the genetic susceptibility exacerbates this effect. The genetic susceptibility has no effect in the absence of risk factor, but the risk factor can act by itself to cause disease, and 3) is the converse of the second. Here the genetic susceptibility has direct effect, and the risk exacerbates this effect. The risk factor has no effect in the absence of the genetic susceptibility, but the genetic susceptibility can raise risk by itself. 4) Neither the genetic susceptibility nor the risk factor can influence the disease risk by itself, but risk is increased when both are present. 5) Either the genetic susceptibility or the risk factor can influence disease risk by itself, and the combined effect of the two may be different from the effect of each acting alone.

Scarr [19] argued that the genotype-environment correlation, rather than gene-environmental interactions, predominates in the construction of experiences. Many environmental opportunities are taken by some individuals and not by others, depending on the individuals characteristics. The selective use of environmental opportunities is better thought of as a genotype-environment correlation than a genotype-environment interaction. The theory of genotype-environment effects has three propositions: passive, evocative and active. Children's genes are necessarily correlated with their environments because parents usually provide both, so that their experiences are constructed from opportunities that are positively correlated with their personal characteristics. People evoke from others responses that are correlated with the person's own characteristics. People actively select environments that are correlated with their interests, talents and personality characteristics [19]. The balance of genotype-environment effects changes from passive to active with development, as children move out from the family to make their own choices of interests and activities. Genetic differences become more important across development, as people make their own environments [19].

Rutter [16] pointed out that prospective longitudinal studies have been crucial in demonstrating the diversity of psychopathological outcomes. Thus, parental mental disorder leads not only to an increased risk for the same type of psychiatric condition but also to a raised risk for a wide range of other psychopathology. Longitudinal data are also needed for the adequate study of "escape" from risk. With virtually all risk factors, it has been found that a substantial proportion of children exposed to the risk survive without serious psychopathological sequelae. This highlights the need to study possible protective as well as risk factors. It is relevant to note that risk mechanisms, often involve indirect effects of one kind or another. Finally, such processes include so-called turning point effects in which risky life trajectories may change direction onto a more adaptive path or vice versa. *Most psychosocial turning points should not be conceptualized in stress terms at all.* Rather, they alter life trajectories because they open up (or close down) important opportunities, because they are accompanied by a lasting change in the environment, because they influence people's selection or shaping of their environment, or because they affect people's control over their lives [16].

In general, gene-environment interactions imply that the effects of experience are modulated by genetic influences, and vice versa. Behavioral geneticists have sometimes assumed that this is the same as a statistical interaction in a multivariate analysis of genetic and environmental factors [12]. A statistical interaction term is an indication of gene-environmental interaction, but such a term will detect only certain sorts of genetic influences on susceptibility to a specific environmental factor [17]. The popular diathesis-stress model of the etiology of psychopathology is also an instance of a hypothesized gene-environment interaction in which environmental stressors have a particularly deleterious effect on only those individuals with a genetic diathesis, or a predisposition to a particular psychopathology [11].

Wahlberg et al. [29] found significant association between communication deviance (scored from audiotaped and transcribed Rorschach Test protocols) in Finnish adoptive parents and thought disorder in genetically high-risk adoptees (HR) but not in low-risk adoptees (LR). This is consistent with the hypothesis of genetic control of sensitivity to the environment. Importantly, there was no difference in communication deviance in the adoptive, rearing parents of HR adoptees versus adoptive parents of LR offspring. This indicates that the adoptees at genetic risk did not have a special impact of increasing the communication deviance of their rearing parents. Communication deviance was stable during adulthood but not from adolescence into adulthood in 12 years follow-up [27]. Also specific categories of subsyndromal thought disorder appear to qualify as vulnerability indicators for schizophrenia. Genetic risk and rearing-parent communication pattern significantly interacted as a joint effect that differentiates adopted-away offspring of schizophrenic mothers from control adopted-away offspring [28].

Adoption studies of schizophrenia can give support to the hypothesis of interaction of genotype and environment. The presumed genotype is perhaps not only "sensitive" to precipitating factors but also to protective environmental factors. In adoption studies, the transmitters of heredity and psychosocial factors can be investigated separately because the biological parents are not the parents who reared the children [12, 22].

⬛ Finnish adoption study

A nationwide Finnish sample of schizophrenics' offspring given up for adoption was compared blindly with matched controls, who were adopted offspring of nonschizophrenic biological parents [24]. Also the biological parents were interviewed and tested. The Finnish adoption study has sought to extend the earlier findings [6, 15] in several ways, including the following: generating a larger sample of adoptees; obtaining standardized personal interviews and tests with all subjects whenever possible; using DSM-III-R criteria for all subjects; carrying out direct investigation of adoptive rearing families with home observations and family-oriented testing; and following up adoptees who were initially not fully into the age of risk for schizophrenia and re-examining them with standardized diagnostic instruments and with psychological tests.

Adoptee diagnostic procedures

The initial evaluations of the adoptees were carried out beginning in 1977. The interviewing psychiatrists were carefully kept blind as to the index/control status of the biological parents. Adoptees were also re-evaluated in a second wave taking place after a median interval of 12 years, with interviews by new research psychiatrists who were blind about all prior assessments of the adoptees and the biological and adoptive relatives. Personal interviews were carried out either initially or at follow-up, or both, with 346 (90.6%) of the adoptees. The follow-up interview schedules included an expanded lifetime version of the PSE, SCID-II, and the SIS. Additionally, for all subjects in the study, Finnish national computerized registers have been searched. The Hospital Discharge Register was systematically surveyed through the end of 2000 for all public and private inpatients, and through November, 2000, the register of reasons for death. Through October, 1994, other register searches have been carried out for diagnoses that justify disability pensions and give information on sick leaves prescribed by a doctor, free medication prescribed for certain illnesses, including psychoses, and information about criminality. The follow-up was (median) 19 years from the initial assessment (and family evaluation). Adoptees were (median) 43 years of age in 2000.

The principal, best estimate, hierarchically most severe lifetime diagnoses were assigned on the basis of meeting DSM-III-R criteria for Axis I or Axis II psychiatric disorders based on all available data for all subjects. Diagnoses were made at three levels of certainty-definite, probable, and possible; the focus in this report is on adoptees with diagnoses at definite and probable certainty levels. As described previously [24], three stringent approaches for assessing and maintaining interrater diagnostic reliability have been carried out, including checks on rater drift over time.

For purposes of the present report, we focus upon DSM-III-R schizophrenia and ten other disorders that have been considered genetically linked to schizophrenia by one or more previous researchers. These constitute what we call the putative "broad" schizophrenia spectrum. Three subgroups, beyond schizophrenia, include other nonaffective psychotic disorders, specifically, schizoaffective disorder, schizophreniform disorder, delusional disorder, and psychosis not otherwise specified (NOS); affective psychoses, that is, bipolar and depressive disorders with psychotic features; and the odd-cluster (A) of personality disorders, namely, schizotypal, schizoid, and paranoid personality disorders, plus avoidant personality disorder.

Adoptive family assessments

Adoptive families have been investigated in their homes, directly and intensively, with tape-recorded procedures that usually took two days (14–16 hours): This started in 1977. Joint interviews with the whole family, joint interviews with the parental couples, Consensus Rorschach, individual interviews with members of adoptive families, Individual Rorschach-test [21]. Experienced psychiatrists interviewed the adoptive families. Total information was used to score family functioning using a 33-item instrument (OPAS) [23]. The OPAS had been developed for evaluation of family relationships during interviews and observation in the family home. Beavers' Family Evaluation Scales [8] was a major source of scales for the study.

The total number of families with OPAS scales scored was 303. Later analyses were performed using 28 OPAS scales (leaving out those three scales that gave poorest reliability score measured by Cronbach's alpha coefficient and two with many missing values.). There were still some missing scores (none in 210 families, 1 – 5 in 66, 6 – 10 in 13, 11 – 20 in 11, and 22 – 24 in three families). In families with missing OPAS scores, the score is substituted from the family with the most similar arithmetic mean for all OPAS categories ("Nearest Neighbor Method" [3]). The inter-rater reliability of the OPAS scales was examined in two separate studies. In the first, the four interviewing psychiatrists rated audiotaped family interviews (N = 40) blindly. In the second reliability study one rater was present when a sample of the families (N = 31) were interviewed by another.

■ Results

Healthy vs. dysfunctional adoptive families

Family's overall health was rated by interviewing psychiatrist using Global Health-Pathology Scale (from 01) healthy or pathology (to 99). (The scale is very similar to the Global Assessment of Relational Functioning, GARF [2]). The median value of the this scale was used as the cut-off point for dividing adoptive families into two groups labeled as "healthy" and "dysfunctional". Age-corrected morbid risks (MR) for schizophrenia were then calculated using Kaplan-Meier procedure [10] in these two groups. MR for schizophrenia in LR adoptees reared in "healthy" families was 0 % (no genetic risk and no environmental risk), but in HR 1.49 ± 1.48 % (genetic risk in the absence of environmental risk). MR for schizophrenia in LR adoptees reared in dysfunctional families was 4.84 ± 2.73 % (environmental risk in the absence of genetic risk), but 13.04 ± 3.86 % in HR adoptees (both genetic risk and environmental risk present).

Specific scales

After several explorative analyses, three specific OPAS scales, Lack of Empathy, Disrupted Communication, and Parent-Offspring Conflict were selected in this analysis. (The same scales as in [25] earlier when partial results were reported). These had been scored on a Likert scale from 1 (healthy) to 5 (severe dysfunction). These were used as dichotomized environmental variables in logistic regression analyses (1 – 2 "healthy, and 3 – 5 "dysfunctional") where Schizophrenia Spectrum diagnosis in adoptees was predicted from (G)enotype and (E)nvironment. Disrupted communication and Parent-Child Conflict were both

Table 1. Prediction of schizophrenia spectrum disorder in adoptees from assessment of family functioning (OPAS) (N = 303)[1] using logistic regression analysis

A Specific Scales of OPAS				
Variable	Regression coefficient	P-value of Wald's test	Odds ratio	95% Confidence interval
Genetic factor[2]				
Mothers mental disorder	1.63	<0.001	5.10	2.18 – 11.93
Environmental factors[3]				
Disrupted Communication	1.34	<0.002	3.81	1.66 – 8.77
Parent-Child Conflict	1.00	0.013	2.74	1.24 – 6.04
Lack of Empathy	(0.29)	0.583	(1.33)	(0.48 – 3.74)
B From variables based on factor scores				
Variable	Regression coefficient	P-value of Wald's test	Odds ratio	95% Confidence interval
Genetic factor[2]				
Mother's mental disorder	1.63	<0.001	5.11	2.19 – 11.89
Environmental factors[3]				
"Critical" Rearing	1.25	0.002	3.50	1.57 – 7.79
"Constricted" Rearing	1.09	0.007	3.30	1.35 – 6.50
"Boundary Problems"	1.04	0.009	2.82	1.30 – 6.18

[1] Missing data were substituted with scores of "nearest neighbor" family
[2] Biological mother's mental disorder (Schizophrenia spectrum disorders /Nonspectrum disorders)
[3] Family functioning in adoptive rearing family

statistically significant independent environmental explanatory variables. Lack of Empathy did not improve the model to predict the adoptee diagnosis. Genetic (indexed by Biological Mother with DSM-III-R diagnosis of Schizophrenia Spectrum) was the strongest explanatory variable (adjusted odds ratio 5.10) (Table 1A). In a stratified logistic regression by genetic risk, adjusted odds ratio was for Disrupted Communication 3.63 (95% confidence interval (CI) 1.37 – 9.64; $p < 0.001$ of Wald's test) in HR adoptee group, as compared to 4.69 (CI 1.03 – 21.41; p = 0.046) in LR group; for Parent/Child Conflict OR 4.42 (1.77 – 10.999), $p < 0.002$ (p = 0.483 in LR), but for Lack of Empathy p = 0.709 in HR (p = 0.599 in LR).

Re-grouping using factor scores

Factor analysis was performed using 28 OPAS scales. Extraction method was principal component analysis with Equamax rotation. Equamax rotation was used to balance the need for interpretable factors with the need for simplified, interpretable variables. In this analysis, three factors were extracted. The result-

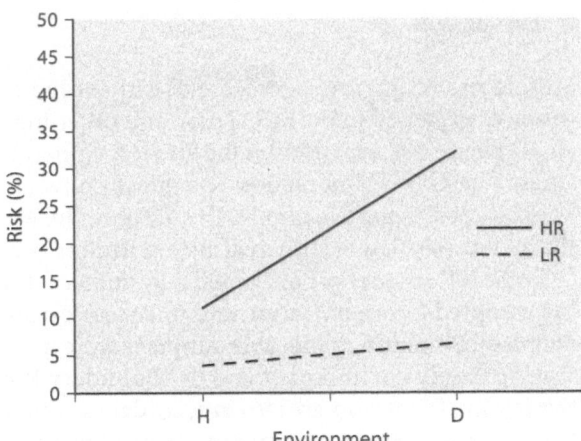

Fig. 1. The observed risk for schizophrenia spectrum disorder in high risk and low risk adoptees in relation to the healthy (H) or disordered (D) "constricted" adoptive family.

ing three factors could be labeled as *Critical* (loading for Criticism scale 0.802, for Intensive, explosive affect 0.735, for Non-acknowledgement 0.689, for Parent-parent conflict 0.688, for Insecurity in family 0.661, Dissatisfaction with family 0.650), *Constricted* (loading for Flat, empty affect scale 0.818, for Narrow range of affect 0.811 and Constricted communication 0.733), and *Boundary Problems* (loading Chaotic, unclear family organization 0.777, for Individual enmeshment scale 0.749, and for Generational enmeshment 0.697). (Only scales each with loadings 0.650 or higher are mentioned). Factor 1 *Critical* seems to assess the same aspects as does Expressed Emotion (EE).

Based on a rotated factor matrix, the score for each subject was computed using standard procedures of factor analysis [20]. To calculate such factor scores, a family's score on each variable included in the factor is multiplied by the factor loading for the particular variable. The sum of these products is the family's factor score. These three factor score variables were dichotomized (using median) to healthy/dysfunctional families for logistic regression analysis and to obtain a measure of risk such as odds ratio (OR). In Table 1 B Spectrum diagnosis in adoptees was predicted from G and E^{1-3} (using variables based on the Factor Scores). There was a strong genetic effect (indexed by Schizophrenia Spectrum diagnosis in Biological Mother). All environmental variables were important explanatory factors. In a stratified logistic regression analysis by genetic risk, genetically vulnerable HR adoptees were more sensitive to "Constricted" family environment (adjusted odds ratio 3.51, CI 1.41 – 8.77; $p < 0.001$ of Wald's test) as compared to LR adoptees ($p = 0.48$) (see also Fig. 1), and to "Boundary Problems" in rearing family (adjusted odds ratio 3.02, CI 1.20 – 7.57; $p < 0.002$) in HR group as compared to LR adoptees ($p = 0.262$), and to "Critical" adoptive family (OR 2.85, CI 1.16 – 6.98; $p = 0.022$) in HR group as compared to LR adoptees OR 8.44 (1.003 – 71.002) $p < 0.05$ of Wald's test).

▪ Discussion

Morbid risk results are in accordance with the hypothesis that Genetics and Environment each add to the MR. These and other findings show that it is individuals at genetic risk who showed the greatest vulnerability to environmental adversities. The G × E interaction was most convincingly demonstrated with the "Constricted" adoptive family. In addition, the MR results are compatible with the hypothesis that healthy rearing environment can have a protective effect.

In the HR adoptee group, genetically vulnerable adoptees were more sensitive to Disrupted Communication and to Parent/offspring Conflict as compared LR adoptees. Similarly, vulnerable adoptees were more sensitive to a "Constricted" rearing family environment and to "Boundary Problems" in the rearing adoptive family. The results are also in accordance with what Gottesman and Bertelsen hypothesized that discordance in identical twins may primarily be explained by the capacity of schizophrenic genotype or diathesis to be unexpressed unless it is released by some kind of environmental, including non-familial stressors [4].

Genotype - environment interaction (G × E) can be defined as a genetic control of sensitivity to environmental factors, or environmental control of gene expression [5]. Thus, some genotypes are more likely than others to develop disease in the event of exposure to certain environmental factors. In the case of genotype-environment interaction, diseases will tend to cluster in families not because of a direct genetic effect, but because relatives are more vulnerable to the risk-increasing effect of a prevalent environmental risk factor [26]. It is possible that neither the genetic susceptibility nor the risk factor can influence the disease risk by itself, but risk is increased when both are present [9]. These and other examples are important in that they illustrate that a genotype associated with a disorder may not indicate any genetic role in the causal pathway to the disorder but may identify who is or is not susceptible to an environmental causal factors [7, 13]. They also point to the same direction as clinical studies of schizophrenic patients and their families [1].

Acknowledgment This study was supported in part by the National Institute of Mental Health, grant MH 39633, from the Public Health Service (Dr. Wynne), by the Scottish Rite Schizophrenia Research Program (Dr. Wynne), and by the National Medical Research Board of Finland (Dr. Tienari, Dr. Moring).

▪ Reference

1. Alanen YO (1997) Schizophrenia: Its Origins and Need-adapted Treatment. Karnac Books, London
2. American Psychiatric Association (1994) Diagnostic and Statistical Manual of Mental Disorders (Fourth edition)
3. Chen J, Shao J (2001) Jackknife variance estimation for Nearest-Neighbor Imputation. Journal of the American Statistical Association 96: 260–269
4. Gottesman II, Bertelsen A (1989) Confirming unexpressed genotypes for schizophrenia. Risks in the offspring of Fischer's Danish identical and fraternal discordant twins. Arch Gen Psychiatry 46: 867–872

5. Kendler KS, Eaves LJ (1986) Models for the joint effect of genotype and environment on liability to psychiatric illness. Am J Psychiatry 143: 279–289
6. Kety SS, Wender PH, Jacobsen B, Ingraham L, Jansson L, Faber B, Kinney D (1994) Mental illness in the biological and adoptive relatives of schizophrenic adoptees. Replication of the Copenhagen study in the rest of Denmark. Arch Gen Psychiatry 51:442-455
7. Kraemer HC, Stice E, Kazdin A, Offord D, Kupfer D (2001) How do risk factors work together? Mediators, moderators and independent, overlapping, and proxy risk factors. Am J Psychiatry 158: 848–856
8. Lewis JM, Beavers WR, Gosset JT, Philips VA (1976) No Single Thread. Psychological Health in Family Systems. Brunner/Mazel, New York
9. Ottman R (1990) An epidemiologic approach to gene-environment interaction. Genet Epidemiol 7: 177–185
10. Parmar Mk, Machin D (1996) Survival Analysis: A Practical Approach. John Wiley & Sons, Chichester-New York
11. Plomin R, DeFries JC, McClearn GE, Rutter M (2000) Behavior Genetics, 4th edn. WH Freeman and Company, New York
12. Pogue-Geile M, Rose R (1987) Psychopathology: a behavior genetic perspective. In: Jacob T (ed) Family Interaction and Psychopathology: Theories, Methods and Findings. Plenum Press, New York, pp 629–650
13. Reiss D (2000) The Relationship Code. Deciphering Genetic and Social Influences on Adolescent Development. Harvard University Press, Cambridge
14. Rosenthal D (1963) The Genain Quadruplets. Basic Book, Inc, Publishers, New York
15. Rosenthal D, Wender PH, Kety SS, Welner J, Schulsinger F (1971) The adopted-away offspring of schizophrenics. Am J Psychiatry 128: 307–311
16. Rutter M (1993) Developmental psychopathology as a research perspective. In: Magnusson D, Caesar P (eds) Longitudinal Research on Individual Development. Present status and future perspective. Cambridge University Press, Cambridge, pp 127–152
17. Rutter M (1997) Nature-nurture integration. The example of antisocial behavior. Am Psychol 32: 390–398
18. Rutter M, Dunn J, Plomin R, Simonoff E, Pickles A, Maughan B, Ormel J, Meyer J, Eaves L (1997) Integrating nature and nurture: implications of person-environment correlations and interactions for developmental psychopathology. Development & Psychopathology 9: 335–364
19. Scarr S (1993) Genes, experience, and development. In: Magnusson D, Caesar P (eds) Longitudinal Research on Individual Development. Present Status and Future Perspectives. Cambridge University Press, Cambridge, pp 26–50
20. SPSS Advanced Models 9.0 (1999) SPSS Inc, New York
21. Tienari P, Lahti I, Sorri A, Naarala M, Wahlberg KE, Ronkko T, Moring J, Wynne LC (1987) The Finnish adoptive family study of schizophrenia: possible joint effects of genetic vulnerability and family interactions. In: Hahlweg K, Goldstein MJ (eds) Understanding Major Mental Disorder: The Contributions of Family Interaction Research. Family Process Press, New York, pp 33–54
22. Tienari P, Wynne LC (1994) Adoption studies of schizophrenia. Ann Med 26: 233–237
23. Tienari P, Wynne LC, Moring J, Lahti I, Naarala M, Sorri A, Wahlberg KE, Saarento O, Seitamaa M, Kaleva M, Läksy K (1994) The Finnish Adoptive Family Study of Schizophrenia: implications for family research. Br J Psychiatry 164: 20–26
24. Tienari P, Wynne LC, Moring J, Läksy K, Nieminen P, Sorri A, Lahti I, Wahlberg KE, Naarala M, Kurki-Suonio K, Saarento O, Koistinen P, Tarvainen T, Hakko H, Miettunen J (2000) Finnish adoptive family study: sample selection and adoptee DSM-III-R diagnoses. Acta Psychiatr Scand 101: 433–443
25. Tienari P, Wynne LC, Moring J, Wahlberg KE, Sorri A, Naarala M, Lahti I (1993) Genetic vulnerability or family environment? Implications from the Finnish Adoptive Family Study of Schizophrenia. Psychiatria Fennica 24: 23–41
26. van Os J, Marcekis M (1998) The ecogenetics of schizophrenia. Schizophr Res 32: 127–135

27.　Wahlberg KE, Wynne LC, Keskitalo P, Nieminen P, Moring J, Läksy K, Sorri A, Koistinen P, Tarvainen T, Miettunen J, Tienari P (2001) Long-term stability of communication deviance. J Abnorm Psychol 110: 443–448

28.　Wahlberg KE, Wynne LC, Oja H, Keskitalo P, Anias-Tanner H, Koistinen P, Tarvainen T, Hakko H, Lahti I, Moring J, Naarala M, Sorri A, Tienari P (2000) Thought Disorder Index of Finnish adoptees and communication deviance of their adoptive parents. Psychol Med 30: 127–136

29.　Wahlberg KE, Wynne LC, Oja H, Keskitalo P, Pykäläinen L, Lahti I, Moring J, Naarala M, Sorri A, Seitamaa M, Läksy K, Kolassa J, Tienari P (1997) Gene-environment interaction in vulnerability to schizophrenia: findings from the Finnish Adoptive Family Study of Schizophrenia. Am J Psychiatry 154: 355–362

30.　Wynne LC 1968) Methological and conceptual issues in the study of schizophrenics and their families. In: Rosenthal D, Kety SS (eds) The Transmission of Schizophrenia. Oxford Pergamon Press, Oxford, pp 185–199

Cognitive epidemiology: psychological and social risk mechanisms for psychosis

J. van Os,* I. Janssen, M. Hanssen, M. Bak, I. Myin-Germeys, M. Marcelis, R. Bijl, W. Vollebergh, P. Delespaul
Department of Psychiatry and Neuropsychology, European Graduate School of Neuroscience, Maastricht University, The Netherlands
*Division of Psychological Medicine, Institute of Psychiatry, London, UK

▓ What phenotype should we identify risk factors for?

Psychosis continuum views

The hypothesis that psychosis exists in nature as a distribution of symptoms is not so bold as it may seem [1]. For example, in the case of depression, both genetic and community studies suggest that the phenotype is more likely to exist as a continuous (albeit skewed, [2]) distribution of symptoms rather than a true disease dichotomy [3–6]. Given the substantial degree of overlap in terms of psychopathology, outcome, risk factors and treatment between depression and psychosis [7], it is unlikely that psychosis, contrary to depression, would have a completely non-continuous, dichotomous distribution. Although possibly more skewed because of their lower prevalence, a degree of continuity in the distribution of symptoms would be expected. This hypothesis, however, has attracted relatively little research effort, especially from the psychiatric profession [8].

The supposition of a psychosis continuum does not necessarily imply that there is a continuum of *disorder*. For example, in the US National Comorbidity Survey, approximately 28% of individuals endorsed psychosis-screening questions. However, when clinicians made diagnoses, the rate of even broadly defined psychosis was only 0.7% [9]. This suggests that the clinical definition of psychosis may represent only a minor selection of the total (not necessarily clinical) phenotypic continuum. The existence of lesser states on a distributed continuum in the population may perhaps, instead of a *forme fruste* of disease, be better thought of as a risk factor for what clinicians would call disorder [10, 11]. In epidemiological terms, this argument can be explored by examining the possible combinations of underlying causes of the presumed psychosis continuum in relation to the predicted distribution of the trait. For example, if psychosis were the result of a single, unconfounded, fully penetrant cause such as a single gene, the distribution would be truly dichotomous. However, it is very unlikely that psychosis is caused by a single factor, and a multifactorial aetiology, similar to that seen in other chronic disorders such as diabetes and cardiovascular disease, is more likely [12]. If there are, for example, five or more different causal factors underlying psychosis, the observed distribution of the trait is highly dependent on the degree to which these causes interact, their prevalence, and the degree to which their effect sizes differ. If the effects of each of the five causes are moder-

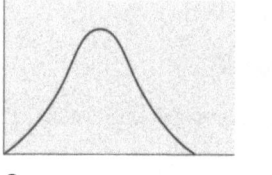 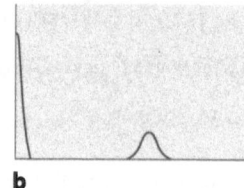 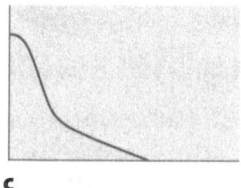

a   b   c

Fig. 1. Possible degrees of continuity of psychosis distributions. In **a**, there is a continuous and normal distribution of psychotic traits in the general population, much as one would expect of, for example, weight or blood pressure. In **b**, there is a clear bimodal distribution, with the great majority of the population having negligible values of the psychosis trait, whereas a very small proportion has extremely high values. In **c**, there is a continuous but only half-normal distribution, with the majority of the population having very low values, but also a significant proportion with non-zero values.

ate, not hugely different in magnitude and contribute additively to the risk function independently of each other, it can be shown that, according to what statisticians call the central limit theorem, psychosis would have to exist in nature as a quantitative trait, as depicted in Fig. 1a [13]. If, on the other hand, the five different causes interacted in such a way that expression of psychosis would *only* occur in the case of joint exposure to all five factors simultaneously (i.e. complete co-participation of the causes), the distribution would much more resemble a dichotomy as depicted in Fig. 1b. If the five causes both contributed independently and also co-participated to a degree, the distribution would lie somewhere between that of Fig. 1a and Fig. 1b (see Fig. 1c), depending on the degree of independent additive action and co-participation of the causes. In the case of large differences in effect size, with one or two very rare but extremely potent causes overshadowing the effect of more prevalent but weak causes, the appearance of the distribution would also be less continuous and more quasi-continuous. It can be surmised that the "real" distribution of psychosis most likely lies somewhere between that of the dichotomous one in Fig. 1b and the continuous one in Fig. 1a, depending on the degree of interaction between the different causes, and differences in their effect size, always assuming that psychosis is subject to more than one causal influence.

Assessment of the distribution of psychosis

From the above, it follows that studying the distribution of psychosis may tell us something about the degree of continuity and underlying causation. However, the resulting distribution very much depends on how the trait is measured. Broadly two approaches can be distinguished. The first approach is to measure in the general population the same symptoms that are seen in patients with psychotic disorders. The implicit assumption of this approach is that experiencing symptoms of psychosis such as delusions and hallucinations is not inevitably associated with presence of disorder. The latter is dependent on symptom factors such as intrusiveness, frequency and comorbidity of symptoms on the one hand, and personal and cultural factors such as coping, illness behaviour, societal tolerance and the development of functional impairments on the other. Thus, even though the prevalence of the clinical disorder is low, the prevalence of the symptoms can conceivably be much higher. The second approach is different, and assumes that in the sub-disorder range along the continuum, the expression of the trait is attenuated and takes on the form of "schizotypal" signs and symptoms. In this context, different schizotypy instruments have been developed, some including items that are close to the "pathological" experiences seen in psychosis (e.g. the Perceptual Aberration Scale [14]), others being more "normalised" (e.g. the Schizotypal Personality Scale [15]), and yet others based on the symptoms seen in relatives of patients with schizophrenia that are the main source for the DSM criteria for schizotypy (e.g. Schizotypal Personality Questionnaire [16]). Lately, these various scales have been combined to generate comprehensive inventories of schizotypal traits [17, 18].

The choice of instruments greatly influences the resulting distribution in prevalence studies. For example, the distribution of the number of delusions and hallucinations per person will be very skewed compared to the sum score of a schizotypy instrument with normalised items, whereas an instrument like the PAS will be somewhere between that of a dichotomous and a truly continuous one. The distribution will also be influenced by the symptom dimension that the instrument is aiming to capture, for example positive or negative dimensions [19].

Are there findings supporting a psychosis continuum?

Prevalence of symptoms of psychosis

Schizotypal signs. The distribution of experiences labelled as "schizotypal" is highly dependent on the instrument used. For example, in a study of a representative sample of 2000 young men in Greece, Stefanis and colleagues (submitted manuscript) found that the distribution of scores on the PAS (more clinical in its approach to schizotypy) was half normal, whereas the distribution of the SPQ total score (more normalised in its approach to schizotypy) was approximately normal (Fig. 2).

These distributions of variably defined schizotypy signs are, in the absence of associations with third aetiological, social impairment or treatment variables, in themselves difficult to interpret. Therefore, as far as the prevalence argument is concerned, studies assessing the prevalence of psychotic symptoms themselves, rather than variably defined attenuated experiences, may be more useful.

Delusions and hallucinations. Many studies have shown that delusional ideation is prevalent in the general population [20, 25]. Similarly, hallucinations also occur in up to around 5 – 10 % of the general population [26–29, 30–35]. However, in patients with psychotic disorder, the positive symptoms of hallucinations and delusions typically occur together [36–38]. This clinical observation is compatible with theories that some delusions arise secondarily in an attempt to explain abnormal perceptual experiences as first suggested by de Clérambault [39] and later elaborated by others [40, 41] and that biased conscious appraisal

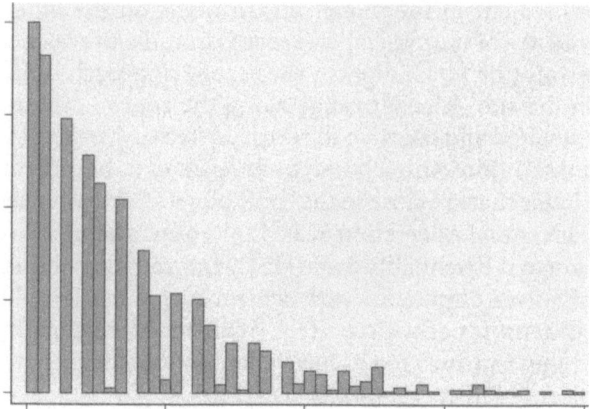

Perceptual aberration scale

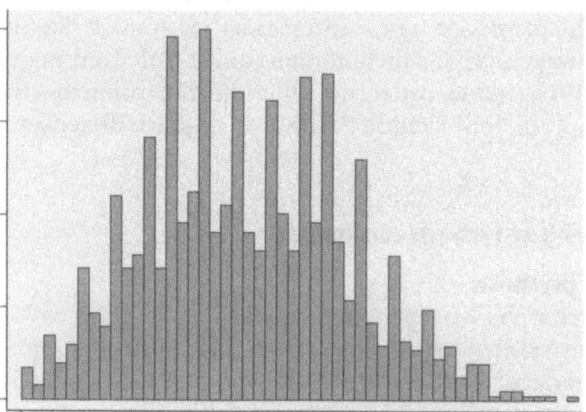

Schizotypal personality questionnaire

Fig. 2. Distributions of schizotypy according to instrument used (data from Stefanis et al., 2000).

processes are critical in judging that these confusing experiences are in fact externally caused [42]. Observational studies suggest that there is also an association between the presence of these psychotic experiences in non-clinical samples. In the study by Verdoux and colleagues, in addition to endorsing items on the PDI, 16 % of subjects with no history of psychiatric disorder reported that they had experienced auditory hallucinations during their lifetime [23]. In the Johns and colleagues' study, there was an association between reports on the PSQ of hallucinations and other psychotic experiences [35].

Data on psychotic symptoms collected as part of the Dutch NEMESIS study [43] suggest a psychosis continuum in the general population [44–46]. In this study, a representative general population sample of 7076 men and women was interviewed using the Composite International Diagnostic Interview (CIDI). For the 17 CIDI core positive psychosis items, the authors studied the four possible ratings on each of these items: i) a rating of "true", psychiatrist verified, presence of hallucinations and/or delusions, ii) a rating indicating that the symptom was present but the respondent did not appear to be bothered by it, iii) a rating indicating that the symptom was the result of drugs or physical disorder, iv) a rating indicating that the symptom *appeared* to be present but the interviewer was uncertain because there could have been a plausible explanation. Although all symptom ratings were strongly associated with the presence of DSM-III-R psychotic disorder in terms of relative risk, the authors found that of the 1237 individuals with any type of positive psychosis rating (17.5%), only 26 (2.1%) had a DSM-III-R diagnosis of non-affective psychosis. In addition, all four positive symptom ratings were elevated in both cases and non-cases of any DSM-III-R psychiatric disorder, although more so in the former (odds ratio 3.2, 95% CI: 2.8-3.7). The presence of any rating of hallucinations was strongly associated with the presence of any rating of delusion, supporting Maher's hypothesis of psychological mechanisms of delusion formation. Associations between hallucinatory and delusional experiences were apparent not only in individuals with any CIDI DSM-III-R lifetime diagnosis (OR = 5.5, 95% CI: 4.4-6.9) but also in individuals without a CIDI lifetime diagnosis (OR = 4.3, 95% CI: 2.9-6.3), suggesting continuity of psychological mechanisms of delusions across patient and non-patient groups. Although psychotic symptoms in this sample were much more common than psychotic disorders, the distribution of individual total psychotic symptom scores in the sample was very skewed. These findings therefore suggest that both symptoms and underlying psychological mechanisms of psychosis occur as part of a continuous, albeit very skewed, distribution that shows only very partial overlap with clinical disorder.

Similarity in underlying dimensional representation
The above findings suggest that the positive symptoms of psychosis are prevalent in the general population, but give little information about other symptoms and how different symptoms might cluster together. One way to further test the hypothesis of a psychosis continuum would be to investigate to what degree non-clinical, or attenuated, "schizotypal" phenomena show a similar pattern of correlation with each other into different symptom dimensions as their equivalents do in clinical psychotic disorders such as schizophrenia. Thus, as mentioned above, complementing the studies of individual symptoms is research into schizotypy, which shares the view that the features of schizophrenia lie on a continuum with normal behaviour and experience [11]. Schizotypy refers to the personality trait of experiencing 'psychotic' symptoms, and psychometric identification of non-clinical schizotypal traits in the normal population provides further evidence for a continuum model of psychosis [10]. Schizotypy, or 'psychosis-proneness', may be a quantitative rather than a qualitative trait, ranging from normality at one end, through eccentricity and different combinations of schizotypal characteristics, to florid psychosis at the other.

A number of scales have been developed to measure schizotypal traits in the normal population. There is growing evidence from factor analytical studies that schizotypy is a multidimensional construct composed of three, and possibly four, dimensions: a positive dimension (aberrant perceptions and beliefs), a negative dimension (introvertive anhedonia), a conceptual disorganisation dimension and an asocial/non-conformity dimension [47]. Although the non-conformity dimension has been fairly consistenly replicated, its presence may reflect a covarying normal personality trait resembling Eysenck's "tough-mindedness" [48], rather than a core component of schizotypy itself [49]. Other authors have proposed a slightly different three-factor model, with a third factor of social impairment [50, 51]. Several authors have drawn attention to the striking resemblance between the exploratory and confirmatory factorial solutions of the signs and symptoms of schizotypy and those observed in schizophrenia. Thus, the dimensions of positive, negative and disorganisation symptoms reported in schizophrenia [36–38] are comparable to similarly construed dimensions in schizotypy [18, 47, 52–56]. These findings suggest that psychosis may exist as a continuum of variation along various comorbid symptom dimensions [57].

Familial clustering and longitudinal associations

If there is variation on a continuum, one would expect lesser states on the continuum to show familial and longitudinal continuity. In other words, one would expect i) that the families of probands with clinical psychotic disorder have higher rates of psychosis-like symptoms and/or schizotypy, and ii) that individuals with high levels of psychosis-like symptoms and/or schizotypy have a higher risk of developing clinical psychotic disorder. Family studies have shown that schizotypy co-occurs with schizophrenia in the same family more often than would be expected by chance [58–60]. This suggests that the same social and/or genetic factors that contribute to schizophrenia also contribute to schizotypy, i.e. that the two conditions are at least in part aetiologically continuous.

Similarly, follow-up studies of subjects with elevated schizotypy scores have demonstrated high rates of clinical psychosis and related disorders [61, 62]. A fascinating study of a birth cohort of children from New Zealand showed that children who had reported psychotic symptoms at age 11 years had a more than 16-fold higher risk of developing schizophreniform disorder by age 26 years [63]. This suggests that lower states on the continuum are a risk factor for more elevated states, and that transitions over the continuum occur with time.

Associations with demographic risk factors

Samples of patients who receive a diagnosis of schizophrenia for the first time (incident cases) show, as a group, a characteristic pattern of associations with a range of demographic variables [64–67]. Thus, incident patients are more likely to be young, single and unemployed. They also have a lower mean level of education and are more likely to reside in urban environments [9, 68–70]. The characteristic age-related variation in the incidence of schizophrenia is mirrored in a similar age-related expression of variably defined schizotypy [71, 72], delusional ideation measured with the PDI [22], and delusions and hallucinations in the absence of a clinical psychotic disorder [45]. Verdoux and colleagues speculated that early adulthood, when levels of psychosis-like experiences are highest, may be a critical developmental phase for the expression of the trait psychosis, other factors determining at what level of the continuum the expression will occur [73]. With regard to the other demographic factors that are associated with schizophrenia, similar associations have been reported for non-clinical psychotic and psychosis-like symptoms [45, 46]. Although it is not known whether these factors are causally related to the incidence of psychotic disorder or the result of premorbid drift, the similarity of the pattern of associations between psychotic disorder and mental states that occupy a lower position on the distribution is again suggestive of a continuum of psychotic experiences.

The population variation argument

Arguably the closest one can get to proof of a psychosis continuum using epidemiological methods is that of similar variation of (relatively prevalent) psychotic experiences and (rare) psychotic disorder through different populations. For example, if the rate of some rare psychotic disorder is higher in population A than in population B, whereas their levels of more prevalent psychotic symptoms are the same, a likely explanation is that i) some rare cause for a rare disorder is more prevalent in population A, and ii) psychosis-like experiences in the population are qualitatively distinct from the disorder. Thus, populations A and

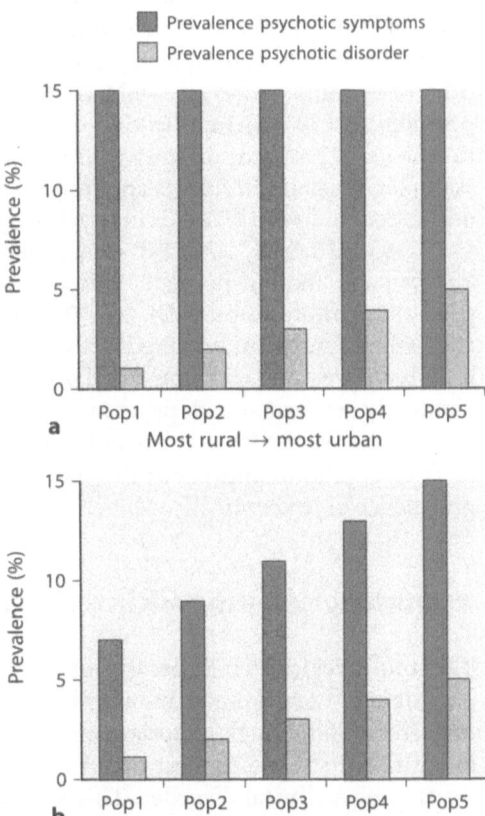

Fig. 3. Testing hypotheses on continuity between psychotic symptoms and psychotic disorders. **a** The prevalence of psychotic disorder increases in populations living in progressively more urbanised areas, but the prevalence of symptoms remains constant. This suggests that there is no continuity between symptoms and disorder. **b** The prevalence of symptoms increases simultaneously with the prevalence of symptoms. If it can be shown additionally that symptoms are associated with disorder in each population, the situation in **a** suggests that symptoms are continuous with the disorder.

B are essentially similar, except for the distribution of some rare cause affecting a few individuals. There is variation *within* populations. If, however, not only the rate of disorder, but also the rate of symptoms is higher in population A than in population B, a likely explanation would be that the i) population level of vulnerability differs *between* population A and population B, and ii) psychosis-like experiences are, at least in part, on a quantitative continuum with disorder. A graphical representation of this argument, using hypothetical data, is depicted in Fig. 3.

If one can define populations with predictable differences in the rate of psychotic disorder, the hypothesis of population variation can be examined by measuring simultaneously psychotic experiences and psychotic disorder in these populations. In a previous study, we used predictable differences in rates of psychotic disorder across different levels of urbanicity to examine the continuum hypothesis [46]. Urban and rural populations have different rates of psychotic illness. If psychosis exists as a continuous phenotype in nature, then urban-rural population differences in the rate of psychotic disorder should be accompanied by similar differences in the rate of abnormal mental states characterised by psychotic or psychosis-like symptoms. In our study, a random sample of 7076 men and women aged 18 to 64 years were interviewed by trained lay interviewers with the Composite International Diagnostic Interview (CIDI). Around half of those with evidence of psychosis according to the CIDI were additionally interviewed by clinicians. We subsequently investigated associations between a five-level urbanicity rating and i) any DSM-III-R diagnosis of psychotic disorder (sample prevalence: 1.5%), ii) any rating of hallucinations and/or delusions (sample prevalence 4.2%), and iii) any rating of psychotic or psychosis-like symptoms (sample prevalence: 17.5%). The results showed that level of urbanicity was not only associated with DSM-III-R psychotic disorder (adjusted OR over five levels = 1.47, 95% CI: 1.25, 1.72), but also, independently, with any rating of delusion and/or hallucination (adjusted OR = 1.28, 95% 1.17, 1.40 – clinician-assessed psychotic symptoms only: OR = 1.30, 95% CI: 1.03, 1.64), and any rating of psychosis-like symptom (adjusted OR = 1.18, 95% CI: 1.13, 1.24). Ratings of both lay interviewer- and clinician-rated psychotic symptoms were strongly and independently associated with psychotic disorder, regardless of the level of urbanisation. The results from this study therefore strongly suggest that community level of psychotic and psychosis-like symptoms is inextricably linked to the prevalence of psychotic disorder.

■ Risk factors for psychosis in the general population

The studies reviewed indicate that hallucinations and delusions are dimensional phenomena lying on continua with normal experiences. Although the great majority of individuals experiencing these "symptoms" are not in need of care, longitudinal studies suggest they may nevertheless have an increased risk of developing a clinical disorder. This section considers the aetiological implications of the results of these studies.

What factors drive variation in the continuum?

The view that psychotic symptoms vary along quantitative dimensions facilitates psychosocial research into the factors that drive such variation. There is a growing body of research on the role of social factors, emotions, perceptions and inferential processes in relation to the onset and persistence of psychotic symptoms [42, 74], and the coping mechanisms that people use to deal with them [75, 76]. Calls have been made to extend the search for psychosocial mechanisms underlying specific psychotic symptoms, such as possible individual-level or contextual-level social factors [77, 78] deficits in theory of mind [79], impaired self-monitoring [80], reasoning bias [81] and dysfunctional attributions [82] to samples at lower levels of the continuum [83]. As described earlier, there is some evidence that psychological mechanisms associated with psychotic symptoms also operate in non-patient samples, and further study of these could greatly contribute to our understanding of psychosis. The study of psychosocial mechanisms of psychotic symptoms would be particularly important in view of the current interest in preventing individuals from making "transitions" from non-clinical to clinical psychotic states. It then becomes crucially important to understand what actually causes individuals on some position at the hypothesised continuum to become a clinical "case". As far as the patient-non patient distinction is concerned, it may be important to consider two interacting risks: one that determines which position a person is going to occupy along the psychosis continuum, and one that determines whether a person at a certain point of the continuum is going to develop illness behaviour. Thus, two persons at different positions on the continuum may experience differences in the number, intrusiveness or frequency of symptoms, or the degree of other comorbid symptom dimensions such as negative symptoms, thought disorder or cognitive impairment [9]. Because of this, the person at the highest position may have a higher risk of becoming a mental health patient. Conversely, however, at each point of the continuum, two persons with the same level of psychotic symptoms may differ in that one copes well and does not develop illness behaviour, whereas the other may develop functional impairments and need for care [8]. Further research is needed to clarify these relationships [84].

Epidemiological research into the psychosocial mechanisms that contribute to psychosis transitions

Coping

Given the strong associations, discussed above, between experiences of psychosis in the general population and "cases" of psychotic disorder, it becomes important to understand what actually causes some individuals with psychotic experiences to develop a need for care. It may be that an individual becomes much more likely to develop need for care if the psychotic experiences simply exceed a "critical" value. However, experiences of psychosis vary in terms of frequency, degree of conviction, preoccupation, influence on behaviour, distress and secondary attributions, all of which may be of crucial importance in producing illness and help-seeking behaviour. There is evidence to suggest that the implausibility of the psychotic experiences and the associated degree of conviction may not be related to illness status [74]. However, degree of preoccupation and distress do seem to be important factors [22, 25]. For example, in studies of predisposition to hallucinations in student samples [29, 30] hardly any subjects reported that they had been troubled by hearing voices, whereas patients with schizophrenia most commonly experience stressful auditory verbal hallucinations [85]. Another important determinant of patient status may be the level of functional coping that the person mobilises in the face of stressful (psychotic) experiences [8, 86–89]. It has been suggested that the level of depression and distress associated with symptoms is driven by appraisals of controllability and rank, making certain individuals feel subordinated to their voices and less in control [90, 91]. It is therefore attractive to hypothesise that individuals with more "symptomatic" coping types, characterised by going along with and indulging in the content of psychotic symptoms rather than develop active coping efforts, are more likely to develop a need for care in the context of psychotic symptoms.

In a recent study [92], a general population sample was followed to identify individuals who had at least one incident experience of psychosis and no previous diagnosis of psychotic disorder. It was hypothesised that only part of these individuals would display a need for care in relation to their psychotic symptoms. It was further hypothesised that need for care status would be associated with a more dysfunctional, "symptomatic" coping style associated with less experience of control, and less functional, "active" coping associated with more experience of control. To this end, a previously described method to assess coping with and experience of control over psychotic experiences was used [76, 84]. In the study, 7076 individuals form the general population were interviewed three times over a period of 3 years (number interviewed on the third occasion: 4818). Forty-seven individuals experienced psychosis with no previous diagnosis of psychotic disorder. They were interviewed by telephone to assess need for care in relation to psychotic symptoms. Need for care was associated with severity of psychotic experiences rather than distress or total level of coping used. Also, individuals with need for care more often resorted to a *symptomatic coping* style (giving in to symptoms; OR = 6.07, 95 % CI: 1.94, 18.95), which was associated with less perceived control over their psychotic experiences (OR = 0.79, 95 % CI: 0.63, 0.98). Any type of coping was associated with level of distress, severity of hallucinations and presence of suspiciousness in both groups, but the effect of suspiciousness was larger in those in need for care (OR = 2.27, 95 % CI: 1.33, 3.87). This study therefore suggests that a symptomatic coping style predicts decreased experience of control and results in need for care. Attribution of locus of control and a more submissive style vis à vis the psychotic experience may contribute to becoming a mental health patient.

Neuroticism and stress-sensitivity

The personality factor neuroticism, which may reflect instability, vulnerability to stress, or anxiety-proneness [93–95] has been shown to robustly predict later onset of depression in short-term and long-term prospective studies [96–98].

Neuroticism therefore figures prominently in aetiological theories of depression [99]. Extraversion, on the other hand, may have a risk-reducing effect in relation to depression [100, 101].

However, more recent work suggests neuroticism may also be involved in the aetiology of psychotic symptoms. In as much as neuroticism reflects habitual cognitions of feeling overwhelmed in the face of external, "uncontrollable" events, or the tendency to worry over experiences, it can easily be imagined that such cognitive styles associated with neuroticism may give rise to attributions of "omnipotency" of psychotic experiences such as hearing voices [102], or enhanced levels of "meta-worry" and distress associated with psychotic experiences [103]. Alternatively, higher levels of neuroticism may predispose to development of anxiety and depression given the presence of a psychotic experience, thereby increasing the risk of social impairment and patient status. Patients with schizophrenia, their first degree relatives, and individuals with schizotypy have been reported to score high on measures of neuroticism, but in the absence of longitudinal studies it is unclear whether this represents a consequence of the illness or a personality risk factor [104–106]. In a recent study, associations between childhood neuroticism and extraversion on the one hand, and adult schizophrenia were investigated in a general population birth cohort of 5362 individuals [107]. Neuroticism and extraversion rated at the age of 16 years were examined in relation to adult schizophrenia in a national birth cohort of 5362 individuals. It was found that neuroticism increased the risk for schizophrenia later independent of the level of affective symptoms in adult life (odds ratio over three levels: 1.93, 95% CI: 1.09–3.43), whereas extraversion reduced the risk (OR: 0.44, 95% CI: 0.23–0.84). These results therefore suggest that depression and schizophrenia may share personality risk-increasing and risk-reducing factors, and that cognitive styles associated with particular personality traits may determine whether isolated experiences progress to full-blown psychotic illness [107].

In as much as neuroticism reflects stress-sensitivity, recent findings from our group using the Experience Sampling Method (ESM is a structured diary technique assessing thoughts, current context and mood in daily life), suggest that the vulnerability for schizophrenia is in part reflected in small increases in dysfunctional reaction patterns to daily life stress [108]. Patients with psychotic illness (n = 42), first-degree relatives (n = 47) and control subjects (n = 49) were studied with the Experience Sampling Method to assess 1) appraised subjective stress of daily events and smaller disturbances in daily life and 2) emotional reactivity conceptualised as changes in both negative affect and positive affect. Multilevel regression analyses showed that an increase in subjective stress was associated with an increase in negative affect and a decrease in positive affect in all groups. However, the groups differed quantitatively in their pattern of reactions to stress. Psychotic patients reacted with more intense emotions to subjective appraisals of stress in daily life than controls. The decrease in positive affect in the relatives was similar to that of the patients, whilst the increase in negative affect in this group was intermediary to that of patients and controls. These findings suggest that higher levels of familial risk for psychosis were associated with higher levels of emotional reactivity to daily life stress in a dose-response fashion. Subtle alterations in the way persons interact with their environment may constitute part of the vulnerability for psychotic illness [108].

Attributions of hallucinatory experiences

As discussed above, in patients with psychotic disorder, the positive symptoms of hallucinations and delusions typically occur together [36–38]. Observational studies suggest that also in non-clinical samples experience of hallucinations is strongly associated with delusional ideation [45]. This clinical observation is compatible with theories that some delusions arise secondarily in an attempt to explain abnormal perceptual experiences, as first proposed by de Clérambault [39] and later elaborated by others [40, 41], and that biased conscious appraisal processes are critical in judging that these confusing experiences are in fact externally caused [109].

Although it is known that experience of hallucinations and delusional ideation are strongly associated in clinical and non-clinical samples, there is not much empirical work on possible factors mediating this relationship. We studied, using a longitudinal design in a sample of adolescents with experiences of hearing voices, the factors that may influence delusion formation given the presence of a hallucinatory experience [110, 111]. The choice of an adolescent sample was made as recent population-based work suggests that among children the prevalence of hallucinatory phenomena is around 8% [112]. Around a third such children presents with a DSM-III diagnosis, which, although representing twice the diagnostic rate of children in the non-hallucinatory group [112], is low enough to suggest that for the majority of hallucinating children in the general population these experiences are non-pathological. A small group, however, is at risk of subsequent psychotic disorder in adult life. In a recent follow-up of 761 children, self-reported psychotic symptoms at age 11 years increased the odds for psychotic illness at age 26 years 16.4 times, but the actual number of children that developed a psychotic disorder was very small. These childhood self-reported psychotic experiences had predictive value independent of childhood psychiatric diagnosis [63]. Other work also suggests that childhood hallucinations may increase the risk for later psychotic disorder [113]. For these reasons, the study of delusion formation in a sample of adolescents may be rewarding prompting us to examine prospectively what factors are associated with formation of delusions in adolescents who were hearing voices [110, 111]. Eighty adolescents (mean age 12.9 years, SD = 3.1) who reported hearing voices were examined at baseline and followed-up three times over a period of three years. 50% were receiving professional care, but 50% were not in need of care. Baseline measurement of voice appraisals, attributions, psychopathology, global functioning, dissociation, stressful life events, coping mechanisms and receipt of professional care were used as predictors of delusion formation, measured as a score of 6 or greater on the extended BPRS items: "suspiciousness", "unusual thought content" and "grandiosity". The results showed that thirteen children (16%) displayed evidence of delusional ideation at at least one of the three follow-up periods, of which 7 (9%) *de novo*. Adjusting for presence of baseline delusional ideation, delusion formation over the follow-up period was associated with baseline voice appraisals and attributions such as tone of the voice (Hazard ratio voice "variably friendly and hostile" compared to "always friendly": HR = 6.8, 95% CI: 1.1, 41.0), perceived location of the voice (outside vs. inside head: HR = 2.9, 95% CI: 1.0, 8.7), and whether the voice resembled that of a parent (HR = 3.5, 95% CI: 1.0, 12.0); baseline BPRS anxiety/depression (HR = 6.4, 95% CI: 1.9, 21.4), baseline BPRS disorganisation (HR = 5.0, 95% CI: 0.98, 26.1) and the baseline amount of reported recent stressful life events (HR continuous life events score: 1.8, 95% CI: 1.0, 3.3). In addition, in older children, the perceived influence of the voices on emotions and behaviour was strongly associated with delusion formation (HR = 5.1, 95% CI: 1.0, 25.9). The results suggest that delusion formation in children hearing voices may be responsive to triggering events and facilitated by feelings of anxiety/depression. The results also highlight the role of attributions associated with external sources, authority figures, perceived influence or "power" over the person, as well as emotional appraisal processes and cognitive disorganisation [110].

Discrimination
There are consistent reports of high rates of affective and non-affective psychosis in some ethnic minority groups [114–116]. These populations are subjected to racial discrimination [117, 118] and there are claims that living in a racist society is the cause of the increased rates of psychosis [119].

There is evidence that subtle, psychosis-like phenomena such as delusional ideation and isolated hallucinations are prevalent in the general population [22, 23, 33, 34], and constitute a risk factor for the development of clinical psychotic disorder [63, 120, 121]. Recent research indicates that high-risk migrant groups, such as African-Caribbean people living in the UK [116, 122], have higher rates of these phenomena [123, 124]. An explanation integrating these findings is that chronic exposure to social adversity and discrimination may give rise to a paranoid attributional style, and higher rates of psychosis-like phenomena, which put individuals at risk of developing clinical psychotic states [125–127]. A direct link between experience of discrimination and psychosis needs to be made if such a hypothesis is to be entertained.

In a previous study, we hypothesised that baseline experience of discrimination would i) result in a higher incidence of psychotic disorder and ii) would be a stronger, independent predictor of psychosis than minority status [128]. We tested this hypothesis using data from a longitudinal, random population sample of 7076 individuals interviewed for the presence of psychiatric symptoms and psychotic disorder [129]. Close to 5000 people were interviewed with the Composite International Diagnostic Interview (CIDI) at baseline, and one and three years later. At baseline, subjects were asked about their experience of discrimination on the basis of age, sex, handicap, appearance, ethnic group and sexual orientation. Ethnic minority status was defined using the subject's and parents' place of birth. At year three, individuals with CIDI evidence of psychotic symptoms were interviewed by clinicians to identify new cases of psychosis. The predictors of developing psychotic symptoms severe enough to warrant treatment over the follow-up period were calculated using regression analysis. It was found that baseline experience of discrimination strongly predicted new onset of psychosis at year 3. This association remained after adjustment for age, sex, minority status, urban residence, level of CIDI paranoid symptoms at baseline, level of education, unemployment and single marital status. Minority status increased the risk for psychosis; this effect was largely confined to young men. Entering minority status and discrimination jointly in the equation attenuated the effect size of minority status much more (28%) than that of discrimination (8%), leaving only discrimination as significant independent predictor. These findings therefore suggest that experience of discrimination is robustly associated with onset of psychotic symptoms and may explain in part the high observed rates of schizophrenia in some minority populations [128].

▦ Conclusion

In this chapter, we sought to show how use of the epidemiological method can be extended to investigate psychosis not only as a dichotomous entity, but as a distribution of experiences that are not necessarily associated with disability, analogous to recent findings in affective disorder [6]. The view that there may be a psychosis continuum is compatible with increasing evidence that a range of psychosocial factors drive variation in the continuum. These factors can be identified using the approach of "cognitive epidemiology", as illustrated in this chapter.

▦ References

1. Hafner H (1989) Application of epidemiological research toward a model for the etiology of schizophrenia. Schizophr Res 2: 375–383
2. Weich S (1997) Prevention of the common mental disorders: a public health perspective [editorial]. Psychol Med 27: 757–764
3. Kendler KS, Gardner CO (1998) Boundaries of major depression: an evaluation of DSM-IV criteria. Am J Psychiatry 155: 172–177
4. Anderson J, Huppert F, Rose G (1993) Normality, deviance and minor psychiatric morbidity in the community. Psych Med 23: 475–485
5. Whittington JE, Huppert FA (1996) Changes in the prevalence of psychiatric disorder in a community are related to changes in the mean level of psychiatric symptoms. Psychol Med 26: 1253–1260
6. Henderson S, Korten A, Medway J (2001) Non-disabled cases in a national survey. Psychol Med 31: 769–777
7. Van Os J, Jones P, Sham P, Bebbington P, Murray RM (1998) Risk factors for onset and persistence of psychosis. Soc Psychiatry Psychiatr Epidemiol 33: 596–605
8. Claridge G (1997) Final remarks and future directions. In: Claridge G (ed) Schizotypy. Implications for Illness and Health. Oxford: Oxford University Press, pp 301–317
9. Kendler KS, Gallagher TJ, Abelson JM, Kessler RC (1996) Lifetime prevalence, demographic risk factors, and diagnostic validity of nonaffective psychosis as assessed in a US community sample. The National Comorbidity Survey. Arch Gen Psychiatry 53: 1022–1031
10. Claridge G (1997) Theoretical background and issues. In: Claridge G (ed) Schizotypy. Implications for Illness and Health. Oxford: Oxford University Press, pp 3–19

11. Claridge G (1994) Single indicator of risk for schizophrenia: probable fact or likely myth? Schizophr Bull 20: 151–168

12. Jones P, Cannon M (1998) The new epidemiology of schizophrenia. Psychiatr Clin North Am 21: 1–25

13. Kendler KS, Kidd KK (1986) Recurrence risks in an oligogenic threshold model: the effect of alterations in allele frequency. Ann Hum Genet 50: 83–91

14. Chapman LJ, Chapman JP, Raulin ML (1978) Body-image aberration in schizophrenia. J Abnorm Psychol 87: 399–407

15. Claridge G, Broks P (1984) Schizotypy and hemisphere function: I Theoretical considerations and the measurement of schizotypy. Personality and Individual Differences 5: 633–648

16. Raine A (1991) The SPQ: a scale for the assessment of schizotypal personality based on DSM-III-R criteria. Schizophr Bull 17: 555–564

17. Mason O, Claridge G, Jackson M (1995) New scales for the assessment of schizotypy. Personality and Individual Differences 18: 7–13

18. Bentall RP, Claridge GS, Slade PD (1989) The multidimensional nature of schizotypal traits: a factor analytic study with normal subjects. Br J Clin Psychol 28: 363–375

19. Chapman LJ, Chapman JP, Raulin ML (1976) Scales for physical and social anhedonia. J Abnorm Psychol 85: 374–382

20. Cox D, Cowling P (1989) Are You Normal? London: Tower Press

21. Eaton WW, Romanoski A, Anthony JC, Nestadt G (1991) Screening for psychosis in the general population with a self-report interview. J Nerv Ment Dis 179: 689–693

22. Peters ER, Joseph SA, Garety PA (1999) Measurement of delusional ideation in the normal population: introducing the PDI (Peters et al. Delusions Inventory). Schizophr Bull 25: 553–576

23. Verdoux H, Maurice-Tison S, Gay B, Van Os J, Salamon R, Bourgeois ML (1998) A survey of delusional ideation in primary-care patients. Psychol Med 28: 127–134

24. Jackson MC (1997) Benign schizotypy? The case of spiritual experience. In: Claridge G (ed) Schizotypy. Implications for Illness and Health. Oxford: Oxford University Press, pp 137–154

25. Peters E, Day S, McKenna J, Orbach G (1999) Delusional ideation in religious and psychotic populations. Br J Clin Psychol 38: 83–96

26. Romme MA, Honig A, Noorthoorn EO, Escher AD (1992) Coping with hearing voices: an emancipatory approach. Br J Psychiatry 161: 99–103

27. Posey TB, Losch ME (1983) Auditory hallucinations of hearing voices in 375 normal subjects. Imagination, Cognition and Personality 3: 99–113

28. Barrett TR, Etheridge JB (1992) Verbal hallucinations in normals, I: People who hear voices. Applied Cognitive Psychology 6: 379–387

29. Bentall RP, Slade PD (1985) Reality testing and auditory hallucinations: a signal detection analysis. Br J Clin Psychol 24: 159–169

30. Young HF, Bentall RP, Slade PD, Dewey ME (1986) Disposition towards hallucination, gender and EPQ scores: a brief report. Personality and Individual Differences 7: 247–249.

31. Sidgewick H, Johnson A, Myers FWH et al. (1894) Report of the census of hallucinations. Proceedings of the Society for Psychical Research 26: 259–394

32. West DJ (1948) A mass-observation questionnaire on hallucinations. Journal of the Society for Psychical Research 34: 187–196

33. McKellar P (1968) Experience and Behaviour. Harmondsworth: Penguin Press

34. Tien AY. (1991). Distributions of hallucinations in the population. Soc Psychiatry Psychiatr Epidemiol 26: 287–292

35. Johns LC, Nazroo JY, Bebbington P, Kuipers E (1998) Occurrence of hallucinations in a community sample. Schizophrenia Research 29: 23

36. Bilder RM, Mukherjee S, Rieder RO, Pandurangi AK (1985) Symptomatic and neuropsychological components of defect states. Schizophr Bull 11: 409–419

37. Liddle PF (1987) The symptoms of chronic schizophrenia. A re-examination of the positive-negative dichotomy [see comments]. Br J Psychiatry 151: 145–151

38. Peralta V, de Leon J, Cuesta MJ (1992) Are there more than two syndromes in schizophrenia? A critique of the positive-negative dichotomy. Br J Psychiatry 161: 335–343
39. De Clérambault GG (1942) Oeuvre Psychiatrique. In: PUF, pp 457–467
40. Maher BA (1974) Delusional thinking and perceptual disorder. J Individ Psychol 30: 98–113
41. Maher BA (1988) Anomalous experience and delusional thinking: the logic of explanations. In: Oltmanns TF, Maher BA (eds) Delusional Beliefs. New York: Wiley, pp 15–33
42. Garety P, Kuipers E, Fowler D, Freeman D, Bebbington P (2001) A cognitive model of the positive symptoms of psychosis. Psychological Medicine 31: 189–195
43. Bijl RV, van Zessen G, Ravelli A, de Rijk C, Langendoen Y (1998) The Netherlands Mental Health Survey and Incidence Study (NEMESIS): objectives and design. Soc Psychiatry Psychiatr Epidemiol 33: 581–586
44. Van Os J, Verdoux H, Maurice-Tison S, Gay B, Liraud F, Salamon R, Bourgeois M (1999) Self-reported psychosis-like symptoms and the continuum of psychosis. Soc Psychiatry Psychiatr Epidemiol 34: 459–463
45. van Os J, Hanssen M, Bijl RV, Ravelli A (2000) Strauss (1969) revisited: a psychosis continuum in the general population? Schizophr Res 45: 11–20
46. van Os J, Hanssen M, Bijl RV, Vollebergh W (2001) Prevalence of psychotic disorder and community level of psychotic symptoms: an urban-rural comparison. Arch Gen Psychiatry 58: 663–668
47. Vollema MG, van den Bosch RJ (1995) The multidimensionality of schizotypy [see comments]. Schizophr Bull 21: 19–31
48. Eysenck HJ, Eysenck SBG (1973) The Manual of the Personality Questionnaire. Unpublished Manuscript
49. Vollema M (1999) Schizotypy: Toward the Psychological Heart of Schizophrenia. Groningen: Shaker Publishing
50. Venables PH, Rector NA (2000) The content and structure of schizotypy: a study using confirmatory factor analysis [In Process Citation]. Schizophr Bull 26: 587–602
51. Lenzenweger MF (1991) Confirming schizotypic personality configurations in hypothetically psychosis-prone university students. Psychiatry Res 37: 81–96
52. Gruzelier JH (1996) The factorial structure of schizotypy: Part I. Affinities with syndromes of schizophrenia. Schizophr Bull 22: 611–620
53. Vollema MG, Hoijtink H (2000) The multidimensionality of self-report schizotypy in a psychiatric population: an analysis using multidimensional Rasch models [In Process Citation]. Schizophr Bull 26: 565–575
54. Raine A, Reynolds C, Lencz T, Scerbo A, Triphon N, Kim D (1994) Cognitive-perceptual, interpersonal, and disorganized features of schizotypal personality. Schizophr Bull 20: 191–201
55. Claridge GS (1990) Can a disease model of schizophrenia survive? In: Bentall RP (ed). Reconstructing Schizophrenia. London: Routledge, pp 89–120
56. Venables PH, Bailes K (1994) The structure of schizotypy, its relation to subdiagnoses of schizophrenia and to sex and age. Br J Clin Psychol 33: 277–294
57. Van Os J, Verdoux H, Bijl R, Ravelli A (1999) Psychosis as a continuum of variation in dimensions of psychopathology. In: Häfner H, Gattaz WF (eds) Search for the Causes of Schizophrenia. Berlin: Springer, pp 59–80
58. Kendler KS, McGuire M, Gruenberg AM, Walsh D (1995) Schizotypal symptoms and signs in the Roscommon Family Study. Their factor structure and familial relationship with psychotic and affective disorders. Arch Gen Psychiatry 52: 296–303
59. Kendler KS, McGuire M, Gruenberg AM, O'Hare A et al. (1993) The Roscommon Family Study: III. Schizophrenia-related personality disorders in relatives. Arch Gen Psychiatry 50: 781–788
60. Kendler KS, Walsh D (1995) Schizotypal personality disorder in parents and the risk for schizophrenia in siblings. Schizophr Bull 21: 47–52
61. Kwapil TR, Miller MB, Zinser MC, Chapman J et al. (1997) Magical ideation and social anhedonia as predictors of psychosis proneness: a partial replication. J Abnorm Psychol 106: 491–495

62. Chapman LJ, Chapman JP, Kwapil TR, Eckblad M et al. (1994) Putatively psychosis-prone subjects 10 years later. J Abnorm Psychol 103: 171–183
63. Poulton R, Caspi A, Moffitt TE, Cannon M, Murray R, Harrington H (2000) Children's self-reported psychotic symptoms and adult schizophreniform disorder: a 15-year longitudinal study [In Process Citation]. Arch Gen Psychiatry 57: 1053–1058
64. Hafner H, Riecher A, Maurer K, Loffler W, Munk-Jorgensen P, Stromgren E (1989) How does gender influence age at first hospitalization for schizophrenia? A transnational case register study. Psychol Med 19: 903–918
65. Hafner H, Maurer K, Loffler W, Riecher-Rossler A (1991) [Schizophrenia and age]. Nervenarzt 62: 536–548
66. Hafner H, Maurer K, Loffler W, Fatkenheuer B, an der Heiden W, Riecher Rossler A, Behrens S, Gattaz WF (1994) The epidemiology of early schizophrenia. Influence of age and gender on onset and early course. Br J Psychiatry (Suppl 23): 29–38
67. Hafner H, Hambrecht M, Loffler W, Munk-Jorgensen P, Riecher-Rossler A (1998) Is schizophrenia a disorder of all ages? A comparison of first episodes and early course across the life-cycle. Psychol Med 28: 351–365
68. Galdos PM, van Os JJ, Murray RM (1993) Puberty and the onset of psychosis [see comments]. Schizophr Res 10: 7–14
69. Marcelis M, Navarro-Mateu F, Murray R, Selten JP, van Os J (1998) Urbanization and psychosis: a study of 1942–1978 birth cohorts in The Netherlands. Psychol Med 28: 871–879
70. Driessen G, Gunther N, Bak M, van Sambeek M, van Os J (1998) Characteristics of early- and late-diagnosed schizophrenia: implications for first-episode studies. Schizophr Res 33: 27–34
71. Rust J (1988) The Rust Inventory of Schizotypal Cognitions (RISC). Schizophr Bull 14: 317–322
72. Claridge G, McCreery C, Mason O, Bentall R, Boyle G, Slade P, Popplewell D (1996) The factor structure of "schizotypal" traits: a large replication study. Br J Clin Psychol 35: 103–115
73. Verdoux H, van Os J, Maurice-Tison S, Gay B, Salamon R, Bourgeois M (1998) Is early adulthood a critical developmental stage for psychosis proneness? A survey of delusional ideation in normal subjects. Schizophr Res 29: 247–254
74. Garety P, Hemsley DR (1994) Delusions. Investigations into the Psychology of Delusional Reasoning. Oxford: Oxford University Press
75. Carr V (1988) Patients' techniques for coping with schizophrenia: an exploratory study. Br J Med Psychol 61: 339–352
76. Bak M, Van der Spil F, Gunther N, Radstake S, Delespaul P, van Os J (2001) Macs-I. Maastricht assessment of coping strategies: a brief instrument to assess coping with psychotic symptoms. Acta Psychiatr Scand 103: 453–459
77. van Os J, Driessen G, Gunther N, Delespaul P (2000) Neighbourhood variation in incidence of schizophrenia. Evidence for person-environment interaction. Br J Psychiatry 176: 243–248
78. van Os J, McKenzie K (2000) Cultural influences on pathway to care, service use and outcome. In: Gelder M, Andreasen N (eds) The New Oxford Textbook of Psychiatry. Oxford/New York: Oxford University Press, pp 1531–1539
79. Frith CD, Corcoran R. (1996). Exploring 'theory of mind' in people with schizophrenia. Psychol Med 26: 521–530
80. Johns LC, McGuire PK (1999) Verbal self-monitoring and auditory hallucinations in schizophrenia [letter]. Lancet 353: 469–470
81. Garety PA, Hemsley DR, Wessely S (1991) Reasoning in deluded schizophrenic and paranoid patients. Biases in performance on a probabilistic inference task. J Nerv Ment Dis 179: 194–201
82. Bentall RP, Kinderman P, Kaney S (1994) The self, attributional processes and abnormal beliefs: towards a model of persecutory delusions. Behav Res Ther 32: 331–341
83. Garety PA, Freeman D (1999) Cognitive approaches to delusions: a critical review of theories and evidence [see comments]. Br J Clin Psychol 38: 113–154
84. Bak M, van der Spil F, Gunther N, Radstake S, Delespaul P, van Os J (2001) Macs II. Does coping enhance subjective control over symptoms? Acta Psychiatr Scand 103: 460–464

85. Kendell RE (1985) Schizophrenia: clinical features. In: Michels R, Cavenar JO (eds) Psychiatry. London: Basic Books, pp 220–249
86. Nuechterlein KH, Dawson ME (1984) A heuristic vulnerability/stress model of schizophrenic episodes. Schizophr Bull 10: 300–312
87. Romme MA, Escher AD (1989) Hearing voices. Schizophr Bull 15: 209–216
88. Lukoff D, Snyder K, Ventura J, Nuechterlein KH (1984) Life events, familial stress, and coping in the developmental course of schizophrenia. Schizophr Bull 10: 258–292
89. Ventura J, Nuechterlein KH, Hardesty JP, Gitlin M (1992) Life events and schizophrenic relapse after withdrawal of medication. Br J Psychiatry 161: 615–620
90. Birchwood M, Mason R, MacMillan F, Healy J (1993) Depression, demoralization and control over psychotic illness: a comparison of depressed and non-depressed patients with a chronic psychosis. Psychol Med 23: 387–395
91. Birchwood M, Chadwick P (1997) The omnipotence of voices: testing the validity of a cognitive model. Psychol Med 27: 1345–1353
92. Bak M, Hanssen M, Bijl RV, Vollebergh W, Delespaul P, van Os J (2001) When does experience of psychosis result in need for care? A prospective general population study. (Submitted Manuscript)
93. Eysenck HJ, Eysenck SBG (1975) Manual of the Eysenck Personality Questionnaire. London: Hodder & Stoughton
94. Ormel J, Stewart R, Sanderman R (1989) Personality as modifier of the life change-distress relationship. A longitudinal modelling approach. Soc Psychiatry Psychiatr Epidemiol 24: 187–195
95. Horwood LJ, Fergusson DM (1986) Neuroticism, depression and life events: a structural equation model. Soc Psychiatry 21: 63–71
96. Kendler KS, Neale MC, Kessler RC, Heath AC, Eaves LJ (1993) A longitudinal twin study of personality and major depression in women. Arch Gen Psychiatry 50: 853–862
97. Rodgers B (1990) Behaviour and personality in childhood as predictors of adult psychiatric disorder. Journal of Child Psychology and Psychiatry 3: 393–414
98. Fergusson DM, Horwood LJ, Lawton JM (1989) The relationships between neuroticism and depressive symptoms. Soc Psychiatry Psychiatr Epidemiol 24: 275–281
99. Kendler KS, Neale MC, Kessler RC, Heath AC, Eaves LJ (1993) A longitudinal twin study of personality and major depression in women. Archives of General Psychiatry 50: 853–862
100. Enns MW, Cox BJ (1997) Personality dimensions and depression: review and commentary [see comments]. Can J Psychiatry 42: 274–284
101. van Os J, Jones P (1999) Early risk factors for depressive disorder and adult person-environment relationships. Psychol Med 29: 1055–1067
102. Birchwood M, Meaden A, Trower P, Gilbert P, Plaistow J (2000) The power and omnipotence of voices: subordination and entrapment by voices and significant others. Psychol Med 30: 337–344
103. Freeman D, Garety PA (1999) Worry, worry processes and dimensions of delusions: An exploratory investigation of a role for anxiety processes in the maintenance of delusional distress. Behavioural and Cognitive Psychotherapy 27: 47–62
104. Gurrera RJ, Nestor PG, O'Donnell BF (2000) Personality traits in schizophrenia: comparison with a community sample [In Process Citation]. J Nerv Ment Dis 188: 31–35
105. Tien AY, Costa PT, Eaton WW (1992) Covariance of personality, neurocognition, and schizophrenia spectrum traits in the community. Schizophr Res 7: 149–158
106. Maier W, Minges J, Lichtermann D, Heun R, Franke P (1994) Personality variations in healthy relatives of schizophrenics. Schizophr Res 12: 81–88
107. van Os J, Jones PB (2001) Neuroticism as a risk factor for schizophrenia. Psychol Med 31: 1129–1134
108. Myin-Germeys I, van Os J, Schwartz JE, Stone AA, Delespaul P (2001) Emotional reactivity to daily life stress in psychosis. Arch Gen Psychiatry 12: 1137–1144
109. Garety PA, Kuipers E, Fowler D, Freeman D, Bebbington PE (2001) A cognitive model of the positive symptoms of psychosis. Psychol Med 31: 189–195
110. Escher A, Romme M, Buiks A, Delespaul P, van Os J (2001) Formation of delusional ideation in adolescents hearing voices: a prospective study. Br J Psychiatry, in press

111. Escher A, Romme M, Buiks A, Delespaul P, van Os J (2001) Independent course of childhood auditory hallucinations: a sequential 3-year follow-up study. Am J Med Genetics, in press
112. McGee R, Williams S, Poulton R. (2000). Hallucinations in nonpsychotic children [letter; comment]. J Am Acad Child Adolesc Psychiatry 39: 12–13
113. Fennig S, Susser ES, Pilowsky DJ, Bromet EJ (1997) Childhood hallucinations preceding the first psychotic episode. J Nerv Ment Dis 185: 115–117
114. Selten JP, Sijben N (1994) First admission rates for schizophrenia in immigrants to The Netherlands. The Dutch National Register. Soc Psychiatry Psychiatr Epidemiol 29: 71–77
115. Harrison G, Owens D, Holton A, Neilson D, Boot D (1988) A prospective study of severe mental disorder in Afro-Caribbean patients. Psychol Med 18: 643–657
116. van Os J, Castle DJ, Takei N, Der G, Murray RM (1996) Psychotic illness in ethnic minorities: clarification from the 1991 census. Psychol Med 26: 203–208
117. Chahal K, Julienne L (1999) "We can't all be white!" Racist victimisation in the UK. London: YPS
118. Virdee S (1995) Racial Violence and Harassment. London: London Policy Studies Institute
119. Littlewood R, Lipsedge M (1997) Aliens and Alienists. New York: Routledge
120. Chapman LJ, Chapman JP, Kwapil TR, Eckblad M, Zinser MC (1994) Putatively psychosis-prone subjects 10 years later. J Abnorm Psychol 103: 171–183
121. Kwapil TR, Miller MB, Zinser MC, Chapman J, Chapman LJ (1997) Magical ideation and social anhedonia as predictors of psychosis proneness: a partial replication. J Abnorm Psychol 106: 491–495
122. Harrison G, Glazebrook C, Brewin J, Cantwell R, Dalkin T, Fox R, Jones P, Medley I (1997) Increased incidence of psychotic disorders in migrants from the Caribbean to the United Kingdom. Psychol Med 27: 799–806
123. Sharpley MS, Peters ER (1999) Ethnicity, class and schizotypy. Soc Psychiatry Psychiatr Epidemiol 34: 507–512
124. Johns L, Nazroo JY, Bebbington P, Kuipers E (1998) Occurrence of hallucinations in a community sample. Schizophr Res 29: 23
125. McKenzie K, van Os J, Fahy T, Jones P, Harvey I, Toone B, Murray R (1995) Psychosis with good prognosis in Afro-Caribbean people now living in the United Kingdom [see comments]. BMJ 311: 1325–1328
126. Murray RM, Hurchinson G (1999) Psychosis in migrants: the striking example of African-Caribbeans resident in England. In: Gattaz WF, Hafner H (eds) Search for the Causes of Schizophrenia. Vol IV. Balance of the Century. Berlin Heidelberg New York: Springer, pp 129–140
127. Gilvarry CM, Walsh E, Samele C, Hutchinson G, Mallett R, Rabe-Hesketh S, Fahy T, van Os J, Murray RM. (1999). Life events, ethnicity and perceptions of discrimination in patients with severe mental illness. Soc Psychiatry Psychiatr Epidemiol 34: 600–608
128. Janssen I, Hanssen M, Bak M, Bijl RV, Vollebergh W, McKenzie K, van Os J (2001) Evidence that ethnic group effects on psychosis risk are confounded by experience of discrimination. (Submitted Manuscript)
129. American Psychiatric Association (1987) Diagnostic Criteria from DSM-III-R. Washington, DC: American Psychiatric Association

Developmental Disorders of the Brain

Neuropathology of schizophrenia: is there evidence for a neurodevelopmental disorder?

P. Falkai, K. Vogeley, R. Tepest, T. Schneider-Axmann
Department of Psychiatry, University of Bonn, Bonn, Germany

■ Neurodevelopment, neurodegeneration and more: evidence for three neuropathological processes in schizophrenia?

Since the revival of the neuropathology of schizophrenia in the late 1970s, an increasing number of studies have been published describing a wealth of macroscopic changes in most regions of the human brain (see Table 1 for summary).

The number of non-replications often equals the papers with positive findings, especially in those regions, where most of the studies were performed, e.g.,

Table 1. Macroscopic neuropathological findings in schizophrenia

Region/Parameter	Finding	Region/Parameter	Finding
General		**Basal ganglia**	
Brain length	($\downarrow$)	Globus pallidum area/volume	($\downarrow$)
Brain weight	($\downarrow$)	Nucleus accumbens area/volume	$\downarrow$
Ventricular area/volume	$\uparrow$	Caudate-putamen area/volume	$\uparrow$
Cortex thickness	($\downarrow$)	Thalamus	
Temporal lobe		Mediodorsal nucleus area/volume	$\downarrow$
Lobar area/volume	–	Whole and various nuclei area/volume	–
Hippocampal area/volume	–	Cerebellum	
Parahippocampal area/volume	($\downarrow$)	Anterior vermis area	$\downarrow$
Parahippocampal cortical thickness	($\downarrow$)	Brainstem	
Amygdala area/volume	–	Substantia nigra volume	$\downarrow$
Sylvian fissure length, planum		Locus coeruleus volume	–
temporale volume	$\downarrow$	Periventricular grey volume	$\downarrow$
Sulcogyral pattern	(Abnormal)		
Frontal, perietal and occipital lobes			
Cingulate cortical thickness	–		
Insula area/volume	–		
Corpus callosum thickness	($\uparrow$)		
Internal capsule area (volume)	–		

In comparison to controls:
$\downarrow$ = reduced
$\uparrow$ = increased
– = no difference
() = finding not or only partially replicated
Adapted from Arnold SE, Trojanowski JQ (1996) Recent advances in defining the neuropathology of schizophrenia. Acta Neuropathologica 92: 217–231

the temporal lobe. Based on this body of evidence and also taking brain imaging studies into account, there is no doubt that schizophrenia is a brain disorder with replicable morphological changes. They comprise an overall decrease of the whole brain volume, an enlargement of the ventricular system, especially lateral ventricles and a volume decrease of the hippocampal formation. Changes in the frontal lobe seem to be more subtle, but functionally much more relevant as was previously thought. Therefore, schizophrenia seems to be an encephalopathy focusing on the fronto-temporal regions. For the last 20 years, these changes were regarded as a consequence of a disturbed development of the central nervous system. Subtle neurohistological remnants of disturbed neuronal migration [12], lack of astrogliosis as a typical feature for a degenerative process [11] and no evidence for progressive pathology in brain imaging studies [10] were taken as arguments for this view.

However in recent years, the efforts to replicate findings of histological remnants of disturbed development often failed (for discussion see [12]) and there is some accumulating evidence suggesting a low grade inflammatory process in at least a subgroup of schizophrenic patients [3]. Furthermore birth cohort and high-risk studies [9, 17] reveal data, supporting the notion to disentangle the neuropathology of schizophrenia into several aspects. They show that not all children, later developing schizophrenia and demonstrating delayed developmental milestones, will become schizophrenic. Some will develop schizotypy and some will remain healthy. Therefore there has to be a neuropathology of this basic vulnerability to develop schizophrenia, which however is not sufficient for all probands later developing the full picture of the disorder (see Fig. 1).

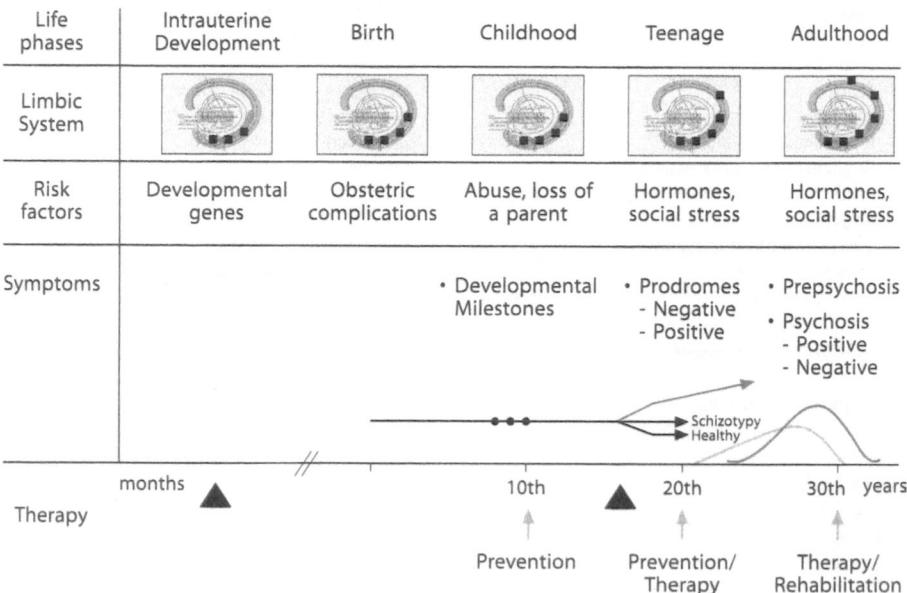

Fig. 1. Pathophysiology of schizophrenia.

Several years before the manifestation of schizophrenia, when patients develop prodromal symptoms, this primary pathology either changes influenced by environmental factors or an additional lesion, e.g., increase of social stress, comes into play leading to a second neuropathological process (Fig. 1). Due to the way neuropathological sampling is performed, it is very unlikely that this second process can be studied post-mortem with the exception of rare cases, where the patients died during the onset of the disorder. Once the full clinical picture of schizophrenia is manifest, the course of this chronic illness is not uniform. Based on long-term outcome, several subtypes can be distinguish. There is increasing evidence pointing to an ongoing disease process in at least a third of the patients suffering from schizophrenia. Especially follow-up brain imaging studies [23, 35] point in this direction (for review see Schröder et al., this book). Therefore there seems to be a third neuropathological process, which is closely linked to the course of schizophrenia and may well reflect the attempts of the brain to beat the disease with its own wepons.

In summary, in order to disentangle the neuropathology of schizophrenia at least three different components or processes have to be taken into account: 1) the neuropathological basis for the predisposition to schizophrenia, 2) the neuropathological events at the disease onset and 3) the neuropathological changes accompanying the disease process. Based on this conceptual frame, the attempt is made to categorize our current knowledge in this respect and furthermore outline what this could mean for further research.

The neuropathological basis of the vulnerability to develop schizophrenia

The predisposition to schizophrenia

About half the risk of developing schizophrenia is explained by genetic and the other half by non-genetic, environmental factors, e.g., obstetric complications [24]. Therefore meaningful biological markers should either be linked to susceptibility genes or specific environmental factors. Currently biological markers adding to the so-called endophenotype seem to be most promising in the search for the molecular basis of schizophrenia. Endophenotypic markers reveal an intermediate phenotype in persons with an increased genetic risk for schizophrenia, which means that this marker gives values in between normal controls and schizophrenic patients. Furthermore these markers should be clearly heritable, meaning that they are much more alike in monozygotic compared to dizygotic twins (for discussion see [25]).

In two subsequent studies disturbed frontal lobe gyrification was described in schizophrenia [36, 37]. Subsequently we have determined the gyrification index in members from multiply affected families with schizophrenia and control subjects (Falkai et al. 2002, in preparation). Family members suffering from schizophrenia (p < 0.0001) as well as their non-schizophrenic relatives (p < 0.001)

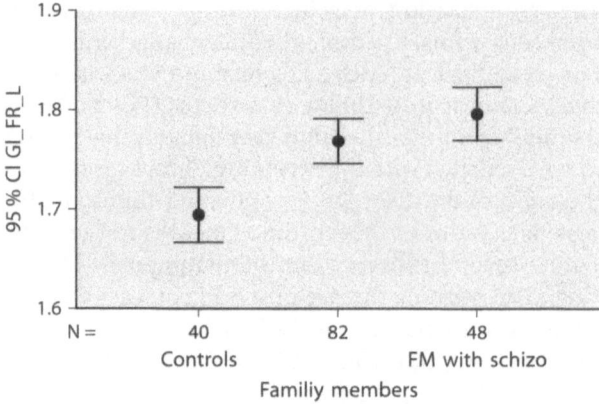

Fig. 2. Gyrification index (GI) frontal left.

demonstrated significantly disturbed gyrification compared to control subjects. In addition, the relatives showed an intermediate phenotype, e.g., values in between that of the family members suffering from schizophrenia and the controls (see Fig. 2). The gyrification index is a reliable measure constituting a ratio between the length of the outer divided by the inner contour on a defined coronal section through the brain [39]. In addition to the families, we determined this gyrification index in the frontal lobe in monozygotic and dizygotic healthy twin pairs and found that the indices were much more alike between monozygotic compared to dizygotic twins pointing to a high degree of heritability of this parameter. Therefore, the frontal gyrification index is a suitable endophenotypic

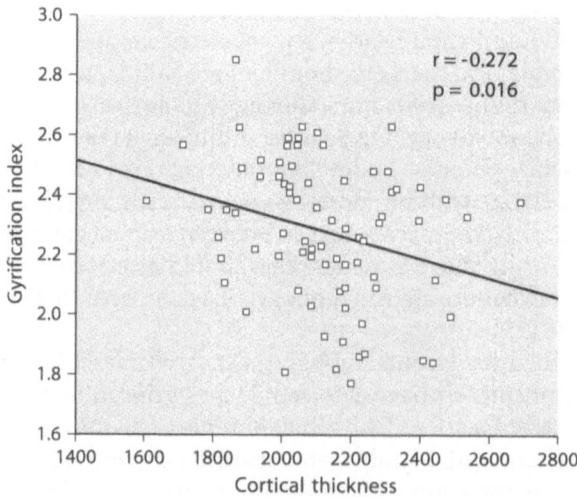

Fig. 3. Gyrification and cortical thickness.

marker forming a suitable link to the genetic basis of schizophrenia. From the literature, it is known that the gyrification index develops in utero and forms a stable marker at the age of one year postpartum and is not influenced by further brain growth or atrophy [2]. Therefore this marker has not only endophenotypic qualities, but in addition mirrors disturbed brain development/maturation up to the age of one year.

What are the changes underlying disturbed gyrification? In several studies we were able to find a significant negative correlation between cortical thickness and the gyrification index, indicating that the more pathological the frontal gyrification, the thinner the underlying cortex is (see Fig. 3).

What is the basis of cortical thinning? Mapping the cytoarchitecture of Brodmann Areas (BA) 9, 10, 22 and 24, a correlation between the neuronal densities and the gyrification index was found only for BA 9, a key area of the dorsolateral prefrontal cortex. Looking at this area a significant increase of neuronal elements was found in schizophrenia compared to control subjects (see Fig. 4).

Volume reduction of the cortex and increase of the density of neuronal elements points towards a subtle disturbance of neuronal migration [22] and/or reduction of non-neuronal elements, e.g., synaptic proteins [32]. Concentrating on the aspect of disturbed neuronal migration, there is some evidence supporting this notion in schizophrenia [1, 12]. Neuronal migration is organized within mainly genetically determined pathways [22]. One of them is the Reelin-Dab1 pathway, whereby Reelin is important for the determination of normal cyto-architectonic lamination. Lack of Reelin leads to significant structural and functional abnormalities [15]. Meanwhile there is substantial literature demonstrating reduced Reelin expression in the cortex of schizophrenic patients [13]. Further research is needed to see whether Reelin and the associated pathway in involved in the pathophysiology of schizophrenia. Beside Reelin, the Wnt-pathway and doubleortin are other interesting candidates, from which we know that reduced expression leads to a deficient neuronal network. These developmentally important proteins form the basis to the neuropathology of the vulnerability to develop schizophrenia.

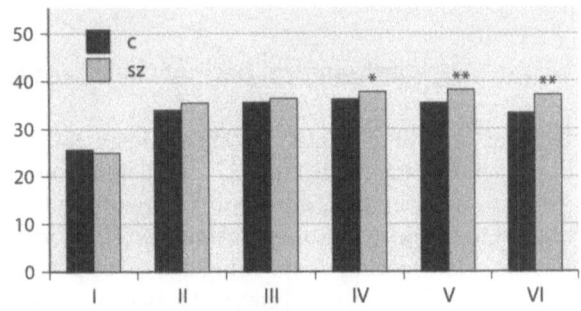

Fig. 4. Cell densities in BA 9 in schizophrenia.

* significant at 0.05 level
** significant at 0.01 level

Developing the full picture of psychosis

Very little information exists about the neurobiological changes accompanying the development of the full clinical picture of schizophrenia. Recent data [35] support the notion that schizophrenia is primarily a disorder of the cortex starting in the parietal region and then spreading to the frontal and temporal areas. Whether the limbic system [5] or the heteromodal association cortices [29] are more involved at the beginning of the disease process is still a matter of discussion. It is proposed that the latter is the origin of first psychotic illness and as the disease progresses further parts of the neuronal network are involved. Comparing schizophrenia with bipolar disorder, there is much more evidence for subcortical than cortical pathology in affective psychosis [33]. It is proposed that affective prodromal symptoms preceding schizophrenia by a mean of four years [14] are based on dysfunction cortical-subcortical circuits mainly responsible for the development and control of emotion. Once cortical regions, especially the parietal lobe, is involved cognitive deficits follow, which are another characteristic of prodromal schizophrenia. If the disease process involves all key regions, thought disorder like delusions of persecution will develop [38]. That is the watershed between affective disorder and schizophrenia, as from this point of the disorder, sufferers have increasing difficulties to realize that their symptoms are part of an illness. The reason for this is that, by then, schizophrenia has taken over most of the cortical regions, which are important for monitoring our "self" [38] meaning that, based on externally generated information and present knowledge, a picture of our own self is generated.

We still do not know what the underlying neurobiology/neuropathology of the events evolving from the deficient neuronal network underlying the vulnerability of schizophrenia is. It is unclear whether the vulnerability factors, e.g., Reelin, change under the influence of environmental factors, e.g., social stress, or if a second hit is necessary to activate the disease process [4]. "The two-hit hypothesis" or see Fig. 1 in this chapter). However, as pointed out above the vulnerability to develop schizophrenia is not sufficient to lead to the disorder in most persons at risk. Therefore, the search for the neuropathology at the onset of the illness will be very important to develop causal therapies.

■ The neuropathological basis of the disease process in schizophrenia

Prospective birth-cohort studies nicely support the neurodevelopmental hypothesis of schizophrenia [17]. It seems clear from these data that the whole group of children later developing schizophrenia reveal a shift of their developmental milestones to abnormal values. These milestones include motoric abilities like first walking or speaking as well as psychic traits like increased fearfulness. These are behavioral correlates of brain development/maturation and their involvement in schizophrenia therefore very much supports the neurodevelopmental hypothesis in this disorder.

On the other hand, further direct neuropathological evidence for a neurodevelopmental process like remnants of disturbed neuronal migration is controversial. Although the original publication by Jakob and Beckmann [16] fostered considerable research efforts in the search for witnesses of disturbed neurodevelopment in schizophrenia, it was subsequently difficult to replicate this and other findings along these lines. First this is due to the fact that is seems unclear what to look for, as the changes in schizophrenia are so subtle that they are easily lost in the normal variability of the human brain. Second, a number of methodological problems often prevent the replication of potentially interesting findings (for review see [10, 12]). Another line of evidence comes from studies looking for signs of degeneration. In a neuropathological process like in Alzheimer's or Huntington's disease neurons are lost and glial cells are activated. The activation of glial cells follows a cascade of events and finally leads to an increase in the number of macroglial cells, e.g., astroglia, which are responsible for the rescue of the neuronal remnants. There is considerable agreement that there is no significant astroglial activation in key limbic areas, e.g., hippocampus or entorhinal cortex in schizophrenia [11]. This is taken as an argument against a degenerative process in schizophrenia. There are however shortcomings to this notion. All studies are performed on tissue of patients, who died after being sick for many years [11]. If there is a degenerative component at the beginning or prior to the onset of the full clinical picture, it might well be missed. Along these lines is a post-mortem study on patients who suffered from Parkinson's disease. There was no change in astroglial, but an increase of microglial cells in the substania nigra, where the main pathological process is situated. This absence of reactive astrocytosis was taken as an indication of a unique inflammatory process in Parkinson's disease [26]. Based on this line of argument we are currently searching for neuropathological evidence of an atypical, possibly low-grade inflammatory process. In a pilot study we found in about twenty percent of patients suffering from schizophrenia increased microglial activation in the hippocampus and frontal cortex based on HLA-DR immunohistochemistry [3]. In a subsequent quantitative study [30] a significant 28% increase of microglial cells in the dorsolateral prefrontal cortex (BA 9), a 57% significant increase in the superior temporal gyrus (BA 22) and a trendwise increase in the anterior cingulate gyrus (BA 24) was found in schizophrenics compared to control subjects. There was no increase in microglial cells and interestingly no reduction of the cortical volume.

What is the meaning of this microglial activation in the key cortical structures in schizophrenia? The most characteristic feature of microglial cells is their rapid activation in response to even minor pathological changes in the CNS. Microglial activation is a key factor in the defense of the neural parenchyma against infectious diseases, inflammation, trauma, ischemia, brain tumors and neurodegeneration. Activated microglia can destroy invading microorganisms, remove potentially deleterious debris, promote tissue repair by secreting growth factors and thus facilitate the return to tissue homeostasis (for review see [20]). Microglial activation is a fine marker for degenerative processes in the cortex, where, e.g. in Alzheimer's disease it correlates to the frequency of plaque pathology [34].

Looking toward infectious diseases, it is interesting to note that in about a third of schizophrenic patients there is evidence for the activation of the immune system as can be seen due to a viral infection [27]. Direct evidence for viral activity was detected in a third of patients with first break schizophrenia [18]. Furthermore, looking for progressive changes in the brain morphology in schizophrenia, the number of *in vivo* imaging studies is growing demonstrating increased ventricular volume and/or cortical atrophy over time [7, 23], for review see Schröder in this book). Rescanning early-onset schizophrenic patients at 2-year intervals at three time points, resulted in a discovery of progressive cortical changes starting in the parietal the brain regions, approaching the temporal and finally the frontal brain areas. This nicely supports the notion of progressive cortical changes in schizophrenia [35].

■ Summary and conclusions

The revival of the neuropathology of schizophrenia in the late 1970s has helped to foster the idea of schizophrenia being a brain disorder. Together with meta-analytically based data from imaging studies, it seems clear today that the volume of the whole brain, especially grey matter, is reduced, the ventricular system increased and the volumes of the hippocampi decreased in schizophrenia. Histological remnants of disturbed neuronal migration, lack of astrogliosis and a lack of progression of the pathological changes in imaging studies support the neurodevelopmental hypothesis of schizophrenia. In recent years however there is increasing evidence for progressive changes in at least a subgroup of patients. Therefore it is proposed that three pathological processes contribute to the neuropathology of schizophrenia: 1) the neuropathological basis of the vulnerability to develop schizophrenia, 2) the changes occurring at the time of the onset of the disorder and 3) the neuropathology of the disease process after the full picture of the disorder developed.

The neuropathological basis of the vulnerability to develop schizophrenia is most probably genetically transmitted and based on a deficiently developed neuronal network. All cascades which are involved in the diverse aspects of the development/maturation of the human brain, like the Reelin-Dab1 pathway, are interesting candidates for susceptibility genes. Changes at the onset of the disorder are difficult to examine post-mortem; however, prospective imaging studies of high-risk individuals give a basis to do so. Studying the process of the disorder over time can well be done post-mortem using promising markers like microglial activation or *in vivo* structural and functional imaging.

All three components of the neuropathology of schizophrenia might well be part of one process, which influenced by environmental factors changes its phenotype over time or each component stems from a different process supporting the "two(several)-hit hypothesis" [4]. This conceptual framework disentangles some of the neuropathological findings seen in schizophrenia and points at the importance of controlling for the different disease stages in any parameter under study. A lot of the variability of biological parameters examined in schizophrenia might well be a consequence of the disease stages not having been taken into account. In a post-mortem study, e.g., we have found, like others, a clearcut reduction of planum temporale asymmetry *in vivo* in chronic schizophrenia [10]. When trying to replicate this finding in first-break schizophrenia we failed [19].

Acknowledgment Kindly supported by the Vada and Theodore Stanley Foundation.

▓ References

1. Akbarian S, Kim JJ, Potkin SG, Hetrick WP, Bunney Jr WE, Jones EG (1996) Maldistribution of interstitial neurons in prefrontal white matter of the brains of schizophrenic patients. Arch Gen Psychiatry 53 (5): 425–436
2. Armstrong E, Schleicher A, Omran H, Curtis M, Zilles K (1995) The ontogeny of human gyrification. Cereb Cortex 5 (1): 56–63
3. Bayer TA, Buslei R, Havas L, Falkai P (1999) Evidence for activation of microglia in patients with psychiatric illnesses. Neuroscience Letters 271: 126–128
4. Bayer TA, Falkai P, Maier W (1999) Genetic and non-genetic vulnerability factors in schizophrenia: the basis of the "two hit hypothesis". J Psychiatr Res 33 (6): 543–548
5. Bogerts B (1997) The temporolimbic system theory of positive schizophrenic symptoms. Schizophr Bull 23 (3): 423–435
6. Bogerts B, Falkai P (1995) The neuropathology of schizophrenia. In: Hirsch SR, Weinberger DR (eds) Schizophrenia. Blackwell Scientific Publishers, chapter 15, pp 276–293
7. DeLisi LE (1999) Defining the course of brain structural change and plasticity in schizophrenia. Psychiatry Res 92 (1): 1–9
8. DeLisi LE, Sakuma M, Ge S, Kushner M (1998) Association of brain structural change with the heterogeneous course of schizophrenia from early childhood through five years subsequent to a first hospitalization. Psychiatry Res 84 (2-3): 75–88
9. Erlenmeyer-Kimling L, Adamo UH, Rock D, Roberts SA, Bassett AS, Squires-Wheeler E, Cornblatt BA, Endicott J, Pape S, Gottesmann II (1997) The New York High-Risk Project. Prevalence and comorbidity of axis I disorders in offspring of schizophrenic parents at 25-year follow-up. Arch Gen Psychiatry 54 (12): 1096–1102
10. Falkai P, Bogerts B, Schneider T, Greve B, Pfeiffer U, Pilz K, Gonsiorczyk C, Majtenyi C, Ovary I (1995) Disturbed planum temporale asymmetry in schizophrenia. A quantitave post-mortem-study. Schizophrenia Res 14: 161–176
11. Falkai P, Honer WG, Bogerts B, Majtenyi C, Bayer TA (1999) No evidence for astrogliosis in brains of schizophrenic patients. A post-mortem study. Neuropathol Appl Neurobiol 18: 17–22
12. Falkai P, Schneider-Axmann T, Honer WG (2000) Entorhinal cortex pre-alpha cell clusters in schizophrenia: quantitative evidence of a developmental abnormality. Biol Psychiatry 47 (11): 937–943
13. Fatemi (2000)
14. Häfner H, Maurer K, Loffler W, an der Heiden W, Munk-Jorgensen P, Hambrecht M, Riecher-Rossler A (1998) The ABC Schizophrenia Study: a preliminary overview of the results. Soc Psychiatry Psychiatr Epidemiol 33 (8): 380–386
15. Hong SE, Shugart YY, Huang DT, Shahwan SA, Grant PE, Hourihane JO, Martin ND, Walsh CA (2000) Autosomal recessive lissencephaly with cerebellar hypoplasia is associated with human RELN mutations. Nat Genet 26 (1): 93–96
16. Jakob H, Beckmann H (1986) Prenatal developmental disturbances in the limbic allocortex in schizophrenics. J Neural Transm 65 (3-4): 303–326
17. Jones PB, Tarrant CJ (1999) Specificity of developmental precursors to schizophrenia and affective disorders. Schizophr Res 39 (2): 121–125; discussion 161
18. Karlsson H, Bachmann S, Schröder J, McArthur J, Torrey EF, Yolken RH (2001) Retroviral RNA identified in the cerebrospinal fluids and brains of individuals with schizophrenia. Proc Natl Sci USA, Vol. 98, Issue 8: 4634–4639

19. Kleinschmidt A, Falkai P, Huang Y, Schneider T, Fürst G, Steinmetz H (1994) *In-vivo* morphometry of planum temporale asymmetry in first-episode schizophrenia. Schizophrenia Res 12: 9–18

20. Kreutzberg GW (1996) Microglia: a sensor for pathological events in the CNS. Trends Neurosci 19: 312–318

21. Lambert de Rouvroit C, Goffinet AM (1998a) The reeler mouse as a model of brain development. Adv Anat Embryol Cell Biol 150: 1–106

22. Lambert de Rouvroit C, Goffinet AM (2001) Neuronal migration. Mechanisms of Development 105: 47–56

23. Lieberman J, Chakos M, Wu H, Alvir J, Hoffman E, Robinson D, Bilder R (2001) Longitudinal study of brain morphology in first episode schizophrenia. Biol Psychiatry 49 (6): 487–499

24. Maier W, Lichtermann D, Rietschel M, Held T, Falkai P, Wagner M, Schwab S (1999) Genetics of schizophrenic disorders. New concepts and findings. Nervenarzt 70 (11): 955–969

25. Malhotra AK, Goldman D (1999) Benefits and pitfalls encountered in psychiatric genetic association studies. Biol Psychiatry 45: 544–550

26. Mirza B, Hadberg H, Thomsen P, Moos T (2000) The absence of reactive astrocytosis is indicative of a unique inflammatory process in Parkinson's disease. Neuroscience Vol 95, No. 2, 425–432

27. Müller N, Ackenheil M (1998) Psychoneuroimmunology and the cytokine action in the CNS: implications for psychiatric disorders. Prog Neuropsychopharmacol Biol Psychiatry 22 (1): 1–33

28. Munn NA (2000) Microglia dysfunction in schizophrenia: an integrative theory. Med Hypotheses 54 (2): 198–202

29. Pearlson GD, Petty RG, Ross CA, Tien AY (1996) Schizophrenia: a disease of heteromodal association cortex? Neuropsychopharmacology 14 (1): 1–17

30. Radewicz K, Garey LJ, Gentleman SM, Reynolds R (2000) Increase in HLA-DR immunoreactive microglia in frontal and temporal cortex of chronic schizophrenics. J Neuropathol Exp Neurol 59 (2): 137–150

31. Rakic P (2000a) Molecular and cellular mechanism of neuronal migration: relevance to cortical epilepsies. Adv Neurona 84: 1–14

32. Selemon LD, Goldman-Rakic PS (2000) The reduced neurophil hypothesis: a circuit based model of schizophrenia. Biol Psychiatry 47 (7): 681–683

33. Soares JC, Mann JJ (1997) The anatomy of mood disorders – review of structural neuroimaging studies. Biol Psychiatry 41 (1): 86–106

34. Thal DR, Arendt T, Waldmann G, Holzer M, Zedlick D, Rüb U, Schober R (1998) Progression of neurofibrillary changes and PHF-ϑ in end-stage Alzheimer's disease is different from plaque and cortical microglial pathology. Neurobiology of Aging 19, 6: 517–525

35. Thompson PM, Vidal C, Giedd JN, Gochmann P, Blumenthal J, Nicolson R, Toga AW, Rapoport JL (2001) Mapping adolescent brain change reveals dynamic wave of accelerated gray matter loss in very early-onset schizophrenia. Proc Natl Acad Sci USA 98, 20: 11650–11655

36. Vogeley K, Bussfeld P, Newen A, Hermann S, Happe F, Falkai P, Maier W, Shah N, Fink GR, Zilles K (2001) Mind reading: neural mechanisms of theory of mind and self-perspective. NeuroImage 13: 1–12

37. Vogeley K, Schneider-Axmann T, Pfeiffer U, Tepest R, Bayer TA, Bogerts B, Honer WG, Falkai P (2000) Disturbed gyrification of the prefrontal region in male schizophrenic patients: a morphometric postmortem study. Am J Psychiatry 157 (1): 34–39

38. Vogeley K, Tepest R, Pfeiffer U, Schneider-Axmann T, Maier W, Honer WG, Falkai P (2001) Right frontal hypergyria differentiation in affected and unaffected siblings from families multiply affected with schizophrenia: a morphometric MRI study. Am J Psychiatry 158 (3): 494–496

39. Zilles K, Armstrong E, Schleicher A, Kretschmann HJ (1988) The human pattern of gyrification in the cerebral cortex. Anat Embryol (Berl) 179 (2): 173–179

High-risk studies and neurodevelopmental hypothesis

J. Parnas*, J. W. Carter**

* Cognitive Research Unit, University Department of Psychiatry, Hvidovre
  Hospital, Hvidovre, Denmark, and Danish National Research Foundation:
  Center for Subjectivity Research
** Social Science Research Institute, University of Southern California, LA,
   USA

Introduction

The purpose of this exposition is two-fold: first, to summarize the import of the prospective High-risk (HR) studies (i.e., longitudinal prospective studies of children with a schizophrenic parent) on the current knowledge of the antecedents of schizophrenia, and, second, to address the nature of the neurodevelopmental hypothesis itself in the light of these results. It has to be noted from the outset, however, that any attempt of theoretical generalization from empirical data is immediately vulnerable to critique because of the unsettled, yet crucial epistemological issues. The most significant of such questions is the very notion of schizophrenia (a strange reservation to make nearly 100 years after this concept was created [1]). Conceptual limitations, if not plain incoherence, of the polythetic operational approach to psychiatric classification [2, 3] have transformed schizophrenia into a diagnosis that is essentially made by exclusion. It is more defined by what *it is not*, than by what it actually *is* [4]. Its psychopathological essence is progressively eluding clinical community and is alarmingly ignored in the empirical research [5]. Such psychopathological void is permissive of *any* theoretical position, no matter how remote from clinical and phenomenological realities. In other words, in the absence of a clear phenomenological concept of schizophrenia, it is nearly impossible to entertain a meaningful discussion of its boundaries, pathogenic mechanisms or potential etiological heterogeneity.

The neurodevelopmental hypothesis (NDH): origins and status

The most commonly held pathogenetic view of schizophrenia has been, for the last fifteen years, the so-called "neurodevelopmental hypothesis" [6]. The NDH remains clinically and pathogenetically vague: noxious factors somehow interfere with early (pre- or perinatal) ontogenesis of the brain. The NDH, already implied in the early days of HR research, became explicitly articulated in the 1980s in order to integrate epidemiological risk factors such as obstetric complications and season of birth effect with the familial aggregation of the disease. The findings of structural brain abnormalities [7], maternal influenza during pregnancy [8], increased frequency of minor ectodermic anomalies and soft neurological signs among schizophrenic patients [9], as well as a number of neuropathological findings [10] can all be incorporated in the NDH. A common reading of these associations is that the development of the brain is affected, either already at the stage of the formation of the neural tube or later, but still during quite early (the perinatal, at the latest) ontogenesis of the CNS. The conceptualization of the lesion varies in sophistication from a focal damage to widespread disruptions of neural connections between more or less specified brain areas. The mechanisms are unknown; candidate proposals usually reflect what appears to be at hand of suggestions from the developmental neuroscience (e.g., neural loss, aberrant neuronal migration and alignment, disturbed axonal myelination, synaptic abnormalities, abnormalities in neural, dendritic and synaptic pruning, apoptosis etc. [see (10) for details]).

In a very influential proposal, Weinberger [11], impressed by certain analogies from neurological diseases, in which the symptoms emerge much later than the contraction of the causative brain lesion (e.g., some forms of temporal lobe epilepsy), suggested that in schizophrenia, the hypothetical pathogenetic CNS lesion occurred prenatally. The lesion was assumed to be both *focal* and *static*, the latter signifying that the *very impact of a hypothetical noxious agent was temporally circumscribed*. Such a lesion, though initially latent and phenotypically dormant, was believed to interact with the developmental brain processes, such as myelination. This interaction turned critical and led to the onset of schizophrenia in adolescence, when the dorsolateral prefrontal cortex is assumed to reach its functional maturity. In the Type I/Type II dichotomy of schizophrenia [12], the "negative" or Type II schizophrenia was considered to be of "organic" nature, caused by pre- or perinatal environmental hazards. Although the dichotomy itself was abandoned after a short period of unjustified enthusiasm, the idea of an inherent association between alleged "organicity" of schizophrenia and its neurodevelopmental origins survived and is being vigorously pursued. For years to come, some authors emphasized a sort of mechanic opposition or causal equivalence, rather than interaction, between neurodevelopmental and genetic factors. Thus, Robin Murray and his collaborators endorsed a division of schizophrenia into "sporadic" and "familial" variants, the former being considered as "organic" and the latter as "genetic" [13]. Somewhat later, a "congenital" subtype of schizophrenia was described, akin to Type II, affecting predominantly males, characterized by poor premorbid adjustment, unfavorable outcome, structural brain abnormalities, cognitive deficits, and caused *either* by a genetic defect, an early brain injury or by an indeterminate mixture of both [14]. In more recent, less dogmatic, dimensional permutation of this view (which now also takes into account the empirical association between the familial and neurodevelopmental risk factors), the phenotypic variation of psychosis is seen as a product of differential admixtures of two causally operative processes: the "neurodevelopmental" (in its extreme resulting in an early onset familial male schizophrenia [6, 15]) and the "affective-socially reactive" (in its extreme resulting in a good outcome female disorder with affective symptoms and a family history of affective illness) [16]. The pervasiveness of the idea of an association between "organicity" and the neurodevelopmental factors seems to have transformed the concept of schizophrenia into a disorder akin to mental retardation or organic-like concreteness, a view perpetuated by the neurocognitive models claiming that schizophrenic patients suffer from abnormalities in the mechanism for "meta-representation". The concept of meta-representation implies some kind of higher-level capacity for self-consciousness or meta-awareness, reminiscent, perhaps, of the neurologist Kurt Goldstein's notion of the abstract attitude or Piaget's notion of formal operations. Schizophrenic patients are "unable to reflect upon their own mental activity" [17; p. 557], and, since such persons are unaware of their goals, they would be "slave[s] to every environmental influence or (...) prone to preseverative or stereotyped behavior, because they would not have the insight to recognize that certain goals were unobtainable or inappropriate" [18; p. 151]. In a similar vein, cognitive deficits, such as low IQ, in a pre-schizophrenic are believed to make such a person "less likely to comprehend the complexities of society (...) and lead to misunderstandings, feelings of paranoia and social withdrawal" [19; p. 1321].

Apart from the fact that such interpretations do not match typical clinical reality of schizophrenia [20, 21], they are also reflective of a fairly mechanistic approach to psychopathology *and* neurobiology and a striking *absence* of developmental psychological and phenomenological considerations. A statement to the effect that "it is now established that schizophrenia is a brain disease" is frequently announced, as if signifying some entirely novel conceptualization of this disorder. Yet this statement is only meaningful on the condition of an underlying metaphysical commitment to the Cartesian mind-brain dualism; otherwise it is referentially opaque, if not entirely empty of meaning. Clinical features of schizophrenia are usually considered as essentially disconnected expressions of the eruptions from a malfunctioning modular substrate. Even such a simplistic framework is not free of plainly conflicting theorizing, as is illustrated by two prominent, yet utterly incompatible, views on a putative causal significance of dysfunctional thalamus for the formation of schizophrenic symptoms: "positive psychotic symptoms (...) do not occur (...) dysfunction of thalamus resembles the negative symptoms of schizophrenia" [22; p. 433], and "a person with defective thalamus is likely to (...) experience the striking misperceptions that we refer to as delusions or hallucinations" [23; p. 297]. It may also be pointed out that the concept of "misconnectivity", emerging in the more recent literature on the etiology of schizophrenia [24], is not so much motivated by a *theoretical distance* to the modular-mechanic paradigm, but is rather a product of a harsh disenchantment with the search for a localized lesion. It is therefore not surprising that a jointly static-organic conceptualization of schizophrenia *and* of the NDH becomes developmentally incomprehensible ("how fetal or neonatal lesions produce hallucinations and delusions two or three decades later remains a mystery" [25; p. 6]) and to some researchers looks like "a perspective (...) that imbues the illness with a pessimistic inevitability and therapeutic nihilism" [26; p. 729].

In summary, a mechanic conceptualization of the developmental insult coupled with a mechanic-modular causal account of the schizophrenic symptoms can not account for the evolution of the illness and its intra-individual variability of course [27], nor does it explain deteriorations seen in significant proportions of patients shortly prior to, and after, the onset of schizophrenia [28, 29].

⬜ The High Risk (HR) studies

The virtue of the HR design, despite its typically small sample size, is its prospective longitudinal design and high data quality. Birth-cohort, draft or family studies, due to their large sample sizes and epidemiological generalizability, may therefore be seen as complementary to the HR designs. The major drawbacks of the HR design comprise its vulnerability to changing diagnostic criteria and its historically determined limitations in the nature of the initially collected data.

By now at least 13 HR projects can be identified in the literature, the most prominent being the NY Infant Study (1952), the Copenhagen HR Project (1962), the NYHR Project (1971/1980), and the Jerusalem Infant Development Study (1973). These projects differ in sample-sizes and other important methodological, diagnostic and socio-demographic aspects that cannot be addressed here (see 30, for a recent review). Yet despite these differences the results seem to converge and are largely supported by other investigations such as birth-cohort and family studies.

The overall picture emerging from the HR studies is that impairments are detectable in multiple domains, even though their exact significance and temporal trajectories are not known in detail:

1) During infancy and early childhood, there is evidence of erratic neuro-motor development, with dysfunctions observable in perceptual, cognitive and motor domains [31–33]. There is, however, disagreement as to whether such dysfunctions are related to obstetric complications [30]. In her pioneer study from 1952 of 12 HR infants and 12 controls, Barbara Fish described the so-called "Pandysmaturation Syndrome" (PDM), a triad comprising transient retardations of visual/motor developments, abnormal profile of functioning (analogous to "intratest scatter") and retardation of skeletal growth. The PDM was present in 7 HR and in one control child. All 7 HR-PDM offspring developed adult schizophrenia spectrum disorder [31]. Fish later replicated her findings in the Jerusalem Infant Development Study [31].
2) During school age, there are observations of aggressivity, especially in boys, and introversion, especially in girls, of disturbed interpersonal relations and neophobia [34–36]. In addition, pre-schizophrenic subjects exhibit neurocognitive impairments, such as attentional, working memory and motor deficits [37].
3) Although the developmental trajectories are poorly examined, there is an indication [38] that poor neuro-behavioral functioning in the HR offspring is temporally stable from childhood to adolescence. Moreover, cognitive deficits recorded at school age seem to be predictive of physical anhedonia in adolescence, the latter, in turn, being predictive of adult schizotypal features [39].
4) Clinical observations in adolescence indicate that elevated levels of autistic features such as eccentricity, subtle formal thought disorder and defective emotional rapport are predictive of adult schizophrenia spectrum disorders [36, 40, 41].

5) The analyses of the MMPI measures taken premorbidly [42–44] indicate that pre-schizophrenics exhibit elevated levels of psychotic ideation.

6) The results from the CHRP indicate that birth complications *interact* with genetic disposition in producing enlarged cerebral ventricles in adulthood, whereas enlarged extracerebral CSF space appears to be linked to genetic factors [45]. Both the schizophrenic and the schizotypal subjects exhibit enlarged extra-cerebral space, whereas only schizophrenic subjects exhibit ventricular enlargement [46].

7) Multivariate "omnibus"-analyses from the CHRP [47] demonstrate that the *most powerful* predictor of subsequent schizophrenia in this particular sample is disrupted childhood rearing conditions. This variable outweighs all other significant univariate predictors, thus confirming previous results from that study [48] and re-emphasizing (today usually neglected) possible pathogenetic impact of early psychosocial environment.

8) In view of the recent findings of the predictive value of low IQ in two large cohorts of draftees [19, 49], we have examined the longitudinal data from the CHRP [50] using-path-analytic approach to evaluate possible predictive value of the premorbid IQ. In the model tested, low premorbid IQ was hypothesized to contribute to adult schizophrenia diagnosis, treatment-status and overall functioning. The premorbid IQ (at the age of 15) was predictive of the adult IQ and educational status (age 25). No relation was found between *concurrent* or *antecedent* IQ on the one hand, and psychopathology, treatment severity, or the overall level of social-occupational functioning, on the other hand. *No decline* in IQ was observed in the schizophrenic subjects. No relation was detected between the age of onset of schizophrenia, no matter how defined (i.e., first psychiatric or first psychotic symptom, age at first hospitalization or the so-called "sick" status at an intermediate social worker follow-up in 1967), and the antecedent IQ. It is not entirely clear how to account for the differences between the results from the draft studies and the present results (possible candidates are, of course, different sample sizes, diagnostic criteria and differences in the instruments used to measure IQ). In a sample of 155 first admission cases collected at Hvidovre Hospital, we observed (Handest et al., in preparation) a significant *negative* correlation between the premorbid IQ estimate (as measured by the National Adult Reading Test [NART; 51]) and the total score on the TDI [52], an index of the *formal* thought disorder (N = 131; r = -0.182, p = 0.037). Moreover, the NART-measured IQ varied substantially as a function of the diagnostic criteria that were used to define schizophrenia.

■ The Copenhagen Infant Follow-up Study (CIFS)

The CIFS is an ongoing new, "second-generation" HR study. It began in 1989–1991, as a research project that was established and led by a child psychiatrist (Dr. Lene Lier) in Copenhagen, to assist pregnant women with major psychiatric illness. In total 50 mothers with a schizophrenia spectrum disorder and 50 mothers with affective disorders entered the study. The assessments consisted of a systematic collection of prenatal/pregnancy and obstetric data, and the subsequent assessment of the offspring at delivery and neonatal period (e.g., Apgar score and neuro-irritability, i.e., excessive excitability, inability to calm down, and marked irregularities in sleeping/eating rhythm). All the offspring were followed-up with videotaped neurodevelopmental assessments (Griffith's Scale) at regular time intervals from the age of 6 months to 3 years. In addition, assessments of attention, checking-back (social referencing), and attachment (Ainsworth's strange situation) were performed at appropriate ages. The subjects (now 10-12 years old) are currently being reassessed with a variety of psychopathological, behavioral and neurocognitive measures.

Comparisons of the developmental trajectories (Parnas et al., in preparation) of 20 HR offspring for schizophrenia (HRS) and 20 HR offspring for affective disorders (HRA) over three assessments at the ages of 6, 18, and 30 months, revealed that on all three occasions HRS performed worse than HRA on neurodevelopmental assessments, in addition to performing worse on naturalistic scorings of social referencing taken at the age of 18 months and of attention at the age of 30 months (Fig. 1). The developmental trajectories of the HRS offspring were markedly intra- and inter-individually scattered, closely reminiscent of the PDM, described by Fish [31]. The HRS offspring were rated as being much more neuro-irritable at birth. They also had lower birth-weight than HRA (3069 g. [sd. 691] vs. 3504 g. [sd. 606], $p < 0.05$). Although gestational age did not discriminate between the risk groups, it was significantly associated with subsequent developmental achievements. Multivariate analyses (with attention and total development scores at 30 months and social referencing at 18 months as outcome measures, and birth weight, gestational age and risk status as predictors) singled

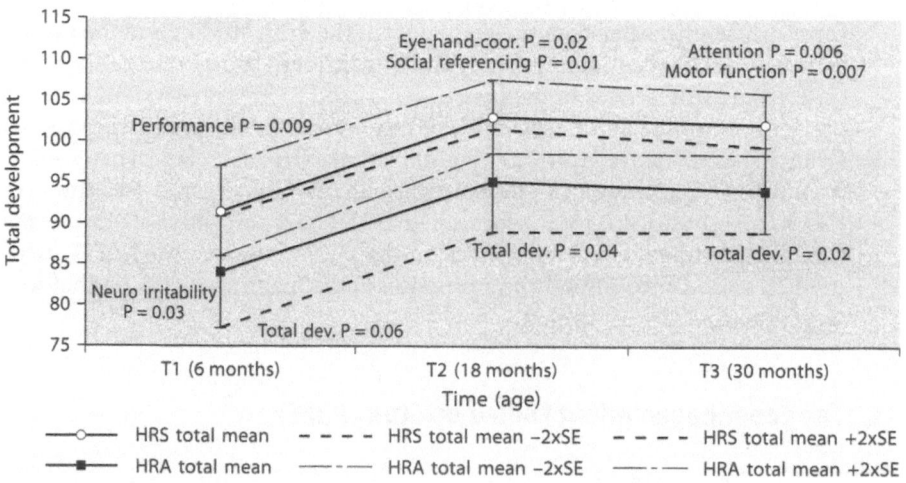

Fig. 1. Copenhagen Infant Follow-up Study. The standard errors (SE) are larger for HRS children than for HRA children. The total development is at all 3 ages larger for HRA than for HRS children. The P-values stems from Mann-Whitney U-test for comparing in the HRS and HRA.

out: a) birth weight (p = 0.016), in conjunction with neuro-irritability (p = 0.0001), as significant predictors of the total developmental score at the age of 30 months; b) neuro-irritability at birth as a predictor of the attentional deficit at the age of 30 months (p = 0.0002); c) genetic risk for schizophrenia in predicting deviant social referencing at the age of 18 months (p = 0.015).

The role of low birth weight has been emphasized in the literature as one of the most important indices of abnormal developmental processes in schizophrenia [53]. We can – although analyses are based on a small, yet closely investigated, sample – conclude the following: the HRS offspring exhibit significantly more developmental problems than the HRA offspring. In this early ontogenetic course, it appears that major developmental achievements are closely associated with perinatal and prenatal factors, such as birth weight. Neuro-irritability at birth may be the earliest schizotaxic indicator, transforming itself in early childhood into more global difficulties in attentional and neuro-motor functioning. The HRS exhibit diminished social referencing, that is perhaps a precursor of deficient emotional attachment, later associated with poor interpersonal rapport, characteristic of adult schizophrenia.

▨ The pathogenetic import of the HR studies

1) Perhaps the single most important scientific impact of the prospective high-risk studies was to document that schizophrenia is *not* a disease process that unexpectedly affects a person in late adolescence or early adulthood as a process in the sense of Jaspers, but is rather an end-state of a gradual evolution that begins in infancy and early childhood. Thus the Kraepelinian-like picture of an illness with adolescent onset and a subsequent typically progressive deterioration can be safely refuted. Here, a common objection is that many, if not a majority, of schizophrenic patients are premorbidly inconspicuous. We think that this apparent neurobehavioral inconspicuousness is an artifact of retrospective collections of crude anamnestic data. The data from the CHRP suggest premorbid deviances in the vast majority of subjects who later develop schizophrenia [36].

2) The premorbid neuro-behavioral deviances *cut across functional domains*, i.e., the data suggest that pre-schizophrenics during their childhood are not only impaired in cognitive and affective domains but also exhibit a generally unstable perceptual-motor performance. The deficits tend to oscillate across time and individuals, pointing more towards instability in *functional* patterns of organization rather than towards a focal lesional defect. In other words, such findings are not supportive of a localized, modular pathology (Note that Jerry Fodor, the major architect of the concept of "modularity of mind", has recently abandoned this idea [54]). Neuropsychological studies of adult schizophrenic patients also demonstrate widespread, multi-domain deficits, largely inconsistent with a notion of localized defect [24, 55, 56].

3) The version of the NDH proposed by Weinberger [11], which claimed a focal static lesion acquired prenatally and dormant until the interaction with late

maturational brain processes set in and so accounted for the adolescent illness onset, is incompatible with the available evidence: first, the deviances are panmodal (see 2 above) and manifest *throughout* the pre-onset life-span of pre-schizophrenics, and, second, an increase of the extra-cerebral CSF space and reduction of gray matter volumes [57] have been observed in the schizophrenics and schizotypal subjects and their biological relatives, thus, necessarily implying a pathological process operative in the *brain during its post-natal growth*. A likely explanation of these cortical changes is a reduction of the neuropile and/or reduction of the neuronal size [10].

4) The results from the HR studies (in particular the CHRP) are more supportive of gene-environment *interactions* than of a mechanic equivalence between the neurodevelopmental and genetic factors: these were observed for perinatal complications and early psychosocial deprivation.

5) Generally, a lack of consistent findings of gliosis is considered as an argument against a simple neuro-degenerative process (involving neuronal death) in the early developmental stages of schizophrenia [10, 58]. Yet, subgroups of patients exhibit significant deteriorations around the onset of psychosis [27, 28], perhaps reflective of more subtle degenerative processes [10, 26].

6) As it is the case with the premorbid neurobehavioral profiles, the evolution of psychotic symptoms also vary across individuals and time [59]. *A pure neuro-anatomical* version of the NDH is incompatible with such phenotypic intra-individual temporal variability [27].

▓ Suggestions for future research

The NDH remains vaguely formulated. Serious conceptual obstacles, alluded to in the introduction, seem to prevent the progress. Psychiatric research, notably in schizophrenia, continues to be technology driven and is short of psychopathological theorizing and phenomenological scrutiny, the elements that are indispensable both as points of departure for integrative efforts and as constrains for empirical investigations. A systematic connection between disparate observations can only be established with reference to a manner or rule of their correlation. Unless such a rule is founded on phenomenological considerations, all of the so-called "bio-psycho-social" integrations will remain merely additive listings of isolated insights or facts.

Currently, and perhaps also due to this conceptual cul-de-sac, a tremendous investment is being made in studying neuro-psychological dysfunctions in adult schizophrenic probands and their relatives with easily available, computer-implemented comprehensive test-batteries. However, a tendency to substitute the clinical and social concept of schizophrenia by that of a neuro-cognitive disorder [60–62] does not seem to carry much promise for solving the mystery of schizophrenia. Most likely, adult neuro-cognitive disturbances represent an important but contingent phenotype, only modestly related to psychiatric symptoms [63]. This phenotype cannot be "of essence" because it is frequently absent in quite typical cases of schizophrenia [64, 65].

A suggestion is emerging from the first-onset studies using in-depth interviews, that vulnerability to schizophrenia may be linked to an unstable sense of selfhood [20, 34, 66–68]. The sense of selfhood and a correlated, automatic intentional attunement to the world (disturbed in the schizophrenic autism [69, 70]) are developmentally founded on quite early sensori-motor and cross-modal sensory integrations ([27]; see 71 for a developmental overview). Spatio-temporally precise ontogenetic formations of cortico-cortical connections, dependent on a variety of organism-environment interactions, constitute a neurobiological prerequisite of such integrations [27]. A variety of adversities may be hypothesized to disrupt such connectivity and so result in an unstable functional organization of the CNS, phenotypically manifest, e.g., as perceptual-motor wavering in the HR infants. Such instabilities may entail an initiation of subtle distortions of intentionality and selfhood. In this way we can perhaps reformulate the NDH to include the possibility of *phenomenological causation*: abnormal organization of the structures of consciousness (intentionality and selfhood) may promote and constrain evolutions of symptoms, evolutions that allow for interactions with environmental factors and that do not need to be understood in linear and mechanical terms. If the brain is seen as a self-organizing, ecologically embedded system and consciousness as its global emergent property [72], then psychotic decompensations may be envisaged as progressive organizations of novel coherence patterns with various degrees of stability and temporal constancy, organizations that articulate themselves around fundamental alterations of self-world relatedness [20].

References

1. Jansson L, Handest P, Nielsen J, Sæbye D, Parnas J (2002) Exploring the boundaries of schizophrenia: a comparison of ICD-10 with other diagnostic systems. World Psychiatry
2. Parnas J, Bovet P (1995) Research in psychopathology: epistemological issues. Compr Psychiatry 36: 167–181
3. Parnas J, Zahavi D (2002) The role of phenomenology in psychiatric classification and diagnosis. In: Maj M, Ibor L (eds) Psychiatric Diagnosis and Classification. World Psychiatric Association's series in Evidence and Experience in Psychiatry, NY, John Wiley & Sons, pp 137–162
4. Maj M (1998) Critique of the DSM-IV operational criteria for schizophrenia. Br J Psychiatry 172: 458–460
5. Andreasen NC (1998) Understanding schizophrenia: a silent spring? Am J Psychiatry 155: 1657–1659
6. Davies N, Russell A, Jones P, Murray RM (1998) Which characteristics of schizophrenia predate psychosis? J Psychiatr Res 32: 121–131
7. Cannon TD, Marco E (1994) Structural brain abnormalities as indicators of vulnerability to schizophrenia. Schizophr Bull 20: 89–102
8. Mednick SA, Machon RA, Huttunen MO, Bonnet D (1988) Adult schizophrenia following prenatal exposure to an influenza epidemic. Arch Gen Psychiatry 45: 189–192
9. Green MF, Satz P, Christenson C (1994) Minor physical anomalies in schizophrenia patients, bipolar patients, and their siblings. Schizophr Bull 20: 433–440
10. Harrison PJ (1999) The neuropathology of schizophrenia. A critical review of the data and their interpretation. Brain 122: 593–624

11. Weinberger DR (1987) Implications of normal brain development for the pathogenesis of schizophrenia. Arch Gen Psychiatry 44: 660–669
12. Crow TJ (1980) Molecular pathology of schizophrenia: more than one disease process? Br Med J (Clin Res) 280: 66–68
13. Murray RM, Lewis SW, Reveley AM (1985) Towards an etiological classification of schizophrenia. The Lancet 1: 1023–1026
14. Murray RM, O'Callaghan E, Castle DJ, Lewis SW (1992) A neurodevelopmental approach to the classification of schizophrenia. Schizophr Bull 18: 329–332
15. O'Connell P, Woodruff PW, Wright I, Jones P, Murray RM (1997) Developmental insanity or dementia praecox: was the wrong concept adopted? Schizophr Res 23: 97–106
16. Curtis VA, van Os J, Murray RM (2000) The Kraepelinian dichotomy: evidence from developmental and neuroimaging studies. J Neuropsychiatry Clin Neurosci 12: 398–405
17. Mlakar J, Jensterle J, Frith C (1994) Central monitoring deficiency and schizophrenic symptoms. Psychol Med 24: 557–564
18. Frith C (1992) The Cognitive Neuropsychology of Schizophrenia. Hove, UK: Erlbaum
19. David AS, Malmberg A, Brandt L, Allebeck P, Lewis G (1997) IQ and risk for schizophrenia: a population-based cohort study. Psychol Med 27: 1311–1323
20. Parnas J, Sass L (2002) Solipsism, self and schizophrenic delusions. Philosophy, Psychiatry, Psychology (in press)
21. Sass LA (1992) Madness and Modernism. Insanity in the Light of Modern Art, Literature, and Thought. New York, Basic Books
22 Bogerts B (1993) Recent advances in the neuropathology of schizophrenia. Schizophr Bull 19: 431-445
23. Andreasen NC, Arndt S, Swayze V, Cizaldo T, Flaum M, O'Leary D, Ehrhardt JC, Yuh WTC (1994) Thalamic abnormalities in schizophrenia visualized through magnetic resonance image averaging. Science 266: 294–298
24. Andreasen NC, Paradisio S, O'Leary DS (1998) "Cognitive Dysmetria" as an integrative theory of schizophrenia: a dysfunction in cortical-subcortical-cerebellar circuitry? Schizophr Bull 24: 203–218
25. Murray RM (1994) Neurodevelopmental schizophrenia: the rediscovery of Dementia Preacox. Br J Psychiatry 165 (suppl 25): 6–12
26. Lieberman JA (1999) Is schizophrenia a neurodegenerative disorder? A clinical and neurobiological perspective. Biol Psychiatry 46: 729–739
27. Parnas J, Bovet P, Innocenti G (1996) Schizophrenic trait features, binding and cortico-cortical connectivity: a neurodevelopmental pathogenetic hypothesis. Neurology, Psychiatry and Brain Research 4: 185–196
28. DeLisi LE (1999) Regional brain volume change over the life-time course of schizophrenia. J Psychiatr Res 33: 535–541
29. Madsen AL, Karle A, Rubin P, Cortsen M, Andersen HS, Hemmingsen R (1999) Progressive atrophy of the frontal lobes in first-episode schizophrenia: interaction with clinical course and neuroleptic treatment. Acta Psychiatr Scand 100: 367–374
30. Erlenmeyer-Kimling L (2001) Neurobehavioral deficits in offspring of schizophrenic parents: liability indicators and predictors of illness. Am J Med Genet 97: 65–71
31. Fish B, Marcus J, Hans S L, Auerbach J G, Perdue S (1992) Infants at risk for schizophrenia: sequelae of a genetic neurointegrative defect. Arch Gen Psychiatry 49: 221–235
32. Walker E, Lewine R J (1990) Prediction of adult-onset schizophrenia from childhood home movies of the patients. Am J Psychiatry 147: 1052–1057
33. Yoshida K, Marks MN, Craggs M, Smith B, Kumar R (1999) Sensorimotor and cognitive development of infants of mothers with schizophrenia. Br J Psychiatry 175: 380–387
34. Hartmann E, Milofsky E, Vaillant G et al. (1984) Vulnerability to schizophrenia. Prediction of adult schizophrenia using childhood information. Arch Gen Psychiatry 41: 1050–1056
35. Olin SS, Mednick SA, Cannon TD, Jacobsen B, Parnas J, Schulsinger F, Schulsinger H (1998) Schoolteacher ratings predictive of psychiatric outcome 25 years later. Br J Psychiatry 172 (Suppl 33): 7–13

36. Tyrka AR, Cannon TD, Mednick SA, Haslam N, Schulsinger F, Schulsinger H, Parnas J (1995) The latent structure of schizotypy: premorbid indicators of a taxon of individuals at risk for schizophrenia-spectrum disorders. J Abnorm Psychol 104: 173–183
37. Erlenmeyer-Kimling L, Rock D, Roberts SA, Janal M, Kestenbaum C, Cornblatt B, Adamo UH, Gottesman II (2000) Attention, memory, and motor skills as childhood predictors of schizophrenia-related psychoses: The New York High-Risk Project. Am J Psychiatry 157 (9): 1416–1422
38. Hans SL, Marcus J, Neuchterlein KH, Asarnow RF, Styr B, Auerbach JG (1999) Neurobehavioral deficits at adolescence in children at risk for schizophrenia. Arch Gen Psychiatry 56: 741–748
39. Freedman LR, Rock D, Roberts SA, Cornblatt BA, Erlenmeyer-Kimling L (1998) The New York High-Risk Project: attention, anhedonia and social outcome. Schizophr Res 30: 1–9
40. Parnas J, Schulsinger F, Schulsinger H, Mednick SA, Teasdale TW (1982) Behavioral precursors of schizophrenia spectrum: a prospective study. Arch Gen Psychiatry 39: 658–664
41. Parnas J, Jørgensen Aa (1989) Premorbid psychopathology in schizophrenia spectrum. Br J Psychiatry 155: 623–627
42. Carter JW, Parnas J, Cannon TD, Schulsinger F, Mednick SA (1999) MMPI variables predictive of schizophrenia in the Copenhagen High-Risk Project: a 25-year follow-up. Acta Psychiatr Scand 99:432-440
43. Gore R (1997) Childhood Precursors of Adult Reality Distortion: A Prospective Study. Dissertation Presented to The Faculty of the Graduate School University of Southern California, pp 1–70
44. Bolinskey PK, Gottesman II, Nichols DS, Shapiro BM, Roberts SA, Adamo UH, Erlenmeyer-Kimling L (2001) A new MMPI-derived indicator of liability to develop schizophrenia: evidence from the New York High-Risk Project. Assessment 8: 127–143
45. Cannon TD, Mednick SA, Parnas J, Schulsinger F, Praestholm J, Vestergaard AA (1993) Developmental brain abnormalities in the offspring of schizophrenic mothers: 1. Contributions of genetic and perinatal factors. Arch Gen Psychiat 50: 551–564
46. Cannon TD, Mednick SA, Parnas J, Schulsinger F, Praestholm J, Vestergaard AA (1994) Developmental brain abnormalities in the offspring of schizophrenic mothers: 2. Structural characteristics of schizophrenia and schizotypal personality disorder. Arch Gen Psychiatry 51: 955–962
47. Carter JW, Schulsinger F, Parnas J, Cannon T, Mednick SA (2002) A multivariate prediction model of schizophrenia. Schizophr Bull (in press)
48. Parnas J, Teasdale TW, Schulsinger H (1985) Institutional rearing and diagnostic outcome in children of schizophrenic mothers: a prospective high-risk study. Arch Gen Psychiatry 42: 762–769
49. Rabinowitz J, Reichenberg A, Weiser M, Mark M, Kaplan Z, Davidson M (2000) Cognitive and behavioural functioning in men with schizophrenia both before and shortly after first admission to hospital. Br J Psychiatry 177: 26–32
50. Parnas J, Cannon T, Jacobsen B, Schulsinger H, Schulsinger F, Mednick SA (1993) Life-time DSM-IIIR diagnostic outcomes in offspring of schizophrenic mothers: The results from the Copenhagen High Risk Study. Arch Gen Psychiatry 50: 707–714
51. Russell AJ, Munro J, Jones PB, Hayward P, Hemsley DR, Murray RM (2000) The National Adult Reading Test as a measure of premorbid IQ in schizophrenia. Br J Clin Psychol 39: 297–305
52. Johnston MH, Holzman PS (1979) Assessing Schizophrenic Thinking: A Clinical and Research Instrument for Measuring Thought Disorder. San Francisco, Jossey-Bass
53. Kunugi H, Nanko S, Murray RM (2001) Obstetric complications and schizophrenia: prenatal underdevelopment and subsequent neurodevelopmental impairment. Br J Psychiatry 178 (suppl 40): 25–29
54. Fodor J (2001) The Mind Doesn't Work That Way. Cambridge MA, MIT Press
55. Mohamed S, Paulsen J S, O'Leary D, Arndt S, Andreasen N (1999) Generalized cognitive deficits in schizophrenia. A study of first-episode patients. Arch Gen Psychiatry 56: 749–754
56. Parnas J, Vianin P, Sæbye D, Jansson L, Larsen AV, Bovet P (2001) Visual binding abilities in the initial and advanced stages of schizophrenia. Acta Psychiatr Scand 103: 171–180

57. Cannon TD, van Erp TGM, Huttunen M, Lönnqvist J, Salonen O, Valanne L, Poutanen V, Standertskjöld-Nordenstam C, Gur RE, Yan M (1998) Regional gray matter, white matter, and cerebrospinal fluid distributions in schizophrenic patients, their siblings, and controls. Arch Gen Psychiatry 55: 1084–1091
58. Woods BT (1998) In schizophrenia a progressive neurodevelopmental disorder? Toward a unitary pathogenetic mechanism. Am J Psychiatry 155: 1661–1670
59. Parnas J (1999) From predisposition to psychosis: progression of symptoms in schizophrenia. Acta Psychiatr Scand 99 (suppl 395): 20–29
60. Tsuang MT, Stone WS, Faraone SV (2000) Toward reformulating the diagnosis of schizophrenia. Am J Psychiatry 157 (7): 1041–1050
61. Tsuang MT, Stone WS, Seidman LJ, Faraone SV, Zimmet S, Wojcik J, Kelleher JP, Green AI (1999) Treatment of nonpsychotic relatives of patients with schizophrenia: four case studies. Biol Psychiatry 45: 1412–1418
62. Faraone SV, Green AI, Seidman LJ, Tsuang MT (2001) "Schizotaxia": clinical implications and new directions for research. Schizophr Bull 27 (1): 1–18
63. Nieuwenstein MR, Aleman A, de Haan EHF (2001) Relationship between symptom dimensions and neurocognitive functioning in schizophrenia: a meta-analysis of WCST and CPT studies. J Psychiatr Res 35: 119–125
64. Palmer BW, Heaton RK, Paulsen JS, Kuck J, Braff D, Harris MJ, Zisook S, Jeste DV (1997) Is it possible to be schizophrenic yet neuropsychologically normal? Neuropsychology 11 (3): 437–446
65. Weickert TW, Goldberg TE, Gold JM, Bigelow LB, Egan MF, Weinberger DR (2000) Cognitive impairments in patients with schizophrenia displaying preserved and compromised intellect. Arch Gen Psychiatry 57: 907–913
66. Parnas J, Jansson L, Sass LA, Handest P (1998) Self-experience in the prodromal phases of schizophrenia: a pilot study of first admissions. Neurology, Psychiatry and Brain Research 6: 107–116
67. Møller P, Husby (2000) The initial prodrome in schizophrenia: searching for naturalistic core dimensions of experience and behavior. Schizophr Bull 26: 217–232
68. Parnas J (2000) The self and intentionality in the pre-psychotic stages of schizophrenia. In: Zahavi D (ed) Exploring the Self: Philosophical and Psychopathological Perspectives on Self-experience. Philadelphia, John Benjamins Publishing Company, pp 115–147
69. Parnas J, Bovet P (1991) Autism in schizophrenia revisited. Compr Psychiatry 32: 7–21
70. Stanghellini G (2000) At issue: vulnerability to schizophrenia and lack of common sense. Schizophr Bull 26: 775–787
71. Rochat P (2001) The Infant's World. Cambridge: Harvard University Press, pp 28–80
72. Varela FJ, Thompson E, Rosch E (1991) The Embodied Mind. Cognitive Science and Human Experience. Cambridge MA, MIT Press

Are structural cerebral changes progressive in schizophrenia?

J. Schröder, C. Bottmer, J. Pantel
Section of Geriatric Psychiatry, University of Heidelberg, Germany

Introduction

Structural cerebral changes in schizophrenia were first described as early as 1927 when Jacobi and Winkler reported ventricular enlargement in patients with chronic schizophrenia using pneuencephalography [21]. Similar findings were obtained by Huber [19] and Haug [16]. These early observations were confirmed by a large number of neuroimaging studies using computed tomography (CT) or – in the last decade – magnetic resonance imaging (MRI). It is generally accepted that a certain proportion of patients with schizophrenia show an enlargement of the CSF spaces at the expense of whole brain volume. In addition, decreased volumes of the frontal and temporal lobes, the medial temporal substructures and thalamic nuclei, and the cerebellum were also frequently described [45].

The question, however, whether these changes are static or progressive in the clinical course remained unresolved. This question is not only of heuristic, but also of potential clinical importance. If schizophrenia involved progressive changes of distinct cerebral sites, examination of the particular neurobiological features of the respective sites or analyses of their potential prognostic importance could facilitate both the development of new prognostic and therapeutic approaches.

A number of CT or MRI studies have investigated cerebral changes in the course of schizophrenia. The aim of the present paper is to summarize these studies and to discuss the findings with respect to methodological issues of the neuroimaging methods involved, the heterogeneity of schizophrenia in terms of symptoms and stages, as well as potential environmental factors.

Longitudinal neuroimaging studies

To date, at least 30 longitudinal studies on structural cerebral changes in schizophrenia involving CT or MRI have been conducted. Studies differed significantly with respect to important methodological features, in particular the resolution capacity of the imaging methods employed, duration of the follow-up interval, patients' symptoms, and stage of the disease. Therefore, the following summary was structured according to the kind of parameters studied (global or regional changes) rather than the imaging method used. We first refer to those studies investigating parameters sensitive to global cerebral changes such as ventricular size; studies investigating more focal changes are discussed thereafter.

Global cerebral changes

CT studies investigating ventricle to brain ratio

Most early CT studies investigated the ventricle-brain ratio (VBR), a parameter sensitive to generalized brain changes. Nasrallah et al. [32] found no significant VBR changes in chronic male patients during a follow-up interval of 36 months. Three other studies [18, 20, 50] assessing chronic patients up to 108 months after initial scanning confirmed these nil-findings. Kemali et al. [26] who included both patients and controls described very heterogeneous findings at follow-up: while VBRs were relatively stable in the healthy controls, the percent change in the patients' group varied greatly, yielding significant results with a longitudinal VBR increase. However, this last difference became nonsignificant when two outliers with VBR increases of greater than 200% were excluded. Woods et al. [53] employed a unique correction method to overcome the difficulties arising from area measurement of a volumetric variable. The group reported a median VBR increase of 25% in 8 of the 9 patients investigated, this result reaching statistical significance.

All of the early studies cited above on chronic schizophrenia used CT with planimetric measurements being performed on the slice showing the ventricles at their largest. Within-subject differences in angular positioning and slicing thus have to be considered all the same as limitations due to the low resolution capacity of CT when discussing diverging findings. Definition of the VBR varied between studies with both whole brain area [50] or whole intracranial area [25] being used as a denominator for calculating the ratio. This is of primary importance, since whole brain area but not whole intracranial area may also be afflicted by the disease process. Moreover, statistical issues need to find consideration. Sample sizes were rather small and healthy controls not studied in the majority of publications. Finally, with VBR calculated on the basis of whole brain area, possible structural changes over time enter the ratio twice, thus, increasing the risk of type I errors. In an effort to overcome these methodological problems, Davis and colleagues [6] assessed ventricular size as an absolute measure. The authors found poor outcome chronic patients to have significantly increased ventricles over time as opposed to no changes in patients with a good outcome and healthy subjects.

CT studies on first-episode patients have found no significant longitudinal VBR increase. Despite presenting with the same methodological difficulties as studies involving chronic patients the research work of Sponheim et al. [47], Jaskiw et al. [23] and Vita et al. [49] came to converging findings. Sponheim et al. actually found VBR to decrease over time; after post hoc visual inspection, however, they came to the conclusion that differences in the scanning process may have introduced an error in VBR measurement. The authors developed a composite VBR (CVBR) derived by superimposing several scans in order to estimate the largest cross-sectional area of the body of the lateral ventricles and thus overcome the problem of the subject's positioning in the scanner. The corrected measure did not change longitudinally. Similarly, the other two groups were not able to detect significant changes in VBR over time.

MRI studies

MRI studies including chronic patients have been presented by Nair et al. [34], Gur et al. [15], Garver et al. [13] and Mathalon et al. [33]. The former report similar results as Davis et al. [6] with a subgroup of patients experiencing marked ventricular expansion, whereas other patients showed a rate of change not differing significantly from healthy controls. As opposed to the CT study by Davis et al., Nair et al. were not able to correlate pronounced expansion with clinical or demographic variables nor with duration of illness. This especially deserves emphasis with regard to the notion that few first-episode studies were able to detect changes at follow-up, whereas positive findings have been reported by some studies dealing with chronicity of the illness. However, Nair et al. concluded that the lack of an association between illness duration and VBR suggests the existence of subtypes to be responsible for the given results. Gur et al. included 20 first-episode and 20 chronic patients as well as 17 healthy controls, but found no significant differences regarding the global measures of ventricles or whole brain volumes, neither between the two stages of illness nor between scanning sessions. In an interesting approach, Garver et al. investigated ventricular and total brain volume with respect to the acuity of the disease. Twenty-five subjects with chronic psychosis were examined during two different illness states, i.e., in (partial) remission under neuroleptic treatment and while experiencing acute psychotic exacerbation. Regardless of the scanning interval and order, patients when suffering from florid psychosis showed larger brain volumes and smaller ventricles as compared to times of remission. Potential medication effects – which may well involve lateral ventricle volumes through an enlargement of the adjacent basal ganglia – were not thoroughly addressed.

Garver et al. concluded that exacerbation of psychosis is associated with brain swelling accompanied by slight encroachment upon ventricular volumes. At times of remission, individuals suffering from schizophrenia exhibit rates of ventricular expansion comparable to those of healthy subjects. While this finding appears to be generally consistent with Gur et al. [15], who found volume reductions at follow-up to be significantly correlated with greater improvement across most symptoms in the previously treated patients, similar associations were not reported by others.

Among the first to report MRI findings on first-episode patients were DeGreef et al. [7] and Keshavan et al. [27]. While the latter examined total brain volume in order to assess global cerebral changes, the former used the measures of ventricular volume, as well. Neither group found evidence for progressive ventricular enlargement or cortical volume decrease, respectively, yet it has to be mentioned that in both studies sample sizes were relatively small and only one included controls. The same applies to the study of Zipursky et al. [54] who reported a longitudinal reduction of total brain grey matter which did not significantly differ between patients and controls. A large first-episode study by DeLisi et al. [8–10] compared rates of volumetric changes between patients and controls over a 4-5 year period, stating that volumes of both hemispheres as well as – on coronal slices only – of the left cerebral ventricle are affected. Further changes were reported by Rapoport et al. [40–42] who enrolled 46 adolescents with schizophrenia, finding total cerebral volume, total grey matter, lateral ventricles and VBR to significantly differ between patients and controls over time. In these studies the expected effect emerged with patients having cortical volume decreases accompanied by ventricular volume increases.

An association between progressive whole brain changes with an unfavorable clinical course was emphasized by DeLisi et al. [8, 9], Lieberman et al. [31] and Puri et al. [39]. In accordance with DeLisi et al., Liebermann et al. assessed ventricular as well as cortical volumes in a large sample of first-episode patients longitudinally finding ventricular volumes to increase in poor outcome but not in good outcome patients or controls. Moreover, good outcome patients exhibited a significant increase in cortical volumes as compared to poor outcome patients. Puri et al. reported no significant differences in mean ventricular volumes between 24 first-episode patients and twelve controls at follow-up. However, a subgroup of patients experienced ventricular increase of greater than one standard deviation while another subgroup was found to have decreased ventricles to a comparable extent after a mean interval of 8 months.

▓ Regional volumetric changes

While a variety of cerebral structures including the hippocampal formation, the cerebellum, and the basal ganglia have been investigated, the majority of studies focused on the frontal and temporal lobes. Nearly all studies included a healthy control group for comparison; the neuroimaging methods used are roughly comparable with slice thickness ranging between 1.5 and 5 mm. Yet, differences in definition of the respective regions of interest (ROI) and other methodological issues render direct comparison of studies difficult. Large structures frequently subject to investigation like the frontal or temporal lobes yield a diversity of findings.

Keshavan et al. [27] published results of MRI of eleven first-episode patients scanned twice a mean of 10 months apart. No significant changes with respect to prefrontal cortex grey matter, white matter or total volume emerged from their analyses. In contrast, a decrease of frontal lobe volumes was reported by our own group [1]. However, both studies lack a control group for comparison. Gur et al. [15] assessed twenty first-episode as well as twenty chronic patients and seventeen controls twice within a period of 12 to 68 months. The authors found frontal lobes to decrease in the first hospitalized subjects, only, but not in the other two groups. This finding is opposed to that of Zipursky et al. [54] stating frontal lobe grey matter to decrease in volume in first-episode patients and controls, equally, at 60 months follow-up. Mathalon et al. [33] – enrolling 24 chronic patients and an equally large number of healthy subjects rescanned after 7 to up to 90 months – have recently published further data on regions corresponding to the frontal lobes. The authors described volumetric decreases of right frontal grey matter in patients to be more pronounced than in controls. Finally, Rapoport et al. [40–42] who investigated adolescents re-analyzed frontal grey matter after 3 – 5 years. The group demonstrated that the percentage of grey matter decrease was signif-

Table 1. Imaging studies examining global cerebral changes in schizophrenia over time

Study	Method	Subjects	State	Time interval	Results*
Nasrallah et al., 1986	CT: VBR	11 male pat.	Chronic	36 months	No significant changes
Illowsky et al., 1988	CT: VBR	13 pat.	Chronic	84–108 months	No significant changes
Vita et al., 1988	CT: VBR	15 pat.	Chronic	23–65 months	No significant changes
Kemali et al., 1989	CT: VBR	18 pat. 8 cont.	Chronic	36–38 months	VBR increases (up to 223%) in 11 of the patients
Woods et al., 1990	CT: VBR	9 pat.	Chronic	12–54 months	VBR increases in 8 of the patients
Hoffman et al., 1991	CT: VBR	19 pat.	Chronic	24–48 months	No significant changes
Sponheim et al., 1991	CT: VBR Composite VBR	15 pat.	First-episode	12–33 months	VBR decrease No significant changes in cVBR
Jaskiw et al., 1994	CT: VBR	7 pat.	First-episode	62–92 months	No significant changes
Vita et al., 1994	CT: VBR	9 pat. 22 cont.	First-episode	24–46 months	No significant changes
Davis et al., 1998	CT: total ventricular & regional ventric. Size	53 male pat. 13 male cont.	Chronic	Mean: 60 months	Bilat. increase in poor outcome patients for total size; increase of lateral vent. in poor outcome pat. for regional comparisons, left > right
DeGreef et al., 1991	MRI Total brain volume Ventricular volume	13 pat. 8 cont.	First-episode	12–24 months	No significant changes

Cont. Table 1.

Study	Method	Subjects	State	Time interval	Results*
Keshavan et al., 1994	MRI Total brain volume	11 pat.	First-episode	Mean: 10 months	No significant changes
DeLisi et al., 1995, 1997	MRI Ventricular volume Hemispheric volume	50 pat. 20 cont.	First-episode	48–60 months	Hemispheres decrease in pat. Left ventricles increase on coronal view in pat (Comparison of rates of change)
Nair et al., 1997	MRI Ventricular volume	18 pat. 5 cont.	Mixed sample	13–45 months	Ventricles increase in subgroup of pat. only
Rapoport et al., 1997, 1999	MRI Cerebral volume Ventricular volume	16 adolescent pat., 24 cont.	Adolescents	18–60 months	Cerebrum decreases in pat. Ventricles increase in pat.
Gur et al., 1998	MRI Total brain volume Ventricular volume	40 pat. 17 con.	20 first-episode 20 chronic	12–68 months	No significant changes
Garver et al., 2000	MRI Total brain volume Ventricular volume	25 pat. schizophrenia spectrum disorders	Chronic	9–49 months	Brain volumes increase during exacerbation compared to (partial) remission Ventricle volumes decrease during exacerbation compared to (partial) remission
Lieberman et al., 2001	Ventricular volume Cortical volume	51 pat. 13 cont.	First-episode	12–72 months	Ventricular volumes increase in poor outcome pat, no changes in good outcome pat. and cont. Cortical volumes increase in good outcome pat., no changes in poor outcome pat.
Puri et al., 2001	MRI Ventricular volume	24 pat. 12 cont.	First-episode	Mean: 8 months	No significant changes. Ventricular increase/decrease in subgroups of patients
Zipursky et al., 2001	MRI Total brain grey matter	17 pat. 10 cont.	First-episode	60 months	Total grey matter decrease in pat. and cont., equally

* stating presence/absence of significant Diagnosis · Time interaction unless specified differently.
  stating presence/absence of main effect Time in studies lacking a control group.

icantly higher in the patients than in the healthy controls. The only CT study on frontal lobe changes [32] investigated the size of cortical fissures and sulci in twenty-one first-episode schizophrenic patients, ten patients with other psychiatric disorders and nine healthy controls. At reinvestigation after 5 years, the indirect measures of frontal lobe atrophy appeared to be more pronounced in the patients with schizophrenia.

Data on temporal structures varies greatly. Gur et al. [15], DeLisi et al. [8, 9], and Zipursky et al. [54] – although differing reasonably in methodology – came to basically converging results, with temporal lobe and right temporal grey matter volumes, respectively, decreasing equally in patients and controls. While these three samples mainly comprised first-episode patients, Mathalon et al. [33] found a significant bilateral temporal grey matter reduction in chronic patients suggesting progression of volume reduction with prolonged disease process. The findings of Hirayasu et al. [17] state a decrease in left superior temporal gyrus in patients, but not so in controls in a rather small sample of first-episode subjects. Moreover, Pantelis et al. [38] conducted an interesting study investigating a high-risk sample of eighteen subjects nine of whom became psychotic during the follow-up interval of 12 months and nine who remained stable. At follow-up, those patients who developed schizophrenia showed decreased volumes of the medial temporal regions, whereas no corresponding changes were observed in the non-psychotic group. Finally, research into childhood-onset schizophrenia has presented with significant longitudinal differences between patients and controls. Jacobsen et al. [22] examining ten adolescents with childhood-onset schizophrenia and seventeen controls reported smaller right temporal lobe and superior temporal gyrus volumes in the patients at follow-up. Similar findings were reported by Rapoport et al. [40–42]. Thompson et al. [48] analyzed MRI of each 12 patients with childhood onset schizophrenia and controls which were obtained over a 5 year interval. For analysis, a pixel-based approach was used. Initial MRIs only showed changes of the parietal lobes. At follow-up, changes had spread to the anterior parts of the brain, engulfing the supplementary motor area, the sensorimotor and frontal cortices, and the temporal lobe. Potential medication effects could not be verified. With respect to the clinical course, negative symptoms on follow-up were significantly correlated with frontal lobe changes. This intriguing study clearly suggests that brain changes in childhood onset schizophrenia originate in the parietal cortex. The temporal and frontal cortices are only secondarily involved in the course of the disease. While childhood onset schizophrenia strikes the brain in a period crucial for brain development and maturation, brain development is not completed by age 18 but continues into the fifth decade of life [2].

With respect to the medial temporal substructures, a significant progression of hippocampal volume reduction was not confirmed in adults with schizophrenia [8, 9, 17], but was present in childhood-onset schizophrenia [14]. On the contrary, Lieberman et al. [31] found the hippocampus to increase in poor outcome patients over time. Other structures investigated up to now were the parietal and occipital lobes and the cerebellum. While parietal and occipital changes were neither detected by Rapoport et al. [40–42] nor Zipursky et al. [54], Thompson et al.

Table 2. MRI studies examining regional volumetric changes in schizophrenia over time

Study	ROI	Subjects	State	Time interval	Results*
Chakos et al., 1994	Caudate nucleus	29 pat. 10 cont.	First-episode	18 months	5.7% increase in pat., 1.6% deecrease in cont.
Keshavan et al., 1994	Caudate nucleus Prefrontal cortex	11 pat.	First-episode	Mean: 10 months	Caudate increases (right, left and total) No significant changes in prefrontal cortex (grey matter, white matter, total)
DeLisi et al., 1995, 1997	Cerebellum Temporal lobes, Hippocampus, Caudate nucleus, Corpus callosum Asymmetries	50 pat. 20 cont.	First-episode	48–60 months	Right cerebellar hemisphere decreases in pat. No significant changes regarding temporal lobes, hippocampus, caudate, corpus callosum or asymmetries (Comparison of rates of change).
Rapoport et al., 1997, 1999	Frontal grey matter Temporal grey matter Parietal grey matter Occipital grey matter Caudate Putamen Globus pallidus	16 adolescent pat., 24 cont.	Adolescents	18–60 months	Frontal grey matter decrease in pat. Temporal grey matter decrease in pat. Parietal grey matter decrease in pat. Occipital grey matter: no significant changes Caudate decrease in pat. > cont. Putamen: no significant changes Globus pallidus: no significant changes
Gur et al., 1998	Frontal lobes Temporal lobes	40 pat. 17 cont.	20 first-episode 20 chronic	12–68 months	Frontal lobes decrease in 1.-ep pat. only Temporal lobes decrease in pat. and controls
Jacobsen et al., 1998	Temporal lobe structures	10 adolescent pat., 17 cont.	Adolescents	24 months	Right temporal lobe, STG and left hippocampus decrease in pat. > cont.
Giedd et al., 1999	Amygdala Hippocampus	23 adolescent pat., 36 cont.	Adolescents	24–48 months	No significant changes regarding amygdala Differential hippocampal volume change between pat. and cont.
Hirayasu et al., 1999	STG Hippocampus/amygdala	9 pat. 7 cont.	First-episode	12–22 months	Left STG decreases in pat. No significant changes in hippocampus/amygdala

Cont. Table 2.

Study	ROI	Subjects	State	Time interval	Results*
Pantelis et al., 2000	Medial temporal regions	18 pat. (9 pat. later psychotic, 9 pat. later non-psychotic)	High-risk	12 months / at onset of psychosis, resp.	At follow-up, those pat. who were psychotic showed decreased temporal volumes, whereas there were no changes in the non-psychotic group.
Bachmann et al., 2001	Frontal lobes Temporal lobes Cerebellum	14 pat.	First-episode	12–15 months	Bilateral frontal and temporal lobe decrease No significant changes regarding cerebellum
Lang et al., 2001	Caudate Putamen Globus pallidus	30 pat. 23 cont.	First-episode	12 months	No significant changes
Lieberman et al., 2001	Caudate Hippo-campus	51 pat. 13 cont.	First-episode	12–72 months	Caudate increase in pat., decrease in cont. Hippocampus increase in poor-outcome pat.
Mathalon et al., 2001	Frontal regions Temporal regions	24 pat. 25 cont.	Chronic	7–90 months	Right frontal grey matter decrease in pat > cont. Bilateral temporal grey matter decrease in pat >cont.
Thompson et al., 2001	Frontal lobe grey matter Temporal lobe g. m. Parietal lobe g. m.	12 pat. 12 cont.	Adolescents	27–55 months	At 2 year follow-up, grey matter decrease in parietal regions in pat. At 5 year follow-up, grey matter decrease in temporal lobes & dorsolat. prefront. cortices in pat.
Zipursky et al., 2001	Frontal lobe grey matter Temporal lobe g. m. Occipital lobe g. m.	17 pat. 10 cont.	First-episode	60 months	Bilateral frontal, right temporal and occipital grey matter decrease in pat. and cont., equally

* stating presence/absence of significant Diagnosis · Time interaction unless specified differently.
  stating presence/absence of main effect Time in studies lacking a control group.

[48] found parietal lobes to decrease over time in 12 patients with early-onset schizophrenia. DeLisi et al. [8, 9] reported longitudinal cerebellar changes in schizophrenia exceeding those observed in healthy controls. However, this finding was not replicated by others [1].

Further studies focused on the basal ganglia as an important site for neuroleptic drug treatment. Chakos et al. [4] found the volume of the caudate nucleus to increase over time in first episode patients who received initial treatment with conventional neuroleptic drugs. This effect was dose-dependent and associated with younger age at study intake. Consistent findings were reported by Lieberman et al. [31] and Keshavan et al. [27]; moreover, a direct effect of conventional neuroleptics on the D2-dopamine receptor system with receptor upregulation was also described in functional imaging studies [46]. That this effect refers to the binding of conventional neuroleptics at the D2-dopamine receptor system is further supported by the observation that treatment with atypical compounds does not increase [40, 41] – and may even normalize [5, 28] – caudate volumes.

▦ Discussion

The present review demonstrates that currently available longitudinal neuroimaging studies on structural cerebral changes in schizophrenia differ widely in terms of imaging methods employed, patients' characteristics, and sample sizes. Accordingly, it appears rather difficult to draw any definite conclusion from the available studies. However – keeping these limitations in mind – two main hypotheses can be formulated based on the data available: first, there is no convincing evidence that schizophrenia is generally accompanied by a progressive global cerebral tissue loss; and second, regional changes of frontal and temporal volumes may occur in subgroups of patients and/or may be related to certain stages of the disease.

Progression of global cerebral changes

While potential global cerebral tissue losses have been investigated in a considerable number of studies, results appear to be rather inconsistent: eight studies described a progressive enlargement of the ventricular space indicating cerebral tissue losses; 12 studies did not confirm this finding. The diversity of findings may be influenced by both, methodological difficulties and factors intrinsic to the disease. Methodological difficulties involve the imaging techniques used which range from early CT to advanced MRI techniques, the latter guaranteeing a better spatial resolution and higher neuroanatomical accuracy. A further variation arises from the fact that some studies compared absolute values, e.g., volumes in ccm, while others – in particular the early CT studies – used relative measures such as VBR. Moreover, healthy control groups were mainly included in the more recent MRI but not early CT studies.

Further methodological differences between studies are related to sample selection. This involves not only different stages of the disease (e.g., first episode versus chronic patient samples) but also factors related to course and outcome. Two large MRI studies – each involving 50 patients – described pronounced global changes in patients with poor outcome; a finding which clearly corresponds to the diversity of the clinical courses following an initial episode of schizophrenia which may vary greatly from a single remitting episode to a recurrent form of the disease or a chronic state. Similarly, pronounced deficits in the poor outcome patients were found for a number of cerebral changes, including neurological soft signs, regional glucose uptake, or benzodiazepine receptor distribution (see 45 for review). One may argue that global cerebral changes in poor outcome patients may also be attributed to unfavorable peristatic factors such as malnutrition or alcohol consumption, influencing bodily hydration and serum protein concentration rather than reflecting specific disease effects. In addition, potential state-related changes of brain volumes were described by Garver et al. [13] with a reversible increase during acute exacerbation. While the study did not control a number of potential confounding factors including medication effects, this observation may well provide an additional explanation for the diversity of findings since the state of disease at examination was not adequately controlled for in the majority of studies.

Treatment-related changes were up to now verified in the basal ganglia with volume increases of this structure under treatment with conventional neuroleptics. This effect was reversible after switch to atypical neuroleptics [5, 28] and corresponds to the finding of D2-dopamine receptor up-regulation in both animal and functional neuroimaging studies [46].

Apart from unfavorable peristatic but potentially reversible factors underlying cerebral volume changes in schizophrenia, non-reversible mechanisms such as excessive neuronal apoptosis and/or neuritic pruning as well as neurodegenerative pathology or activation of endogenous retroviruses have been discussed to be etiologically relevant [24, 40, 52]. Accordingly, a comparison between the progression of global cerebral volume loss in schizophrenia and changes observed in well-characterized neurodegenerative disorders – such as Alzheimer's disease – would be of interest. MRI studies which investigated the progression of global cerebral volume changes in Alzheimer's disease found an average annual volume decrease ranging between 2 and 3 % in these patients [12, 37, 44]. However, it is rather difficult to compare those findings with the magnitude of changes observed in schizophrenic samples, since most studies in schizophrenia do not explicitly report the relevant figures. The few studies which did found an average annual volume decrease of the cerebral hemispheres ranging between approximately 0.3 % [8] and 1.3 % [40]. The greater respective values obtained in Alzheimer's disease would argue against an aggressive neurodegenerative pathology affecting the whole brain in schizophrenia.

In conclusion, the presently available neuroimaging studies do not convincingly support the hypothesis that schizophrenia is generally associated with a global cerebral tissue loss. Nevertheless, global cerebral tissue loss may be characteristic for a subset of patients with poor outcome or worse illness course. Inconsistencies of the findings may be related to the fact that studies investigating global cerebral changes do not adequately address the hypothesis that structural brain changes in schizophrenia occur in neuroanatomically distinct regions rather than affecting the brain as a whole. A selective vulnerability of yet to be defined distinct brain regions would correspond more convincingly to symptoms and course as well as etiology of this heterogeneous disorder. Furthermore, aspects of stage and course of the disease need to be taken into consideration since progressive tissue loss might only be observable during certain disease stages and the dynamics of the supposed changes might not necessarily follow a linear fashion.

Timing and progression of regional changes: childhood-onset schizophrenia as a model?

Fifteen studies investigated progression of regional cerebral changes in schizophrenia, with a particular focus on the frontal and temporal lobes. Longitudinal frontal lobe differences were reported by Gur et al. [15], Madsen et al. [32] and Mathalon et al. [33]. Following Gur et al., these changes are more pronounced in first-episode patients emphasizing the potential impact of stage and course of the disease. The fact that in particular smaller studies [27, 54] failed to detect the respective changes underlines the importance of adequate sample sizes and corresponds to earlier results from cross-sectional studies (review in [45]) indicating that frontal lobe changes occur in the majority but not all patients with schizophrenia. An association between frontal lobe changes and an ongoing illness course has been indicated by our own group [45] finding a significant correlation between duration of illness and hypofrontality in patients using positron emission tomography. While negative symptoms shared by most patients with schizophrenia are generally associated with frontal lobe dysfunction, yet the latter being a rather large structure, further studies differentiating between substructures at the level of Brodman areas are needed to validate the above findings.

Progressive temporal lobe changes – mainly affecting the grey matter – were identified in five out of seven studies. That this finding may contribute to the pathogenesis of positive symptoms is emphasized by a study [38] of individuals at high risk for schizophrenia which found decreased volumes of medial temporal substructures in those probands who developed psychosis during the follow-up period. This finding corresponds to results from the Edinburgh high risk project [30] demonstrating that probands with an increased genetic liability take an intermediate position with respect to volumes of the amygdala-hippocampus complex when compared to healthy controls and first episode patients with schizophrenia. However, a corresponding correlation between temporal lobe changes and progression of positive symptoms was only reported by 2 of the longitudinal studies cited above [15, 22].

The parietal and occipital lobes and the cerebellum were among other cerebral sites investigated. Of the five studies [1, 9, 41, 47, 54], only two reported progressive changes in the parietal cortex in adolescent patients [47] or in the cerebellum [9].

In contrast to the studies cited above, childhood-onset schizophrenia provides the unique opportunity to investigate the onset and progression of cerebral changes during a critical period of brain development. Although brain development may continue into the fifth decade of life [2], it can be assumed that these processes have their greatest dynamics in adolescence. In addition, childhood-onset schizophrenia is generally considered to be a severe form of the disorder that nonetheless appears to be clinically and neurobiologically continuous with the later onset illness [40–42].

Cross-sectional studies confirmed smaller volumes of the frontal and parietal lobes in childhood-onset schizophrenia [40–42]. Using sophisticated MRI-based visualization techniques, Thompson et al. [48] described a spatio-temporal pattern of grey matter loss with an early involvement of the parietal cortices followed by an anterior progression of changes into temporal, sensorimotor, and dorsolateral prefrontal areas. Faster loss rates of frontal cortex were strongly correlated with more severe negative symptoms. These intriguing results raise the prospect of a staging model of progressive brain changes in the disease and facilitate the interpretation of cross-sectional findings in adult schizophrenia which in general revealed more pronounced changes of the respective sites with chronicity of the disorder.

In conclusion, the neuroimaging studies discussed above indicate that schizophrenia is not generally associated with progressive global cerebral tissue losses. However, progressive volume reductions may affect distinct anatomical sites such as the frontal and temporal cortices. These changes may reflect the diversity of psychopathological symptoms and courses of this heterogeneous disorder and appear to be compatible with both neurodevelopmental insults [52] as well as nongenetic triggers [24] identified previously. Taking into account the psychopathological and course-related heterogeneity of the disorder, future studies may rather focus on the investigation of subgroups of patients defined by clinical and/or neurobiological parameters.

▪ References

1. Bachmann S, Bottmer C, Pantel J, Amann M, Essig M, Schad LR, Schröder J (2001) MRI-volumetric changes of first-episode schizophrenic patients at 14 months follow-up. Schizophrenia Res 49 (Supp): 150
2. Bartzokis G, Beckson M, Lu PH, Nuechterlein KH, Edwards N, Mintz J (2001) Age-related changes in frontal and temporal lobe volumes in men: a magnetic resonance imaging study. Arch Gen Psych 58: 461–465
3. Cannon TC, Mednick SA, Parnas J (1989) Genetic and perinatal determinants of structural brain deficits in schizophrenia. Arch Gen Psychiatry 46: 883–889
4. Chakos MH, Lieberman JA, Bilder RM, Borenstein M, Lerner G, Bogerts B, Wu H, Kinon B, Ashtari M (1994) Increase in caudate nuclei volumes of first-episode schizophrenic patients taking antipsychotic drugs. Am J Psychiatry 151: 1430–1436
5. Corson PW, Nopoulos P, Miller DD, Arndt S, Andreasen NC (1999) Change in basal ganglia volume over 2 years in patients with schizophrenia: typical versus atypical neuroleptics. Am J Psych 156 (8): 1200–1204
6. Davis KL, Buchsbaum MS, Shihabuddin L, Spiegel-Cohen J, Metzger M, Frecska E, Keefe RS, Powchik P (1998) Ventricular enlargement in poor-outcome schizophrenia. Biol Psychiatry 43: 783–793
7. DeGreef G, Ashtari M, Wu H, Borenstein M, Geisler S, Lieberman JA (1991) Follow up MRI study in first episode schizophrenia. Schizophrenia Res 5: 204–206
8. DeLisi LE, Hoff AL, Schwartz JE, Shields GW, Halthore SN, Gupta SM, Henn FA, Anand AK (1991) Brain morphology in first-episode schizophrenic-like psychotic patients: a quantitative magnetic resonance imaging study. Biol Psychiatry 29: 159–175

9. DeLisi LE, Sakuma M, Tew W, Kushner M, Hoff AL, Grimson R (1997) Schizophrenia as a chronic active brain process: a study of progressive brain structural change subsequent to the onset of schizophrenia. Psychiatry Res Neuroimaging 74: 129–140

10. DeLisi LE, Tew W, Xie SH, Hoff AL, Sakuma M, Kushner M, Lee G, Shedlack K, Smith AM, Grimson R (1995) A prospective follow-up study of brain morphology and cognition in first-episode schizophrenic patients: preliminary findings. Biol Psychiatry 38: 349–360

11. Falkai P, Bogerts B, Rozumek M (1988) Limbic pathology in schizophrenia: the entorhinal region – a morphometric study. Biol Psychiatry 24: 515–521

12. Fox NC, Freeborough PA (1997) Brain atrophy progression measured from registered serial MRI: validation and application to Alzheimer's disease. J Magn Reson 7: 1069–1075

13. Garver DL, Nair TR, Christensen JD, Holcomb JA, Kingsbury SJ (2000) Brain and ventricle instability during psychotic episodes of the schizophrenias. Schizophrenia Res 44: 11–23

14. Giedd JN, Jeffries NO, Blumenthal J, Castellanos FX, Vaituzis AC, Fernandez T, Hamburger SD, Liu H, Nelson J, Bedwell J, Tran L, Lenane M, Nicolson R, Rapoport JL (1999) Childhood-onset schizophrenia: progressive brain changes during adolescence. Biol Psychiatry 46: 892–898

15. Gur RE, Cowell P, Turetsky BJ, Gallacher F, Cannon T, Bilker W, Gur RC (1998) A follow-up magnetic resonance imaging study of schizophrenia. Arch Gen Psychiatry 55: 145–152

16. Haug JO (1962) Pneumoencephalographic studies in mental disease. Acta Psychiatr Scand 38 (suppl 165): 1–114

17. Hirayasu Y, Shenton ME, Salisbury DF, Frumin M, Fischer IA, Farrell D, Yurgelun-Todd D, Zarate C, McCarley RW (1999) Progressive change in posterior superior temporal gyrus in schizophrenia. Biol Psychiatry 45: 117S

18. Hoffman WF, Ballard L, Turner EH, Casey DE (1991) Three-year follow-up of older schizophrenics: extrapyramidal syndromes, psychiatric symptoms, and ventricular brain ratio. Biol Psychiatry 30: 913–926

19. Huber G (1957) Pneumoencephalographische und psychopathologische Bilder bei endogenen Psychosen. Springer, Berlin

20. Illowsky BP, Juliano DM, Bigelow LB, Weinberger DR (1988) Stability of C.T. scan findings in schizophrenia: results of an 8 year follow-up study. J Neurol Neurosurg Psychiatry 51: 209–231

21. Jacobi W, Winkler H (1927) Encephalographische Studien an chronisch Schizophrenen. Arch Psychiatrie Nervenkr 81: 299–332

22. Jacobsen LK, Giedd JN, Castellanos X, Vaituzis AC, Hamburger SD, Kumra S, Lenane MC, Rapoport JL (1998) Progressive reduction of temporal lobe structures in childhood-onset schizophrenia. Am J Psychiatry 155: 678–685

23. Jaskiw GE, Juliano DM, Goldberg TE, Hertzman M, Urow-Hamell E, Weinberger DR (1994) Cerebral ventricular enlargement in schizophreniform disorder does not progress: a seven year follow-up study. Schizophrenia Res 14: 23–28

24. Karlsson H, Bachmann S, Schröder J, McArthur J, Torrey EF, Yolken RH (2001) Retroviral RNA identified in the cerebrospinal fluids and brains of individuals with schizophrenia. Proc Natl Acad Sci USA 98: 4634–4639

25. Kemali D, Maj M, Galderisi S, Milici N, Salvati A (1989) Ventricle-to-brain ratio in schizophrenia: a controlled follow-up study. Biol Psychiatry 26: 753–756

26. Kemali D, Maj M, Galderisi S, Milici N, Salvati A, Starace F, Valente A, Pirozzi R (1986) Clinical, biological and neuropsychological features associated with lateral ventricular enlargement in DSM-III schizophrenic disorder. Psychiatry Res 21: 137–149

27. Keshavan MS, Bagwell WW, Haas GL, Sweeney JA, Schooler NR, Pettegrew JW (1994) Changes in caudate volume with neuroleptic treatment. Lancet 344: 1434

28. Lang DJ, Kopala LC, Vandorpe RA, Rui Q, Smith GN, Goghari VM, Honer WG (2001) An MRI study of basal ganglia volumes in first-episode schizophrenia patients treated with risperidone. Am J Psychiatry 158: 625–631

29. Lawrie SM, Whalley HC, Abukmeil SS, Kestelman JN, Donnelly L, Miller P, Best JJK, Owens DGC, Johnstone EC (2001) Brain structure, genetic liability, and psychotic symptoms in subjects at high risk of developing schizophrenia. Biol Psychiatry 49: 811–823

30. Lawrie SM, Whalley HC, Kestelman JN, Abukmeil SS, Byrne M, Hodges A, Rimmington JE, Best JJK, Owens DGC, Johnstone EC (1999) Magnetic resonance imaging of brain in people at high risk of developing schizophrenia. Lancet 353: 30–33

31. Lieberman J, Chakos M, Wu H, Alvir J, Hoffman E, Robinson D, Bilder R (2001) Longitudinal study of brain morphology in first-episode schizophrenia. Biol Psychiatry 49: 487–499

32. Madsen AL, Karle A, Rubin P, Cortsen M, Andersen HS, Hemmingsen R (1999) Progressive atrophy of the frontal lobes in first-episode schizophrenia: interaction with clinical course and neuroleptic treatment. Acta Psychiatr Scand 100: 367–374

33. Mathalon DH, Sullivan EV, Lim KO, Pfefferbaum A (2001) Progressive brain volume changes and the clinical course of schizophrenia in men. Arch Gen Psychiatry 58: 148–157

34. Nair TR, Christensen JD, Kingsbury SJ, Kumar NG, Terry WM, Garver DL (1997) Progression of cerebroventricular enlargement and the subtyping of schizophrenia. Psychiatry Res: Neuroimaging 74: 141–150

35. Nasrallah HA, Olson SC, McCalley-Whitters M, Chapman S, Jacoby CG (1986) Cerebral ventricular enlargement in schizophrenia: a preliminary follow-up study. Arch Gen Psychiatry 43: 157–159

36. Nasrallah HA, Schwarzkopf SB, Olson SC, Coffman JA (1991) Perinatal brain injury and cerebellar vermal lobules I-X in schizophrenia. Biol Psychiatry 29: 567–574

37. O'Brien JT, Paling S, Barber R, Williams ED, Ballard C, McKeith IG, Gholkar A, Crum WR, Rossor MN, Fox NC (2001) Progressive brain atrophy on serial MRI in dementia with Lewy bodies, AD and vascular dementia. Neurology 56: 1386–1388

38. Pantelis C, Velakoulis D, Suckling J, McGorry P, Phillips L, Yung A, Wood S, Bullmore E, Brewer W, Soulsby B, McGuire P (2000) Left medial temporal volume reduction occurs during the transition from high-risk to first-episode psychosis. Schizophrenia Res 41 (Suppl): 35

39. Puri BK, Hutton SB, Saeed N, Oatridge A, Hajnal JV, Duncan L, Chapman MJ, Barnes TR, Bydder GM, Joyce EM (2001) A serial longitudinal quantitative MRI study of cerebral changes in first-episode schizophrenia using image segmentation and subvoxel registration. Psychiatry Res 106 (2): 141–150

40. Rapoport JL, Castellanos FX, Gogate N, Janson K, Kohler S, Nelson P (2001) Imaging normal and abnormal brain development: new perspectives for child psychiatry. Australian and New Zealand Journal of Psychiatry 35: 272–281

41. Rapoport JL, Giedd JN, Blumenthal J, Hamburger S, Jeffries N, Fernandez T, Nicolson R, Bedwell J, Lename M, Zijdenbos A, Paus T, Evans A (1999) Progressive cortical change during adolescence in childhood-onset schizophrenia: a longitudinal magnetic resonance imaging study. Arch Gen Psychiatry 56: 649–654

42. Rapoport JL, Giedd J, Kumra S, Jacobsen L, Smith A, Lee P, Nelson J, Hamburger S (1997) Childhood-onset schizophrenia: progressive ventricular change during adolescence. Arch Gen Psychiatry 54: 897–903

43. Roberts GW, Colter N, Lofthouse R, Bogerts B, Zech M, Crow TJ (1986) Gliosis in schizophrenia: a survey. Biol Psychiatry 21: 1043–1050

44. Schönknecht P, Pantel J, Essig M, Amann M, Schad LR, Schröder J (2001) Progression of hippocampal but not of global cerebral atrophy is correlated with rate of clinical deterioration in the course of Alzheimer's disease. The World Journal of Biological Psychiatry 2 (Suppl. 1): 124

45. Schröder J (1998) Subsyndrome der chronischen Schizophrenie. Springer, Berlin

46. Schröder J, Silvestri S, Bubeck B, Karr M, Demisch S, Scherrer S, Geider FJ, Sauer H (1998) D₂ Dopamine receptor up-regulation, treatment response, neurological soft signs, and extrapyramidal side effects in schizophrenia. Biological Psychiatry 43: 660–665

47. Sponheim SR, Iacono WG, Beiser M (1991) Stability of ventricular size after the onset of psychosis in schizophrenia. Psychiatry Res Neuroimaging 40: 21–29

48. Thompson PM, Vidal C, Giedd JN, Gochman P, Blumenthal J, Nicolson R, Toga AW, Rapoport JL (2001) Mapping adolescent brain change reveals dynamic wave of accelerated grey matter loss in very early-onset schizophrenia. Proc Natl Acad Sci USA 98: 11650–11655

49. Vita A, Giobbio GM, Dieci M, Garbarini M, Morganti C, Comazzi M, Invernizzi G (1994) Stability of cerebral ventricular size from the appearance of the first psychotic symptoms to the later diagnosis of schizophrenia. Biol Psychiatry 35: 960–962
50. Vita A, Sacchetti E, Valvassori G, Cazullo CL (1988) Brain morphology in schizophrenia: a 2–5 year CT scan follow-up study. Acta Psychiatr Scand 78: 618–621
51. Whalley HC, Kestelman JN, Rimmington JE, Kelso A, Abukmeil SS, Best JJK, Johnstone EC, Lawrie SM (1999) Methodological issues in volumetric magnetic resonance imaging of the brain in the Edinburgh High Risk Project. Psychiatry Research Neuroimaging 91: 31–44
52. Woods BT (1998) Is schizophrenia a progressive neurodevelopmental disorder? Towards a unitary pathogenetic mechanism. Am J Psychiatry 155: 1661–1670
53. Woods BT, Yurgelun-Todd D, Benes FM, Frankenburg FR, Pope HC, McSparren J (1990) Progressive ventricular enlargement in schizophrenia: comparison to bipolar affective disorder and correlation with clinical course. Biol Psychiatry 27: 341–352
54. Zipursky RB, Christensen BK, Dolman RA, Mikulis DJ (2001) Grey matter deficits are stable in first episode psychosis: a 5-year follow-up study. Schizophrenia Res 49 (Suppl): 170 f

Discussion: developmental disorders of the brain

E. GOUZOULIS-MAYFRANK
Department of Psychiatry and Psychotherapy, University of Aachen, Germany

The three presentations of this session focus on neurodevelopmental aspects of the etiology of schizophrenia. The original neurodevelopmental hypothesis claims a static lesion acquired prenatally, which interacts with the normal brain maturation processes and accounts for the onset of the illness mostly during early adulthood [12]. However, the hypothesized lesion may result in several subtle and uncharacteristic cognitive, emotional and behavioral deviations already in infancy, i.e., several years prior to the onset of clear-cut psychotic symptoms. These childhood prodromal signs of schizophrenia were described by Professor Parnas in his excellent summary of high-risk studies.

The picture emerging from Professor Falkai´s presentation supports the existence of a major neurodevelopmental part of the etiology of schizophrenia resulting from an early disturbance of normal brain development. With his studies on the gyrification index (GI) and the gray level index profile (GLI), Professor Falkai presented a very elegant new tool for the study of the neurodevelopmental hypothesis. He found a higher and abnormal gyrification in the cortex of both affected and unaffected siblings. This finding is likely to reflect a genetic basis of the schizophrenic disorder, or – I would prefer to say – the genetic basis of the vulnerability to the schizophrenic disorder. In addition, this finding is compatible with the neurodevelopmental hypothesis of schizophrenia and the arrest proposed in it.

However, other findings from the literature seem to be in conflict with a simple neurodevelopmental model. Professor Schroeder summarized several brain imaging studies demonstrating progressive ventricular enlargement and reductions of gray matter volume in certain brain regions during the course of schizophrenia. Although these findings were not confirmed in all studies, an additional neurodegenerative origin of schizophrenia must be considered possible. I would also say that the intra- and interindividual temporal variability of the evolution of psychotic symptoms is in conflict at least with the original, simple, focal neuroanatomical version of the neurodevelopmental hypothesis. Finally, Professor Falkai presented some evidence for a microglial activation in a subset of schizophrenic or schizoaffective patients. These finding are also not easily compatible with a simple neurodevelopmental model and they may reflect an additional neurodegenerative process.

One possible explanation is that there may be two independent mechanisms – the "two hit hypothesis" [8] – and this may apply to the same or to different patient populations and might reflect the biological heterogeneity of the schizo-phrenic disorder. Alternatively, as Professor Falkai suggests, common single molecules might be involved in both the neurodevelopmental and the neuro-degenerative processes.

However, there are also other possible factors which might explain the part of the pathologic process which looks "neurodegenerative", but may actually be independent from the pathophysiology of the disorder itself. These factors may include nutritional aspects, influences of the way of life and influences of both prescribed and abused psychotropic substances. For example, Professor Schroeder demonstrated that an increase in basal ganglia volume in schizo-phrenic patients may be attributable to the treatment with classical neuroleptics. So, these aspects have to be addressed carefully when looking at group differ-ences between schizophrenics and controls.

In addition, I think that the currently emerging concepts on the patho-physiology of schizophrenia begin to reflect the accumulating knowledge about the interactions between the developing human brain and several environmen-tal and even social/ psychological factors. Professor Parnas proposed a sophis-ticated model which integrates biological and psychological aspects for our understanding of the origins of schizophrenia. This model has striking similar-ities to the model on psychosocial risk factors of schizophrenia as proposed by Professor Harrison in another session of this symposium.

At this point, I wonder whether it is still reasonable to treat the brain and the environment as two unconnected entities. We know from recent basic research that the brain is not a static organ. In contrast, the brain shows a remarkable degree of adaptation and plasticity in response to experience throughout adult-hood. However, the plasticity of the brain is particularly marked during early childhood. Studies with maternally deprived rodent pups and young primates show that these animals exhibit alterations in neurotransmitter functions such as a hypersensitivity of the dopaminergic system in their adult life [7]. Moreover, maternally deprived young animals exhibit persisting alterations in the density of synaptic connections in several brain regions including the limbic system [3, 5, 9]. These and other findings mean that there is an experience-dependent neu-ronal plasticity, which is most effective during early life: early experiences influ-ence the synaptic connectivity, i.e., the wiring of the brain. In other words, early experiences help to form the experiencing organ itself. So, we can say that the way the world is perceived and experienced in later life is partly a result of our early experiences. This influence may be only observed so far on a psychological basis, but in fact it may also be exerted biologically.

Another example, which may apply even more directly to schizophrenia, derives from animal studies on the prepulse inhibition (PPI) model of schizo-phrenia [10]. The PPI is an operational measure of sensorimotor gating. It is decreased in schizophrenics and this deficit is thought to be related to deficient inhibitory, filter mechanisms of information processing in these patients [2]. The PPI was also found to be reduced in animal studies with acute administration of serotonergic, dopaminergic and antiglutamatergic drugs. In addition, the PPI is reduced after surgical lesions in the neural circuitry of the PPI modulation [10].

Interestingly, animals reared in social isolation, but not having suffered any pharmacological or surgical manipulation, exhibit a similar attenuation of the PPI later in their life, i.e., from puberty on [4]. There seems to be no particular vulnerable period to this effect, but it has to be a significant part if not the entire rearing period for the PPI deficit to emerge in later life [11]. Extensive handling of the young socially deprived animals by the experimenters can prevent the development of a PPI deficit in adulthood. Taken together, these data match the epidemiological data on environmental risk factors for schizophrenia presented by Dr. Harrison and Dr. Mortensen in another session of this symposium. Interestingly, the PPI attenuation in the isolation rearing PPI model is reversed by neuroleptics [1].

In conclusion, the question is not any more, whether schizophrenia is a neurodevelopmental or a neurodegenrative disorder, or a disorder of psychosocial origin. The question is rather how these different aspects of origin interact with each other and how this interaction may account for the phenomenological heterogeneity of the schizophrenic disorder. In my view, this is the way the question has to be studied in the future. From a methodological point of view, it will be difficult to address these complex issues together. But we now know enough to say that some of the most important understanding will come from just such studies.

▪ References

1. Bakshi VP, Swerdlow NR, Braff DL, Geyer MA (1998) Reversal of isolation rearing-induced deficits in prepulse inhibition by seroquel and olanzapine. Biol Psychiatry 43: 436–445
2. Braff D, Grillon C, Geyer MA (1992) Gating and habituation of the startle reflex in schizophrenic patients. Arch Gen Psychiatry 49: 206–215
3. Braun K, Lange E, Metzger M, Poeggel G (2000) Maternal separation followed by early social deprivation affects the development of monoaminergic fiber systems in the medial prefrontal cortex of Octodon degus. Neuroscience 95: 309–318
4. Geyer MA, Wilkinson LS, Humby T, Robbins TW (1993) Isolation rearing of rats produces a deficit in prepulse inhibition of acoustic startle similar to that in schizophrenia. Biol Psychiatry 34: 361–372
5. Helmeke C, Ovtscharoff W Jr, Poeggel G, Braun K (2001) Juvenile emotional experience alters synaptic inputs on pyramidal neurons in the anterior cingulate cortex. Cereb Cortex 11: 717–727
6. Krebs-Thomson K, Giracello D, Solis A, Geyer MA (2001) Post-weaning handling attenuates isolation-rearing induced disruptions of prepulse inhibition in rats. Behav Brain Res 120: 221–224
7. Lewis MH, Gluck JP, Beauchamp AJ, Keresztury MF, Mailman RB (1990) Long-term effects of early social isolation in Macaca mulatta: changes in dopamine receptor function following apomorphine challenge. Brain Res 513: 67–73
8. Maynard TM, Sikich L, Lieberman JA, LaMantia AS (2001) Neural development, cell-cell signaling, and the "two-hit" hypothesis of schizophrenia. Schizophr Bull 27: 457–476
9. Ovtscharoff W Jr, Braun K (2001) Maternal separation and social isolation modulate the postnatal development of synaptic composition in the infralimbic cortex of Octodon degus. Neuroscience 104: 33–40
10. Swerdlow NR, Geyer MA (1998) Using an animal model of deficient sensorimotor gating to study the pathophysiology and new treatments of schizophrenia. Schizophr Bull 24: 285–301

11. Varty GB, Braff DL, Geyer MA (1999) Is there a critical developmental 'window' for isolation rearing-induced changes in prepulse inhibition of the acoustic startle response? Behav Brain Res 100: 177–183
12. Weinberger DR (1986) The pathogenesis of schizophrenia: a neurodevelopmental theory. In: Nasarallah HA, Weinberger DR (eds) Handbook of Schizophrenia. Elsevier, New York, pp 397–406

Environmental Risk Factors

Obstetric complications, maternal psychopathology, and the risk of psychosis

H. Verdoux, A.-L. Sutter
Department of Psychiatry, University Victor Segalen Bordeaux, France

▓ Introduction

The neurodevelopmental model of schizophrenia [28, 29] is now supported by a growing body of evidence suggesting that perinatal environmental risk factors are implicated in the etiology of schizophrenia. The list of putative perinatal risk identified by epidemiological studies has dramatically expanded over the past decade. This list is ranging from exposure from somatic adverse events such as obstetric complications (OCs) [13, 14, 21, 43], viruses [7, 22, 26] or nutritional factors [8, 40], to psychological factors such as maternal stress [42] or maternal depression [19]. The present review will be focused on the links and possible interactions between somatic perinatal risk factors and maternal psychopathology in the association with an offspring's increased vulnerability for psychosis.

▓ Is maternal psychopathology a risk factor for obstetric complications?

Are mothers with schizophrenia at greater risk of obstetric complication?

There is a consensus on the fact that women mothers with schizophrenia are more likely to present with at-risk behavior during pregnancy (such as poor antenatal care, use of drugs) [1], but there is conflicting evidence regarding the increased risk of somatic OCs in women with schizophrenia. A first review of the literature by McNeil [25] concluded that somatic OCs are not more frequent in women with schizophrenia, although these women are more exposed to at-risk behavior during pregnancy. A meta-analysis of 14 case-control studies showed that a parental diagnosis of schizophrenia was associated with an increased risk of OCs, and that this association was stronger if the mother was a parent with an schizophrenia [35]. However, this finding was not supported in a population-based study based upon the Danish database for Epidemiological Research, which did not find evidence that pregnancy or delivery complications were more frequent in women with schizophrenia compared to normal control's [3]. Nevertheless, this same research group reported that women with schizophrenia are at increased risk of poor pregnancy outcome, and that preterm delivery, low birthweight and intra-uterine growth retardation were more frequent in children of a schizophrenia mother [2]. Moreover, neonatal death is much more frequent in these children, in particular, death caused by sudden infant death syndrome [4].

The underlying question regarding the association between maternal schizophrenia and perinatal complication is whether or not maternal psychosis may mediate or confound the relationship between OCs and increased vulnerability for schizophrenia in the offspring [34, 35]. Although children of mothers with psychosis are at increased risk of poor pregnancy outcome, most mothers of subjects with schizophrenia do not present with severe psychiatric disorder. Thus, maternal psychosis is probably not a major confounding or mediating factor in the association between OCs and schizophrenia.

Is maternal depression a risk factor for obstetric complications?

The links between OCs and maternal milder psychiatric disorders are more complex than those between OCs and maternal psychosis. It has been suggested that prenatal maternal depression may at least in part explain the persistence of a (relatively) high prevalence of complicated pregnancies in the general population of developed countries, in spite of the major technical progress in prenatal care over the last few decades [31]. Several studies reported that women with depressive symptoms during pregnancy are at increased risk of pregnancy and delivery complications, such as prematurity, artificial induction of labor, or cesarean section delivery [31, 41]. For example, Hedegaard et al. [17], using a dimensional assessment of psychological distress (GHQ-30) in 6000 pregnant women, found that high scores during pregnancy strongly predicted an increased risk of prematurity, after adjustment for social and somatic confounding factors. However, these findings were not replicated by other studies [6, 33].

Using data from the Camberwell Collaborative Psychosis Study collected in 150 subjects with psychosis and 150 controls, Marcelis et al. [23] found that mothers of subjects with a history of OCs more frequently reported a personal history of mood disorder. The association between maternal history of depression and greater frequency of OCs was observed in subjects with psychosis as well as in normal controls. A weaker association in a similar direction was found between family history of mood disorder and greater risk of OCs. Thus, the association between maternal depression and increased risk of obstetric somatic complications may be related not only to maternal depression during pregnancy, but more generally to maternal vulnerability for depression, independently from the psychiatric status over the index pregnancy.

The mechanisms underlying the association between maternal depression and increased risk of OCs are poorly understood. This association may be mediated by the greater frequency of at-risk behavior in women with depression [31], or by the somatic consequences of maternal depression, such as weight loss. Neurotransmission or hormonal dysregulation may also induce premature induction of labor, or placental abnormalities [15, 24, 30]. Some OCs such as instrumental delivery, or induction of labor, may be due to the direct impact of maternal depression on medical practice: obstetricians and midwives may be more likely to decide to use these medical interventions in depressed women [41].

■ Are mothers with obstetric complications at increased risk of postnatal depression?

This question is mirroring the previous one. The most consistent finding reported by studies exploring the links between OCs and maternal postnatal depression is an increased risk of postnatal depression after delivery complications, especially after cesarean delivery, forceps use, or long labor [5, 11, 16, 41, 46].

However, the association between obstetric complications and postnatal depression has not been confirmed by other studies [9, 32, 38], including studies carried out in large community samples [12, 45]. Using a transversal method Warner et al. [45] investigated the risk factors for postnatal depression in a sample of 2375 women recruited after delivery in the maternity units of Manchester hospitals. Women were interviewed at home 6-8 weeks after delivery to collect information on demographic characteristics, OCs and depressive symptoms. OCs were defined as "complications during pregnancy sufficient to result in hospital admission or investigation", "cesarean section", "low birth weight", or "baby on special care baby unit". No association was found using univariate analyses between these OCs and early postnatal depression assessed using a categorical measure of postnatal depression (score at the Edinburgh Postnatal Depression Scale (EPDS) >12). Forman et al. [12] conducted a prospective study in a sample of 5252 Danish women attending antenatal care at the Aarhus University Hospital. Women were enrolled during the second trimester of pregnancy. Information on demographic characteristics and psychopathology was obtained using self-report questionnaires sent by mail at 16, 30 weeks of gestation, and 4 months after delivery. OCs were collected in a specific registration form completed by the midwives after delivery. Using multivariate analyses, no association was found between OCs and postnatal depression (defined by a score >12 on the EPDS).

These discrepancies may be linked to methodological differences, such as sampling procedure, dimensional vs. categorical evaluation of postnatal depression, assessment and rating of OCs, and adjustment for confounders. In order to clarify this issue, we prospectively investigated in a cohort of pregnant women whether a history of OCs predicted more severe depressive symptomatology in the early postpartum period [44]: 441 consecutive pregnant women attending the State Maternity Hospital in Bordeaux were interviewed during the third trimester of pregnancy, then at 3 days and 6 weeks after birth. Our sample was biased toward the inclusion of women with few severe obstetric complications, since multiple pregnancy, very premature births and cesarean section delivery had been a priori excluded in the design of the study. We used a dimensional assessment of postpartum depressive symptoms (EPDS score). Data on a large range of pregnancy, delivery and neonatal somatic adverse events were collected by interviewing the mothers, and rated using the McNeil-Sjöström scale for OCs. No association was found between delivery complications and the intensity of postpartum depressive symptoms. This latter inconclusive finding may be due to the design of the study that did not allow us to explore the association between depressive symptomatology and cesarean section delivery. On the other hand, we found that exposure to severe OCs during pregnancy was associated with more intense depressive symptoms in the early postnatal period, independent from demographic characteristics, marital adjustment, parity, and a history of depressive or anxiety disorder during pregnancy. At trend level, a history of threatened abortion/premature contractions predicted the intensity of postnatal depressive symptoms.

Women with complicated pregnancy or delivery may be at increased risk of postnatal depression through several mechanisms. Physical exhaustion induced by long or difficult labor may be a risk factor for postnatal depression. Severe pregnancy complications may also increase the risk of postnatal depression by acting as acute or chronic stressors. For example, threatened abortion can be considered as a severe life event for a pregnant woman, owing to the psychological consequences induced by the threat of stillbirth or of giving birth to a premature baby.

■ Does maternal prenatal mental state influence offspring's psychiatric outcome?

The hypothesis that perinatal maternal psychological risk factors may increase the risk of severe mental disorder in the offspring is currently supported by a limited number of studies. The existence of a link between exposure to stress during pregnancy and subsequent schizophrenia was first suggested by a study showing that prenatal death of father was associated with increased risk of schizophrenia [18]. In an ecological population-based study, an increased risk of schizophrenia was found in subjects exposed during the first trimester of pregnancy to a population stress (invasion of the Netherlands by the Nazi army) [42]. Exposure to this stress in the second trimester of pregnancy was a risk factor for schizophrenia only in male subjects. Another population-based study carried out in the Netherlands also found an (non-significant) increased risk of schizophrenia in subjects prenatally exposed to the 1953 Dutch flood disaster [36]. The association between prenatal exposure to maternal stress and later schizophrenia may be mediated by the direct impact of stress, such as fetal hypoxia induced by vasoconstriction [15]; or more indirectly, by increasing the risk of OCs, such as prematurity, or by increasing the risk of maternal prenatal or postnatal depression.

A growing body of evidence suggests that maternal depression has potential deleterious impact on the child's development [27, 37, 39]. However, few studies have investigated the impact of maternal depression on the risk of psychosis in the offspring. Using data from the Finish cohort, Jones and collaborators reported that maternal depression during pregnancy was a risk factor for schizophrenia, independently from a history of OCs [20]. However, the interpretation of this finding is limited by the fact that maternal depression was assessed by a proxy measure, i.e. by asking mothers at 6 – 7 months pregnancy whether they felt in their "usual mind", "depressed" or "very depressed". Furthermore, no information was available on postnatal maternal mental state. To our knowledge, no study has examined the long-term consequences of maternal postnatal depression risk factor, especially with regard to offspring's risk of severe mental disorder in adolescence or adult life.

▓ Conclusion

The causal pathway between OCs, maternal psychopathology and psychological disorder in the offspring is far from being elucidated. The directions of the associations are often bi-directional, or the mediating variables, if any, are not clearly identified (Fig. 1). Prenatal maternal depression may be a risk factor for schizophrenia by a direct negative impact on fetal brain development, or more indirectly by increasing the risk of exposure OCs and/or the risk of developmental abnormalities induced by maternal postnatal depression. OCs may have a direct negative impact on fetal brain development, or may be on the causal pathway between prepartum maternal depression/exposure to stress and increased risk of schizophrenia. OCs may also indirectly increase the risk of child's later psychiatric disorder by acting as a risk factor for postpartum depression. The links between the different risk factors might be more complex, and interactions and circular causation may exist between OCs and maternal depression. For example, a child with brain abnormalities linked to OCs exposure may have a greater vulnerability to the deleterious impact of postnatal depression on his/her devel-

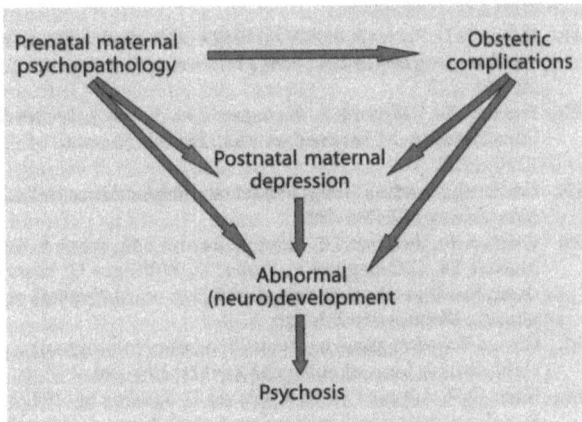

Fig. 1. (Putative) associations between maternal psychopathology and obstetric complications.

opment. These brain abnormalities may also have subtle effects on the child's interactions with his/her mother, which may in turn favor the occurrence of postnatal maternal depression in vulnerable mothers.

It would be an oversimplification to reduce the link between exposure to OCs and subsequent psychosis in the offspring to the fact that maternal vulnerability for psychopathological disturbance may mediate the association between both events. However, reducing the link between OCs and psychosis to the impact of the putative brain lesions induced by OCs might also be an oversimplification of the complex relationships between somatic OCs, maternal psychopathology, child-mother interaction, and child development.

▓ References

1. Bennedsen B (1998) Adverse pregnancy outcome in schizophrenic women: occurrence and risk factors. Schizophr Res 33: 1–26
2. Bennedsen BE, Mortensen PB, Olesen AV, Henriksen TB (1999) Preterm birth and intrauterine growth retardation among children of women with schizophrenia. Brit J Psychiatry 175: 239–245
3. Bennedsen B, Mortensen BB, Olesen AV, Henriksen TB, Frydenberg M (2001a) Obstetric complications in women with schizophrenia. Schizophr Res 47: 167–175
4. Bennedsen B, Mortensen BB, Olesen AV, Henriksen TB (2001b) Congenital malformations, stillbirths, and infant deaths among children of women with schizophrenia. Arch Gen Psychiatry 58: 674–679
5. Boyce P, Todd A (1992) Increased risk of postnatal depression after emergency caesarean section. Med J Aust 157: 172–174
6. Brooke O, Anderson H, Bland J, Peacok J, Stewart C (1989) Effects of birth weight on smoking, alcohol, caffeine, socioeconomic factors, and psychosocial stress. BMJ 298: 795–801
7. Brown A, Cohen P, Greenwald S, Susser E (2000a) Nonaffective psychosis after prenatal exposure to rubella. Am J Psychiatry 157: 438–443
8. Brown AS, van Os J, Driessens C, Hoek HW, Susser ES (2000b) Further evidence of relation between prenatal famine and major affective disorder. Am J Psychiatry 157: 190–195
9. Cox J, Connor Y, Kendell R (1982) Prospective study of the psychiatric disorders of childbirth. Brit J Psychiatry 140: 111–117
10. Done D, Johnstone E, Frith C, Crow T (1991) Complications of pregnancy and delivery in relation to psychosis in adult life: data from the British perinatal mortality survey sample. BMJ 302: 1576–1580
11. Edwards D, Porter S, Stein G (1994) A pilot study of postnatal depression following casearean section using two retrospective self-rating instruments. Journal of Psychosomatic Research 38: 111–117
12. Forman D, Videbech P, Hedegaard M, Salvig J, Secher N (2000) Postpartum depression: identification of women at risk. British Journal of Obstetrics and Gynaecology 107: 1210–1217
13. Geddes J, Lawrie S (1995) Obstetric complications and schizophrenia: a meta-analysis. Brit J Psychiatry 167: 786–793
14. Geddes JR, Verdoux H, Takei N, Lawrie SM, Bovet P, Eagles JM, Heun R, McCreadie RG, McNeil TF, O'Callaghan E, Stober G, Willinger U, Murray RM (1999) Schizophrenia and complications of pregnancy and labor: an individual patient data meta-analysis. Schizophrenia Bulletin 25: 413–423
15. Glover V (1997) Maternal stress or anxiety in pregnancy and emotional development of the child. British Journal of Psychiatry 171: 105–106
16. Hannah P, Adams D, Lee A, Glover V, Sandler M (1992) Links between early post-partum mood and post-natal depression. British Journal of Psychiatry 160: 777–780

17. Hedegaard M, Henriksen T, Secher N (1993) Psychological distress in pregnancy and preterm delivery. BMJ 307: 234–239
18. Huttunen M, Niskanen P (1978) Prenatal loss of father and psychiatric disorders. Archives of General Psychiatry 35: 429–431
19. Jones P, Rantakallio P, Hartikainen A, Isohanni M, Sipila P (1998a) Schizophrenia as a long-term outcome of pregnancy, delivery, and perinatal complications: a 28-year follow-up of the 1966 North Finland general population birth cohort. American Journal of Psychiatry 1998: 355–364
20. Jones PB, Rantakallio P, Hartikainen AL, Isohanni M, Sipila P (1998b) Schizophrenia as a long-term outcome of pregnancy, delivery, and perinatal complications: a 28-year follow-up of the 1966 north Finland general population birth cohort. American Journal of Psychiatry 155: 355–364
21. Könnecke R, Häfner H, Maurer K, Löffler W, an der Heiden W (2000) Main risks factors for schizophrenia: increased familial loading and pre- and peri-natal complications antagonize the protective effect of oestrogen in women. Schizophrenia Research 44: 81–93
22. Kunugi H, Nanko S, Takei N, Saito K, Hayashi N, Kazamatsuri H (1995) Schizophrenia following in utero exposure to the 1957 influenza epidemics in Japan. American Journal of Psychiatry 152: 450–452
23. Marcelis M, Van Os J, Sham P, Jones P, Gilvarry C, Cannon M, Mc Kenzie K, Murray R (1998) Obstetric complications and familial morbid risk of psychiatric disorders. Am J Med Genet Neuropsychiatr Genet 81: 29–36
24. McAnarney E, Stevens-Simon C (1990) Maternal psychological stress/depression and low birthweight. Is there a relationship? Amer J Dis Child 144: 789–792
25. McNeil T (1991) Obstetric complications in schizophrenic parents. Schizophen Res 5: 89–101
26. Mednick SA, Machon RA, Huttunen MO, Bonett D (1988) Adult schizophrenia following prenatal exposure to an influenza epidemic. Archives of General Psychiatry 45: 189–192
27. Murray L (1992) The impact of postnatal depression on infant development. Journal of Child Psychology Psychiatry 33: 543–562
28. Murray R, Lewis SW (1987) Is schizophrenia a neurodevelopmental disorder? Brit Med J 295: 681–682
29. Murray RM (1994) Neurodevelopmental schizophrenia: the rediscovery of dementia praecox. British Journal of Psychiatry 25 (Suppl): 6–12
30. Omer H, Everly G (1988) Psychological factors in preterm labor: critical review and theoretical synthesis. Am J Psychiatry 145: 1507–1513
31. Orr S, Miller C (1995) Maternal depressive symptoms and the risk of poor pregnancy outcome. Review of the literature and preliminary findings. Epidemiological Review 17: 165–171.
32. Paykel ES, Emms E, Fletcher J, Rassaby E (1980) Life events and social support in puberteral depression. British Journal of Psychiatry 136: 339–346
33. Perkin M, Bland J, Peacok J, Anderson H (1993) The effects of anxiety and depression during pregnancy on obstetric complications. Brit J Obst Gyn 100: 629–634
34. Sacker A, Done D, Crow T, Golding J (1995) Antecedents of schizophrenia and affective illness. Obstetric complications. Brit J Psychiatry 166: 734–741
35. Sacker A, Done DJ, Crow TJ (1996) Obstetric complications in children born to parents with schizophrenia: a meta-analysis of case-control studies. Psychol Med 26: 279–287
36. Selten J, van der Graaf Y, van Duursen R, Gispen-de Wied C, Kahn R (1999) Psychotic illness after prenatal exposure to the 1953 Dutch flood disaster. Schizophrenia Research 35: 243–245
37. Sharp D, Hay D, Pawlby S, Schmucker G, Allen H, Kumar R (1995) The impact of postnatal depression on boy's intellectual development. Journal Child Psychology Psychiatry 36: 1315–1336
38. Stein A, Cooper P, Campbell E, Day A, Altham P (1989) Social adversity and perinatal complications: their relation to postnatal depression. British Medical Journal 298: 1073–1074
39. Stein A, Gath D, Bucher J, Bond A, Day A, Cooper P (1991) The relationship between postnatal depression and mother-child interaction. British Journal of Psychiatry 158: 46–52
40. Susser E, Lin S (1992) Schizophrenia after prenatal exposure to Dutch hunger winter of 1944–1945. Archives of General Psychiatry 49: 983–988

41. Thalassinos M, Rouillon F, Engelman P, Lempérière T (1988) Etude des relations entre données gynéco-obstétricales et troubles psychiques de la grossesse et du post-partum. J Gynecol Obstet Biol Reprod 17: 879–887
42. van Os J, Selten JP (1998) Prenatal exposure to maternal stress and subsequent schizophrenia. British Journal of Psychiatry 172: 324–326
43. Verdoux H, Geddes JR, Takei N, Lawrie SM, Bovet P, Eagles JM, Heun R, Mccreadie RG, Mcneil TF, O'callaghan E, Stober G, Willinger MU, Wright P, Murray RM (1997) Obstetric complications and age at onset in schizophrenia: an international collaborative meta-analysis of individual patient data. American Journal of Psychiatry 154: 1220–1227
44. Verdoux H, Sutter A, Glatigny-Dallay E, Minisini A (2002) Obstetric complications and the development of postpartum depressive symptoms. Acta Psychiatrica Scandinavica, in press
45. Warner R, Appleby L, Whitton A, Faragher B (1996) Demographic and obstetric risk factors for postnatal psychiatric morbidity. British Journal of Psychiatry 168: 607–611
46. Yoshida k, Marks M, Kibe N, Kumar R, Nakano H, Tashiro N (1997) Postnatal depression in Japanese women who have give birth in England. Journal of Affective Disorders 43: 69–77

Migration and the social epidemiology of schizophrenia

G. Harrison*, W. Eaton**
 * Division of Psychiatry, University of Bristol, Cotham House, Bristol, UK
** Department of Mental Hygiene, School of Hygiene & Public Health, The John
   Hopkins University, Hampton, House, Baltimore, Maryland, USA

▓ Migration and risks of psychotic illness

The observation that some migrant populations experience increased risk of psychotic illness is now one of the most robust in psychiatric epidemiology. Although this association has been reported in studies spanning several decades, until recently it has remained largely ignored by researchers investigating aetiology because individuals prone to schizophrenia may be prone also to migrate. In other words, the association was interpreted as being due to selection biases operating in migrant populations.

Evidence [12] of increased incidence of psychotic disorders among Afro-Caribbean migrants to the United Kingdom, however, has opened up new avenues of research and stimulated the search for causation. This is because the increased risk is observed in *second generation* (i.e. British born) individuals, a finding that narrows and re-focuses the range of interpretative possibilities. It is unlikely, for example, that increased risk in the second generation can be adequately explained by selection factors alone, and the effects of short-term stress-related exposures associated with assimilation and acculturation also appear less important. In addition, the association with 'ethnic status' offers new opportunities to explore the relationship between socio-economic status and psychosis and for untangling the problems of selection versus causation. Compared with other indicators such as social class, an individual's ethnic status cannot be caused by illness processes and may act as a marker for a range of candidate variables in the search for the causes of psychosis.

▓ How robust is the evidence?

We have previously summarised [6] findings from over 16 studies investigating incidence rates of psychotic illness in migrant populations in the last 2 decades. Although selection factors may partly explain some of the observed associations in first generation populations, Selten et al. [30] found increased rates among migrants from the Dutch Antilles and Surinam to the Netherlands in ethnic groupings where about half of the entire population had migrated. In addition, as we have noted, new findings began to emerge from the UK in the late 1980s [2,

10, 12, 17] showing increased rates of psychosis in British-born (second generation) individuals with a family history of migration from the Caribbean.

The finding in the second generation African Caribbean population in the UK has now been replicated several times. Susser [34] has pointed out, however, that the replication of a finding does not necessarily provide us with conclusive evidence. In his classic paper on making judgements about causal inference, Susser points out that replication studies may merely repeat evidence with the same underlying weaknesses of study design and the same flaws in the interpretation of data. To counter this, he suggests that the judgements applied by scientists in the process of making causal inferences require the application of several key criteria. These include: *coherence* (in the sense of reasonableness of the association in biological terms); *specificity of association* (the precision with which the occurrence of one variable will predict the occurrence of another); and *consistency of an observation using diverse methodologies*. If we apply Susser's criteria to the 16 studies noted above, although there are significant variations in the size of the relative risks reported, there is a remarkable consistency of effect across the studies. In addition, the effect is observed in studies that use quite different methodological approaches. Harrison et al. [12] King et al. [17] Harrison et al. [10] and Bhugra et al. [2], for example, calculated rate ratios on the basis of standardised assessments (face-to face) of all first contact cases from a defined catchment area. Other studies [5, 36] used data derived from case records and case registers. Wesseley et al. [37], on the other hand, report data based upon a case controlled design using non-psychotic controls selected from the same treatment facility. These studies, carried out by different groups of investigators in different parts of the United Kingdom, produce findings of remarkable strength and consistency.

But is the association specific to schizophrenia? There is little evidence to suggest that the increased risk is specific to any diagnostic group within the clinical psychotic syndromes. Several authors [10, 12, 17] found higher rates of all psychotic disorders in British-born African Caribbeans, including both non-affective and affective syndromes. Leff et al. [19], and van Os et al. [36] also report increased rates of mania and schizo-mania in this population. Some authors report differences in the syndromal patterning of psychotic illness, including differences in course and outcome, among British-born African Caribbean people. McKenzie et al. [24] , for example, found a lower prevalence of continuous unremitting illness. In a small British population-based survey, Sharpley and Peters [32] found that UK resident African Caribbeans reported hallucinatory phenomena 2.5 times more often than 'white' respondents, and had an excess of delusion-like ideation compared with other population groups. They suggest that the excess of psychosis in the African Caribbean population may be due to an excess of affective disorders that produces an accentuation of these schizotypal phenomena. Alternatively, these population-prevalent schizotypal phenomena could act as independent risk-factors for psychotic illness. These preliminary findings should be treated with great caution however. The cross-cultural equivalence and validity of the survey instruments used in such studies has yet to be established and other follow-up studies of course and outcome [23, 35] report no difference or worse outcomes in African Caribbeans.

Overall, we conclude that the epidemiological evidence for an excess of the clinical psychotic syndromes in the African Caribbean population in the UK is strong, but the question of diagnostic specificity remains unclear, and potentially intriguing differences in syndromal patterning require more research and clarification.

Causal relationships

There are numerous possible explanations, reviewed by Eaton and Harrison [6] and by Sharpley et al. [31], for the association between migration and psychotic illness. For the purposes of this brief overview, we shall focus on key emerging issues. First, however, the issue of confounding and intervening variables needs careful consideration, especially the relationship between migration and social disadvantage. Most of the rates published over the last two decades are adjusted for age and sex, and it is unlikely that observed associations are due to confounding by these basic socio-demographic variables. But none of these studies addresses the issue of confounding due to socio-economic status. In the majority, this omission probably reflects relatively small sample size, the limited power of analyses, and the absence of adequate controls. In addition, the high prevalence of single parent families in African Caribbeans in the UK, and high levels of unemployment among young African Caribbean men [2] makes it difficult for researchers to indicate socio-economic status by occupation. The relationship between migrant status and socio-economic status is of considerable interest however and, despite these methodological hurdles, further research is needed. It is clear, for example, that African Caribbean people living in the UK are structurally disadvantaged in socio-economic terms, compared with the majority population. They have high levels of single parent families (70% in some areas) [28], a factor known to be correlated with childhood success in education and later employment, and greater frequency of living in children's homes and being placed in foster care. In adult life, more live alone [3] and unemployment is much greater [2]. Could the association between migration and schizophrenia be due to social disadvantage?

It is important to distinguish societal inequality at the macro-level from individual disadvantage. In the field of general health, research on social inequalities has mushroomed in recent years but, surprisingly, this area remains relatively unexplored in the field of mental health, and particularly so in schizophrenia research. Historically, the relationship between socio-economic status and schizophrenia has tended to be polarised in the 'either/or' paradigm of the 'drift' (social selection) and 'breeder' (social causation) hypotheses, and there are substantial methodological difficulties involved in untangling reverse causality. For example, it is difficult to measure the effects of downward socio-economic pressure caused by childhood impairments, and prodromal symptoms, in those who will later develop a psychotic illness. Associations between the prevalence of the disease and social class are therefore likely to be related, at least in part, to the effects of early disease processes on the individual's ability to succeed. One approach to this problem has been to study parental social class, but findings are conflicting. Some investigations based upon case-control designs [4, 11] report an association between schizophrenia and having a father in a low social class. Others, notably those investigating carefully defined birth cohorts [15, 20] find an association with *higher* socio-economic parental position. The findings from birth cohorts apply only to relatively early onset cases and may reflect, at least in part, earlier detection of those with parents from higher social classes. But for the moment this issue remains unresolved. Whatever the eventual finding for socio-economic status, the fact that associations with risk of psychosis are so much stronger for migration than any reported for class status suggests that there must be an additional force of risk in these key minority groups. What other factors might be involved?

Embracing a life course model of schizophrenia: biological and social chains of risk

Potential risk factors for psychosis can be classified, crudely, into three domains: genetic factors; foetal and early life-biological exposures; and social-psychological processes in early and later life. Our understanding of the potential interplay between these risk factors has been hampered by a number of important conceptual issues. First, over the last two decades theoretical models of causation have been largely biological in nature, with social and psychological factors sometimes construed as mere 'fall-out' to what is going on in the brain. Psychosocial factors have been incorporated as risk factors into models of course and outcome but usually excluded from models of causation. This bias toward biological causation is understandable in historical terms, given previous methodological errors in much psychosocial research and the potential for stigmatisation and blame of families. But it is difficult to see why 'social' factors that are capable of modifying the course and outcome of a disease process should not be capable of modifying its development and evolution. It seems curious that with accumulating evidence for psychosocial factors in the aetiology of heart disease, some psychiatrists should continue to be so reluctant to consider the role of such factors in the aetiology of *brain* disease. We have noted previously that psychiatrists interested in the social patterning of psychosis have not been very sophisticated about the concepts involved in psychosocial risk; and sociologists, too, have been naïve about potentially important biological mediators and the effects of social class that are not strictly social in nature [6]. We suggest that we abandon these polarised models and recover the principle of bio-psycho-social causation. Two recent theoretical models of causal relationships developed for other chronic diseases, namely the concept of 'allostatic load' [22] and the 'life course approach' [18], offer important insights for schizophrenia researchers.

The concept of allostatic load is important because it provides a theoretical model for how psychosocial stress can be translated into physiologically mediated biological change via a cascade of cause and effect operating over a lifetime. The notion of 'allostasis' refers to physiological systems that 'maintain stability through change', such as the processes involved as the cardiovascular system adjusts to resting and active states. In the field of psychiatry, the concept can be applied to physiological stress mediators such as the secretion of catecholamines, and their effect upon brain function and plasticity. The concept of 'allostatic load' is used to describe the adverse biological effects that result from repeated cycles of allostasis and the inefficient switching on and off of these responses. Examples include accelerated atherosclerotic plaque formation resulting from persistent activation of blood pressure and, in the brain, reduced neuronal excitability and atrophy due to over-activity of excitatory neurotransmitters. We are not suggesting that similar biological pathways are involved in the aetiology of schizophrenia, but that this model provides a conceptual framework for the accumulation of adverse biological outcomes as a result of psychosocial stress factors operating over a lifetime.

The life course model of disease, a development of Barker's [1] disease 'programming' model, also embraces long time periods over which adverse outcomes gradually accumulate. Additionally, this model emphasises the interplay of risk factors in 'chains' of risk. Barker hypothesised that the risk of adult-onset chronic diseases such as CHD, stroke and bronchitis is biologically programmed during gestation and early infancy. 'Programming' described the process whereby a stimulus or insult during critical periods of development (for example, under-nutrition in the case of CHD) has lasting effects on the structure or function of organs, tissues and bodily systems. The life course model extends Barker's approach, hypothesising that adult chronic diseases reflect cumulative lifetime exposures to damaging physical and social environments, rather than the effects of one-time insults. This theoretical framework does not eliminate the notion of an early critical period, but places greater emphasis on a range of biological and social factors operating across the life course.

The life course model is important to schizophrenia researchers because it is proposed that exposures can interact with other exposures (one adverse event leading to another) setting up a 'chain' of risk. There is also interplay between effects and exposures over long time periods. Here, the emphasis is upon non-linear rather than linear, and probabilistic rather than pre-determined conceptualisations of the evolution of illness [16]. An example would be the case of an individual who experiences suspiciousness as an antecedent personality effect of underlying vulnerability to schizophrenia. Their suspiciousness leads to social withdrawal and then to social isolation. In turn, their social isolation diminishes their chances of finding a supportive relationship. The absence of a supportive relationship, linked with social isolation, then strengthens and kindles suspicious and paranoid thinking. If the individual is already socially isolated at the first development of suspiciousness, the whole process would be accelerated. The point is that the antecedent features of psychosis do not simply unfold into environment, but may interact with it, leading to cumulative exposures over time. There are some tentative indications in the literature of this kind of effect modification. For example, in a study of cognitive performance in Swedish male conscripts, Gunnell et al. (8) found that the risk of subsequent schizophrenia was higher in individuals with low scores, but was greater still in those low performing individuals who had better educated parents. It could be hypothesised that poor cognitive performance produces additional internal stress in a family setting of high parental expectations. We shall return to this model later when we consider the stresses associated with formulating a life plan.

A final issue that has hampered the search for aetiological factors in the link between migration and psychosis is the low power of most studies, and their consequent limited ability to analyse effect modification, and multiplication, through interactions between variables. For example, studies examining familial morbid risk and the prevalence of obstetric complications in African Caribbeans in the United Kingdom have small sample sizes and relatively little replication. It would therefore be premature to exclude these factors from aetiological models at this stage. Ideally, sample sizes should confer sufficient power to investigate potential multiplicative effects of provocative and protective agents across the individual's life course.

Psychosis and complex cognitive tasks of formulating a life plan

Within a life course conceptual framework, what are the risk factors that may be operating in migration, and especially in second generation African Caribbeans? Studies carried out so far have failed to identify a role for genetic factors [14, 33] or obstetric complications [13]. Negative findings from these relatively small and low powered studies should not detract from further research into biological factors, but interest has begun to focus on the potential role of psychosocial risk factors.

We have proposed [6] that in late adolescence and early adult life the complex cognitive tasks involved in formulating a 'life plan' may be especially vulnerable to adverse psychosocial processes and may hold the key to understanding the excess of psychotic disorders in some first and second generation migrant populations. This hypothesis ties together several aspects of psychological function that have been linked to risk of schizophrenia including executive function, goal striving and complex social tasks. It also incorporates sociological concepts of cognitive rigidity associated with lower class socialisation, and of so-called 'structural lag'. This model can also accommodate recent epidemiological data on urban/rural differences in risk for schizophrenia [25] and allows for predisposing biological and genetic factors.

Murphy [26] first suggested that elevated rates of schizophrenia in certain situations of low social class and disadvantaged ethnic groups could be explained by the 'schizophrenia-evoking role of complex social tasks'. In attempting to understand what type of 'stress' might be related to schizophrenia, he focussed on stress which demands responses that have no clear precedent... 'it is only when the individual is isolated from, and has not learned the traditional answers, or when events conspire to make him seriously doubt them, that the simplicity of such stress situations is thus changed and one can expect the risk of schizophrenia to increase'. Parker and Kleiner [29] elaborated on this notion to explain variations in rates of schizophrenia among African-American migrants to Philadelphia and other northern urban areas. They focused upon *goal striving stress* in which feelings of success or failure about a given goal depend upon how the person comprehends the result: if he or she feels the failure is due to a fault within the self there may be a loss of self esteem. If they understand the failure as a barrier imposed by external forces, their sense of powerlessness may evoke quite different consequences in terms of psychopathology and risk of psychosis.

For individuals in late adolescence and early adult life, decisions are required in several key domains of social life, namely occupation and social integration through the development and sustainment of supportive relationships. Occupational attainment is heavily influenced by aspirations, which in turn are strongly affected by peer group, and success is determined by ability and equality of opportunity. This process, carried out in what has been called the 'crisis of autonomy' [7], involves estimation of a range of probabilities, and then selecting, prioritising, balancing and integrating subtly different future behaviours. It is one of the most complex cognitive activities a person will engage in throughout their life. It is also closely allied to the notion of executive function.

The likelihood of success in this cognitive task will depend upon the individual's executive and cognitive abilities; the necessary cognitive flexibility to adapt to new information and formulate new strategy; the internal 'balance' between aspiration and innate or potential ability; contextual expectations of performance and achievement; and a facilitative social structure in terms of role models, training and encouragement. Individuals in communities with relative institutional completeness with regard to these facilitative requirements are substantially advantaged compared to those with incomplete or fragmented institutional processes.

It is possible within the above conceptual framework to accommodate a number of observations regarding the risk of schizophrenia in general. Those with fathers in the upper class in Finland, Sweden and Denmark may have higher risks for schizophrenia because parents who have been upwardly mobile during their own generation would have unrealistically high expectations for the mobility of their children. Other, as yet unidentified factors, which limit their ability to achieve (for example, low intellectual performance), may contribute to an unusually large gap between aspirations and achievement. Conversely, at the low end of the socio-economic spectrum, circumstances that act to limit opportunities may increase risk. These risks in the social-psychological landscape of the individual, at either end of the socio-economic spectrum, are likely to be increased in urban as opposed to rural settings, because of lower inter-generational stability and rapidly changing labour markets that accentuate the challenges in choosing new career directions. These risk factors are especially increased for selected migrant groups, where limited opportunities can outweigh expectations, and where there may be substantial institutional fragmentation, both at the micro (family), and macro (community) level.

Several studies in the UK suggest that second generation African Caribbean migrants to the UK (and some first generation migrants in other cultures) experience a high level of exposure to the risk factors embraced in this paradigm. First, African Caribbean children in England achieve less academically and have higher rates of diagnosed learning disabilities compared with the population as a whole [38]. As we have noted, in large metropolitan areas there is evidence of high prevalence of one-parent families, high rates of separation from parents and experience of placement in children's homes [21], all known risk factors for poor educational achievement. More are unemployed in adult life [2]. Despite these factors, Mallett, Leff and Bhugra (personal communication) found that African Caribbean patients expected to reach as high a level of achievement as white patients in the future, even though their current level of employment was significantly lower than whites. By contrast, Asian psychotic patients were reported as having significantly lower expectations than the other African Caribbeans or whites, although their current level of employment was equal to that of whites.

There may also be subtle cultural differences in attributional style among African Caribbeans in the UK, which are capable of heightening risks in the critical period of life-plan formulation. Gilvarry et al. [9] reported no difference in the number of life events experienced in different ethnic groups with chronic psychosis but African and African Caribbean patients were more likely to interpret such events as part of a pattern of continuous adversity experienced on account of their ethnicity. For example, difficulties with housing tended to be attributed to systematic discrimination more than among other ethnic groups. Building upon earlier notions of externalisation of attribution, Sharpley and Peters [32] found that proto-delusional and grandiose ideas were more common among African Caribbean subjects compared with whites. Whilst the mediating processes that converge to produce these potential idiosyncrasies of attributional style are ill understood, it is clear that racism and inequality of opportunity, in a context of social and institutional fragmentation, may be key determining factors.

There are difficulties with this hypothesis, of course, not least the question of why such factors do not produce more neurotic illness in the African Caribbean population. Emerging evidence from population surveys [27], however, suggests that rates of depression may be higher than in previous estimates, and more data are required for rates of common mental disorders in the African Caribbean population.

We conclude that in some migrant groups, of which second generation African Caribbeans in the UK may represent a case study, there may emerge a toxic combination of exposures related to the complex cognitive tasks of formulating a life plan. We assume several variables, probably of small individual effect, with accumulating effect over the life course. We think it likely that there are biological pre-disposing and mediating factors, and that multiplicative effect modification sculpts the profile of risk that eventually gives way to full-blown psychotic disorder.

In future research, large risk sets will be required with sufficient follow-up data to analyse complex inter-relationships of exposures over the life course. Given that individual effect sizes are likely to be small, and interaction tests demand even more power, there are formidable hurdles in terms of sample size and the statistical complexities of multi-level modelling. Well planned and executed case-control studies will assist in resolving some of these studies, but if these questions are to be satisfactorily resolved we shall have to grasp the nettle, as have researchers of coronary heart disease and cancer, of mounting large multi-centre studies capable of investigating birth and historic cohorts over many years.

▮ References

1. Barker DJP (ed) (1992) Fetal and Infant Origins of Adult Disease. London: BMJ Publishing Group
2. Bhugra D, Leff J, Mallett R, Der G, Corridan B, Rudge S (1997) Incidence and outcome of schizophrenia in whites, African-Caribbeans, and Asians in London. Psychological Medicine 27: 791–798
3. Burnett R, Mallett R, Bhugra D et al. (1999) The first contact of patients with schizophrenia with psychiatric services; social factors and pathways to care in a multi-ethnic population. Psychological Medicine II: 581–599
4. Castle DJ, Scott K, Wessely S, Murray RM (1993) Does social deprivation during gestation and early life predispose to later schizophrenia? Social Psychiatry and Psychiatric Epidemiology 28: 1
5. Castle D, Wessely G, Der G, Murray RM (1991) The incidence of operationally defined schizophrenia in camberwell, 1965–84. British J of Psychiatry 159: 790–794
6. Eaton W, Harrison G (2001) Life chances, life planning, and schizophrenia. A review and interpretation of research on social deprivation. International Journal of Mental Health 30 (1): 58–81
7. Erikson EH (1968) Identity: Youth and Crisis. New York: Norton
8. Gunnell D, Harrison G, Fouskakis D, Rasmussen F (in press) Associations between pre-morbid intellectual performance, early-life exposures and early onset schizophrenia: a cohort study. British Journal of Psychiatry
9. Gilvarry C, Walsh E, Samele C et al. (1999) Life events and perceptions of racism in a sample of community care patients with psychotic illness. Social Psychiatry and Psychiatric Epidemiology 24: 49–56
10. Harrison G, Glazebrook C, Brewin J, Cantwell R, Dalkin T, Fox R, Jones P, Medley I (1997) Increased incidence of psychotic disorders in migrants from the Caribbean to the United Kingdom. Psychological Medicine 27: 799–806
11. Harrison G, Gunnell D, Glazebrook C, Page K, Kwiencinski R (2001) Association between schizophrenia and social inequality at birth: case-control study. British Journal of Psychiatry 179: 346–350
12. Harrison G, Owens D, Holton A, Neilson D, Boot D (1988) A Prospective study of severe mental disorder in Afro-Caribbean patients. Psychological Medicine 18: 643–657
13. Hutchinson G, Takei N, Bhugra D, Fahy TA, Gilvarry C, Mallett R, Moran P, Leff J, Murray RM (1997) Increased rate of psychosis among African-Caribbeans in Britain is not due to an excess of pregnancy and birth complications. British J of Psychiatry 171: 145–147
14. Hutchinson J, Takei N, Fahy TA et al. (1996) Morbid risk of schizophrenia in first degree relatives of white and African-Caribbean patients with psychosis. British Journal of Psychiatry 169: 776–780
15. Jones P, Rodgers B, Murray R, Marmot M (1994) Child developmental risk factors for adult schizophrenia in the British 1946 birth cohort. The Lancet 344: 1398–1402
16. Keshavan MS, Hogarty GE (1999) Brain maturational processes and delayed onset in schizophrenia. Development and Psychopathology 11: 525–543
17. King M, Coker E, Leavey G, Johnson-Sabine E (1994) Incidence of psychotic illness in London: comparison of ethnic groups. BMJ 309: 1115–1119
18. Kuh D, Ben-Sholomo Y (1997) A Life Course Approach to Chronic Disease Epidemiology. Oxford University Press
19. Leff J, Fisher M, Bertelsen A (1976) A cross-national epidemiological study of mania. British Journal of Psychiatry 129: 428–442
20. Makikyro T, Isohanni M, Moring J, Oja H, Hakko H, Jones P, Rantakallio P (1997) Is a child's risk of early onset schizophrenia increased in the highest social class? Schizophrenia Research 23: 245–252

21. Maughan B (1989) Growing up in the inner city. Paediatric and Perinatal Epidemiology 3: 195–215
22. McEwen BS (2000) Allostatis and allostatic load: implications for neuropsychopharmacology. Neuropsychopharmacology 22: 1008–1018
23. McGovern D, Hemmings P, Cope R et al. (1994) Long term follow-up of young Afro-Caribbean Britons and white Britons with a first admission diagnosis of schizophrenia. Social Psychiatry and Psychiatric Epidemiology 29: 8–19
24. McKenzie K, van Os J, Fahy TA et al. (1995) Psychosis with good prognosis in Afro-Caribbean people now living in the United Kingdom. BMJ 311: 1325–1328
25. Mortensen PB, Pedersen CB, Westergaard T, Wohlfahrt J, Ewald H, Mors O, Andersen PK, Melbye M (1999) Familial and non-familial risk factors for schizophrenia: a population-based study. New England J of Medicine 340: 603–608
26. Murphy HBM (1972) The evocative role of complex social tasks. In: Kaplan AR (ed) Genetic Factors in Schizophrenia, Charles C Thomas, Chicago, IL, pp 407–422
27. Nazroo J (1997) Ethnicity and Mental Health. London Policy Studies Institute
28. ONS: Social Focus on Families (1997) Office of National Statistics. UK
29. Parker S, Kleiner RJ (1966) Mental Illness in the Urban Negro Community. New York. Free Press
30. Selten JP, Slaets JPJ, Kahn RS (1997) Schizophrenia in Surinamese and Dutch Antillean immigrants to The Netherlands: evidence of an increased incidence. Psychological Medicine 27: 807–811
31. Sharpley M, Hutchinson G, McKenzie K, Murray RM (2001) Understanding the excess of psychosis among the African-Caribbean population in England. British J of Psychiatry 178 (suppl 40): s60–s68
32. Sharpley MS, Peters E (1999) Ethnicity, class and shizotypy. Social Psychiatry and Psychiatric Epdiemiology 34: 507–512
33. Sugarman PA, Craufurd D (1994) Schizophrenia in the Afro-Caribbean community. British J of Psychiatry 164: 474–480
34. Susser M (1977) Judgement and causal inference: criteria in epidiologic studies. Am.J.Epidemiol. 05: 1–15.
35. Takei N, Persaud R, Woodruff P et al. (1998) First episodes of psychosis in Afro-Caribbean and white people. An 18-year follow-up population-based study. British Journal of Psychiatry 172: 147–153
36. Van Os J, Castle D J, Takei N, Der G, Murray RM (1996) Psychotic illness in ethnic minorities: clarification from the 1991 census. Psychological Medicine 26: 203–208
37. Wessely S, Castle D, Der G, Murray R (1991) Schizophrenia and Afro-Caribbeans. A case control study. British Journal of Psychiatry 159: 795–801
38. Wing JK (1979) Mentally retarded children in Camberwell, London. In: Hafner H (ed) Estimating Needs for Mental Health Care, New York, Springer, pp 77–91

Urban/rural life as a risk factor?

P. B. Mortensen, C. B. Pedersen
National Center for Register-based Research, University of Aarhus, Denmark

An elevated prevalence of mental disorders, including schizophrenia, in urban areas has been reported for several decades [9]. Results have varied, however, but recently a number of studies, including studies from our own group [11, 13, 14] have documented an association between urbanicity at birth or upbringing and

Table 1. Adjusted relative risk of schizophrenia in a population-based cohort according to family history, place of birth and season of birth

Variable	RR1	95% CI	RR2	95% CI	RR3	95% CI
Family history[4]						
Parental						
F+, M+	65.49	(24.55–174.73)	59.74	(22.39–159.45)	46.90	(17.56–125.26)
F+, M-	8.34	(5.91–11.76)	7.97	(5.65–11.24)	7.20	(5.10–10.16)
F-, M+	11.33	(8.84–14.53)	10.19	(7.93–13.09)	9.31	(7.24–11.96)
F-, M- (ref.)	1.00	(ref)	1.00	(ref)	1.00	(ref)
F unknown, M+	20.99	(12.59–35.00)	17.12	(10.24–28.64)	14.18	(8.48–23.70)
F unknown, M-	2.48	(2.14–2.88)	2.45	(2.11–2.84)	2.00	(1.72–2.32)
Sibling						
One or more affected	9.04	(6.97–11.72)	7.33	(5.63–9.53)	6.99	(5.38–9.09)
No affected (ref.)	1.00	(ref)	1.00	(ref)	1.00	(ref)
Other factors						
Place of birth						
Capital		(2.21–2.80)	2.49	(2.20–2.80)	2.40	(2.13–2.70)
Capital suburb	1.64	(1.40–1.93)	1.64	(1.40–1.93)	1.62	(1.37–1.90)
Provincial cities	1.57	(1.36–1.81)	1.57	(1.36–1.81)	1.57	(1.36–1.81)
Provincial towns	1.24	(1.10–1.41)	1.24	(1.10–1.41)	1.24	(1.10–1.41)
Rural area (ref.)	1.00	(ref)	1.00	(ref)	1.00	(ref)
Greenland	3.71	(2.03–6.75)	3.71	(2.04–6.76)	3.71	(2.04–6.76)
Abroad	3.52	(2.74–4.52)	3.52	(2.73–4.52)	3.45	(2.69–4.44)
Unknown	1.28	(0.48–3.42)	1.26	(0.47–3.39)	1.22	(0.46–3.27)
Season of birth						
Amplitude[5]	1.12	(1.06–1.18)	1.11	(1.06–1.18)	1.11	(1.06–1.18)

1 *Relative Risk1* adjusted for age-gender interaction, calendar year, age of father and mother.
2 *Relative Risk2* as Relative Risk1 and adjusted for other variables in same category (family history/other factors).
3 *Relative Risk3* as Relative Risk1 and adjusted for all variables in the table.
4 *F+* father affected, *F-* father not affected, *M+* mother affected, *M-* mother not affected.
5 For all three adjustment scenarios (Relative Risk1, Relative Risk2, Relative Risk3) the estimated peak of the sine function was at 6 March (95% confidence interval from 6 February to 5 April).
Table modified from New England Journal of Medicine (1999); 340: 603–608

schizophrenia risk. In this chapter, we will address some of the methodological criticisms that have been raised against these observations, we will review the studies we are currently conducting, and give examples of our research regarding possible causes for urban-rural differences in schizophrenia risk.

A number of studies have associated urbanicity at birth or upbringing with schizophrenia risk. These studies include, for example, studies by Lewis and others studying Swedish data [5], and Marcelis and coworkers studying data from Holland [7]. In our own studies, we started measuring urbanicity of place of birth using a crude categorization of five degrees of urbanization. In Table 1 the results from this publication from 1999 are shown [11]. It shows that family history for schizophrenia is a very strong risk factor, but that urbanicity of place of birth has a dose-response-like relationship with about twice the risk for those born in the Copenhagen area compared to those born in rural areas. We later replicated this in a larger sample including diagnoses according to ICD-10 [14] as well as outpatient contacts, and what we saw here was that we still had a dose-response relationship with a much finer subdivision according to urbanicity of the municipalities of birth (Table 2).

However, a number of methodological criticisms have been raised against the findings of urbanicity and schizophrenia [4, 8]. The most often raised criticism is against the prevalence studies where an increased occurrence in cities could be due to selective migration into or selectively reduced migration out of inner

Table 2. Distribution of 10,264 cases of schizophrenia. 50.7 million person-years at risk and estimates of relative risks for the total study population according to the detailed classification of degree of urbanization of place of birth

Detailed degree of urbanization of place of birth	Cases (n)	Person years	Relative risks	95% CI
Municipalities in the capital region				
Capital (1)	3.210	8,926,711	2.30	(2.04–2.60)
Capital suburb (2)	958	4,552,162	1.73	(1.51–1.98)
>10,000 inhabitants in built-up area (4)	462	2,433,877	1.50	(1.29–1.74)
Other (5)	93	605,615	1.33	(1.06–1.69)
Municipalities where the largest city has more than 10,000 inhabitants				
Largest city has more than 100,000 inhabitants (3)	1,300	6,429,845	1.58	(1.38–1.79)
Largest city has 40,000–99,999 inhabitants (4)	659	3,691,487	1.39	(1.21–1.60)
Largest city has 20,000–39,999 inhabitants (4)	1,102	6,947,291	1.25	(1.10–1.43)
Largest city has 10,000–19,999 inhabitants (4)	688	4,367,539	1.22	(1.06–1.40)
Other municipalities				
50–100 % of inhabitants in built-up[3] area (5)	512	3,450,250	1.14	(0.99–1.32)
33.3–50 % of inhabitants in built-up area (5)	685	4,823,608	1.09	(0.95–1.25)
<33.3 % of inhabitants in built-up area (5)	313	2,351,639	1.00	(0.85–1.17)
Outside built-up area (reference) (5)	282	2,118,632	1.00	(ref)

1. Numerals (1)–(5) refer to the 5-level classification of degree of urbanization: (1) capital; (2) capital suburb; (3) provincial cities with more than 100,000 inhabitants; (4) provincial towns with more than 10,000 inhabitants; (5) rural area.
2. The relative risk was adjusted for age and its interaction with gender, calendar year of diagnosis, ages of the mother and father at the time of child's birth, season of birth, and mental illness in a parent or sibling
3. Built-up areas were defined by cities with more than 2,000 inhabitants

Table modified from Br J Psychiatry (2001); 179: 46–52

city areas of people with mental disorders. This criticism is, of course, to some extent eliminated by using place of birth as an index, but a variant of this criticism could then be that it is the mentally ill parents who have migrated into inner cities, and what we see reflected is an increased genetic loading among those giving birth in city areas. However, in our own studies we have adjusted for mental illness among parents and siblings without any substantial reduction in the effect of urbanicity. Another criticism that has been raised, for example by Schelin and others [15], has been that perhaps diagnostic practice varies, and especially maybe diagnostic delay was longer for individuals living in rural areas. Again, this would, of course, not necessarily be directly related to urbanicity at birth, but we have also tried to model this directly in our data. We have not yet published this, but the preliminary results from this analysis suggest that diagnostic delay cannot explain the urban-rural differences in schizophrenia risk.

Another issue could, of course, be if people living in rural areas have less access to psychiatric inpatient treatment thereby leading to lower first-admission rates. We do not believe this to be the case in Denmark, however, partly because distances are so small, meaning that one would rarely be more than 30 or 40 km away from a psychiatric department. Furthermore, if such differences were the cause of the urban-rural differences we would also expect this to apply to other severe mental disorders. However, we have also unpublished data on bipolar disorder showing no difference in first-admission rates according to urbanicity at birth. So, in summary, our present position is that it is unlikely that findings regarding urban-rural differences are only due to methodological issues.

So, if we accept the notion that factors occurring more frequently in urbanized areas contribute to schizophrenia risk, the next question would be what these factors are, and when and how they act. In order to address the issue of timing of exposure or, put in another way, if there are periods during fetal life or childhood where urbanicity seems to influence schizophrenia risk to a particularly high degree, we conducted a new study that was recently published [13].

The study was, as the other studies we have just mentioned, based on data from the Danish Civil Registration System [6] and from the Danish Psychiatric Case Register [12]. In brief, the Danish Civil Registration System makes it possible to link individuals with their parents, siblings and children, and the CPR-number issued by the Danish Civil Registration System is used uniformly across all Danish registers, making linkage with other registers possible.

We included 8,235 incident cases of schizophrenia in a population-based cohort of 1.89 million dl. Danish people, so the calculations were based on about 27 million person-years at risk (Table 3). Family history was subdivided according to the diagnoses of the relative, and the category schizophrenia, schizophrenia-like psychoses, any other mental disorder leading to hospitalization. What we wanted to do was to estimate the relative importance of urbanicity at birth, at the 5th, 10th, and 15th birthday, respectively. We chose not to look at place of residence later than the 15th birthday because we wanted to avoid as much as we could to get our results influenced by selective migration, and our assumption was that it would very rarely be the children themselves who decided to move before their 15th birthday. First, we wanted to see if there was any particular age

Table 3. Distribution of 8,235 cases of schizophrenia and 27.1 million person-years at risk in a population based cohort of 1.89 million Danish people

Variable	No. of cases	Person-years
Gender		
Male	5,462	14,150,781
Female	2,773	12,964,444
Maternal history		
Schizophrenia	234	86,524
Schizophrenia-like psychoses	257	196,298
Other mental disorders	1,323	2,067,383
Mother not affected	6,421	24,765,019
Paternal history		
Schizophrenia	98	45,980
Schizophrenia-like psychoses	106	96,483
Other mental disorders	888	1,573,112
Unknown father	640	990,119
Father not affected	6,503	24,409,531
History in siblings		
Schizophrenia	284	105,515
Schizophrenia-like psychoses	115	80,535
Other mental disorders	546	705,134
No affected siblings	7,290	26,224,040
Urbanicity at birth		
Capital	2,594	5,008,126
Capital suburb	793	2,328,013
Provincial cities	1,073	3,451,055
Provincial towns	2,375	9,405,666
Rural area	1,400	6,922,365
Urbanicity at age 5 years		
Capital	559	940,862
Capital suburb	635	1,720,492
Provincial cities	449	1,239,834
Provincial towns	836	3,220,339
Rural area	822	4,114,556
Other countries	29	80,010
Unknown	6	7,909
Unaccessible information	4,893	15,775,738
Urbanicity at age 10 years		
Capital	913	1,427,445
Capital suburb	1,139	2,915,199
Provincial cities	660	1,988,951
Provincial towns	1,416	5,369,404
Rural area	1,602	7,224,640
Other countries	47	131,801
Unknown	10	18,555
Unaccessible information	2,448	8,039,228
Urbanicity at age 15 years		
Capital	1,240	2,011,689
Capital suburb	1,559	4,017,883
Provincial cities	896	2,760,442
Provincial towns	2,020	7,629,875
Rural area	2,453	10,547,958
Other countries	57	126,824
Unknown	10	20,553
Total	8,235	27,115,224

Table modified from Arch Gen Psychiatry (2001) 58: 1039–1046

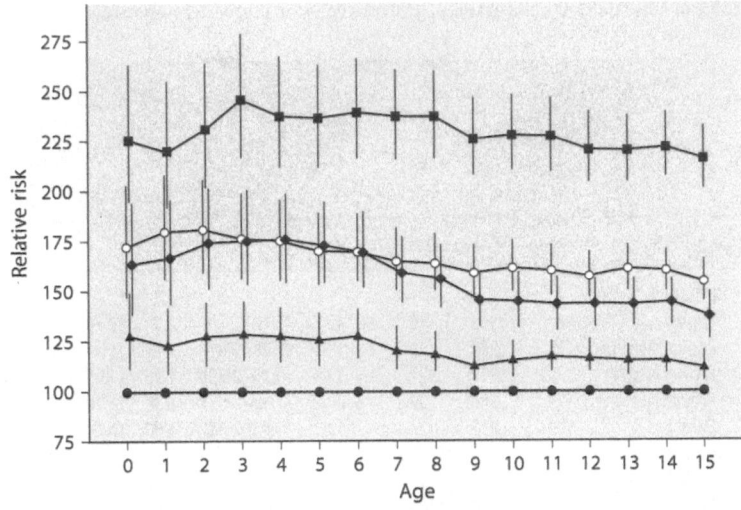

Fig. 1. Risk of schizophrenia according to urbanicity and age at residence. Urbanicity from 0 to 15 years of age enter separately in these 16 models. Age 0 indicates the time at birth, etc. Vertical lines indicate 95% confidence intervals. To avoid the confidence intervals from overlapping graphically, we have moved the age scale for the capital suburb slightly to the left and the age scale for the provincial city slightly to the right. Estimates of relative risks were adjusted for age and its interaction with gender, calendar year of diagnosis, and mental illness in a parent or sibling. Further adjustment for change of the municipality would reduce the effect of urbanicity only slightly (Modified from Arch Gen Psychiatry (2001) 58: 1039–1046)
■ capital, ○ capital suburb, ◆ provincial city, ▲ provincial town, ● rural area

at which urbanicity was more important for schizophrenia risk. However, as shown in Fig. 1, the urban-rural differences were very similar, irrespective of when we measured urbanicity in the interval from birth to the 15th birthday. Of course, this figure did not tell us everything because place of residence at a given age will be very closely related to the place of residence, e.g., one year before or one year after. So, to further address the effect of urbanicity we studied the effect of moving to a higher or lower degree of urbanization at different ages. In Table 4, we compare those who at a given age live at a certain degree of urbanicity and 5 years later continue to live at this degree of urbanicity to those who move to higher or lower degrees of urbanicity, respectively. For example, we see that compared to those born in a rural area and also living in a rural area on their fifth birthday, those who were born in the capital area and still lived there 5 years later had a 2.53 increased risk. What we see in almost every case is that those moving to a higher degree of urbanicity have an increased risk, whereas those moving to a lower degree of urbanicity have a decreased risk, again compared to those who stay on the same degree of urbanicity.

The estimates implied that at any age from birth to the 15th birthday, risk would increase if you moved to a higher degree of urbanicity and be reduced if you moved to a lower degree of urbanicity. These findings gave rise to the hypothesis that urbanicity at any age during upbringing, influences schizophrenia risk, and that the higher the degree of urbanicity during upbringing the

Table 4. Adjusted relative risk of schizophrenia according to urbanicity in a population-based cohort of 1.89 million Danish people

	No. of cases			Relative degree of urbanization at place of residence 5 years later (Second adjustment *)					
	Relative degree of urbanization at place of residence 5 years later								
Urbanicity	Higher	Same	Lower	Higher		Same		Lower	
Birth (Age 0 years)									
Capital	–	503	430	–		2.53	(2.19–2.92)	1.94	(1.68–2.25)
Capital suburb	22	268	56	1.82	(1.18–2.81)	1.74	(1.48–2.05)	1.44	(1.08–1.92)
Provincial city	9	367	124	1.44	(0.74–2.79)	1.92	(1.65–2.24)	1.41	(1.14–1.73)
Provincial town	117	658	332	2.02	(1.63–2.51)	1.35	(1.18–1.55)	1.17	(1.00–1.37)
Rural area	100	315	–	1.83	(1.46–2.30)	1.00	(ref)	–	
Age 5 years									
Capital	–	434	117	–		2.63	(2.33–2.96)	1.53	(1.22–1.90)
Capital suburb	32	514	84	2.04	(1.41–2.95)	1.67	(1.49–1.87)	1.62	(1.26–2.07)
Provincial city	9	375	62	2.16	(1.11–4.21)	1.84	(1.63–2.09)	1.53	(1.16–2.02)
Provincial town	43	707	85	1.78	(1.29–2.46)	1.30	(1.17–1.45)	1.16	(0.90–1.48)
Rural area	116	704	–	1.45	(1.16–1.81)	1.00	(ref)	–	
Age 10 years									
Capital	–	725	179	–		2.41	(2.20–2.64)	1.93	(1.63–2.28)
Capital suburb	58	955	114	2.26	(1.73–2.96)	1.60	(1.47–1.73)	1.41	(1.16–1.73)
Provincial city	7	582	70	1.70	(0.81–3.59)	1.53	(1.39–1.69)	1.45	(1.13–1.86)
Provincial town	53	1,242	115	1.52	(1.14–2.01)	1.18	(1.10–1.28)	1.15	(0.94–1.40)
Rural area	180	1,417	–	1.37	(1.16–1.62)	1.00	(ref)	–	

* Estimates of relative risk were adjusted for gender and its interaction with age, calendar year, and mental illness in a parent or sibling and for change of the municipality
Table modified from Arch Gen Psychiatry (2001) 58: 1039–1046

greater the risk. We therefore tried to model the effect of "the cumulative exposure to urbanicity" during childhood, again finding a strong and consistent dose-
response relationship between how large a proportion of childhood a child had
been living in a city area and their schizophrenia risk. In Table 5, we show the

Table 5. Adjusted relative risk according to a log-linear model for urbanicity during upbringing

Urbanicity from 0 to 15 years	Relative risk (95% CI) per year	Relative risk (95% CI) per 15 year	P-value
Capital	1.07 (1.06–1.08)	2.75 (2.31–3.28)	
Capital suburb	1.04 (1.02–1.05)	1.69 (1.43–1.99)	
Provincial cities	1.04 (1.02–1.05)	1.71 (1.41–2.06)	
Provincial towns	1.02 (1.01–1.03)	1.32 (1.13–1.54)	
Rural area (ref)	1.00	1.00	<0.00001

Risk per 15 years is calculated by raising the relative risk per year to the 15th power
$: Estimates of relative risk was adjusted for age and its interaction with gender, calendar year, mental illness in a par-
ent or sibling, and change of the municipality.
Table modified from Arch Gen Psychiatry (2001) 58: 1039–1046

final result of this model, demonstrating that if dla persons had spent their first 15 years in the capital area they had a 2.7 times increased risk compared to those spending all their childhood in a rural area. One should note in the footnotes for Tables 4 and 5 that we also adjust for change of municipality. We will just briefly explain why we did that, and what it means. In Table 6, estimates of the effect of moving address at different ages are shown. It came as a surprise to us to find that there was a strong effect of moving address, but only if this move included moving to another municipality. Also, there was a strong age-specific effect of this variable with no effect before the 5th birthday, relatively little effect of moving between the 5th and 10th birthday, and 10th and 13th birthday, respectively, and a strong effect of moving, especially moving frequently, from the 13th to the 15th birthday. We do not know the causes underlying this. Many hypotheses, including difficulties in adapting to new peer groups or exposure to new infections to the individual, could be suggested, but at least, it was interesting to us to see that it only had an effect when it included moving municipality which in Denmark would be a move that in most cases also necessitated moving to another school for these children. Also, it was interesting to us that there was this strong age-specific effect which at least would not be predicted if this were only due to special characteristics of parents moving frequently.

Table 6. Adjusted relative risks according to number of changes of municipality in a population – based cohort of 1.89 million Danish people

Number of changes of municipality	No. of cases	Person-years	Relative risk (95% CI)*	
From 0 to 4 years ($p = 0.34$)				
None	1,004	3,890,119	1.00	(ref)
1	328	1,123,412	0.92	(0.82–1.05)
2	131	376,364	0.97	(0.80–1.16)
3+	90	217,165	0.91	(0.73–1.13)
From 5 to 9 years ($p < 0.0001$)				
None	2,390	9,119,282	1.00	(ref)
1	601	1,570,244	1.18	(1.07–1.29)
2	216	433,266	1.29	(1.12–1.49)
3+	135	216,693	1.28	(1.07–1.54)
From 10 to 12 years ($p < 0.0001$)				
None	4,845	17,244,968	1.00	(ref)
1	665	1,455,258	1.16	(1.07–1.26)
2	199	283,956	1.40	(1.21–1.62)
3+	78	91,815	1.36	(1.08–1.70)
From 13 to 14 years ($p < 0.0001$)				
None	6,324	22,485,003	1.00	(ref)
1	696	1,240,162	1.45	(1.34–1.57)
2	184	217,825	1.79	(1.54–2.08)
3+	76	55,656	2.49	(1.97–3.13)

*: Estimates of relative risk were adjusted for age and its interaction with gender, calendar year, urbanicity at birth, mental illness in a parent or sibling, and change of the municipality.
Categories with unaccessible information are not shown.
Table modified from Arch Gen Psychiatry (2001) 58: 1039–1046

We believe that our studies of urban-rural differences would suggest that continuous or repeated exposures during upbringing that occur more frequently in urbanized areas are responsible for the association between urbanization and schizophrenia risk. However, we have tried to systematically test different possibilities for risk factors explaining urban-rural differences, and our first attempt to do so was published last year by Eaton and co-workers [1, 2] in a smaller study looking at pregnancy and birth complications and urbanization at birth. However, this study also found urban-rural differences according to urbanicity at birth, but these differences were not explained by differences in occurrence of pregnancy or birth complications. Also, our findings cannot be explained by differences in seasonality of birth or exposure to influenza epidemics during prenatal life [16]. Also, preliminary findings by Dr. Byrne and others from our group show that urban-rural differences cannot be ascribed to socio-economic differences in the parents [1, 10].

The results just mentioned regarding the dose-response relationship between cumulative exposure to urbanization during upbringing have led us to pursue the possible role of exposure to pollution during upbringing. We have, so far, focused on indicators of traffic density as the main source of pollutants as, for example, lead. We have chosen this because even low-dose lead exposure has been shown to affect the normal intellectual development of children [3], and of course, there is a strong urban-rural difference in exposure to lead, or at least there was until the removal of lead additives to gasoline within the last decade or so. We are currently analyzing this in two ways. First, we are analyzing the address of upbringing by distance to roads classified according to road size, probably reflecting different traffic intensities, as this would correlate with lead exposure. Also, we are analyzing data involving actual measurement and modeling of exposure to a number of air pollutants, including pollution from combustion engines directly on the individual address level. Also, we are attempting to follow-up cohorts where lead exposure has actually been measured during childhood. However, the results of these studies are not available yet.

In summary, we believe there is sufficient evidence that factors related to urbanicity during upbringing may be important risk factors for schizophrenia, and also that any candidate risk factor(s) behind this would be likely to be something that acts continuously or repeatedly during most of the childhood rather than at some specific vulnerable period.

■ References

1. Byrne M, Agerbo E, Eaton WW, Mortensen PB (2001) Socio-economic predictors of schizophrenia. (submitted)
2. Eaton WW, Mortensen PB, Frydenberg M (2000) Obstetric factors, urbanization and psychosis. Schizophr Res 43 (2–3): 117–123
3. Finkelstein Y, Markowitz ME, Rosen JF (1998) Low-level lead-induced neurotoxicity in children: an update on central nervous system effects. Brain Res Brain Res Rev 27 (2): 168–176
4. Freeman H (1994) Schizophrenia and city residence. Br J Psychiatry (Suppl 23): 39–50

5. Lewis G, David A, Andreasson S, Allebeck P (1992) Schizophrenia and city life. Lancet 340 (8812): 137–140
6. Malig C (1996) The civil registration system in Denmark. Technical Papers IIVRS 66: 1–6
7. Marcelis M, Navarro-Mateu F, Murray R, Selten JP, Van Os J (1998) Urbanization and psychosis: a study of 1942–1978 birth cohorts in The Netherlands. Psychol Med 28 (4): 871–879
8. McGuffin P, Gottesman II (1999) Risk factors for schizophrenia [letter; comment]. N Engl J Med 341 (5): 370–371
9. Mortensen PB (2000) Urban-rural differences in the risk for schizophrenia. Int J Ment Health 29 (3): 101–110
10. Mortensen PB, Agerbo E, Eriksson T, Westergaard-Nielsen N (2000) Parental education and socioeconomic variables as predictors of schizophrenia in the offspring. Schizophr Res 41: (1) (Abstract)
11. Mortensen PB, Pedersen CB, Westergaard T, Wohlfahrt J, Ewald H, Mors O et al. (1999) Effects of family history and place and season of birth on the risk of schizophrenia. N Engl J Med 340 (8): 603–608
12. Munk-Jørgensen P, Mortensen PB (1997) The Danish Psychiatric Central Register. Dan Med Bull 44 (1): 82–84
13. Pedersen CB, Mortensen PB (2001) Evidence of a dose-response relationship between urbanicity during upbringing and schizophrenia risk. Arch Gen Psychiatry 58: 1039–1046
14. Pedersen CB, Mortensen PB (2001) Family history, place and season of birth as risk factors for schizophrenia in Denmark: a replication and reanalysis. Br J Psychiatry 179: 46–52
15. Schelin EM, Munk-Jorgensen P, Olesen AV, Gerlach J (2000) Regional differences in schizophrenia incidence in Denmark. Acta Psychiatr Scand 101 (4): 293–299
16. Westergaard T, Mortensen PB, Pedersen CB, Wohlfahrt J, Melbye M (1999) Exposure to prenatal and childhood infections and the risk of schizophreina. Suggestions from a study of sibship characteristics and influenza prevalence. Arch Gen Psychiatry 56: 993–998

Environmental risk factors of psychosis

W. F. GATTAZ, A. L. ABRAHÃO, R. FOCCACIA
Department of Psychiatry, Faculty of Medicine, University of São Paulo, Brazil

The fact that the rates of concordance for schizophrenia among monozygotic twins is far below 100 % proves that non-genetic factors must be operant for the development or not of the disease. The three previous authors presented a number of factors that may increase the risk of psychosis. Dr. H. Verdoux discussed the role of obstetric complications and its interactions with maternal psychopathology (such as stress or depression) during pregnancy. She mentioned further the contribution of intrauterine factors such as growth retardation, viruses, nutrition and low birth weight. Drs. P. Mortensen and G. Harrison presented data on the contribution of urbanicity and migration, respectively, two environmental factors that are complex because they comprise a series of elements, such as cultural, socioeconomic, infectious and pollution influences.

In spite of the heterogeneity of the risk factors discussed by the three authors, they agreed to give them a longitudinal mode of action. Dr. Verdoux stressed the interaction of the different factors over time increasing the risk of psychosis. Dr. Mortensen considered the environmental contribution as "something that acts continuously during most of the childhood rather than at some specific vulnerable period", whereas Dr. Harrison proposed a "life-course model involving multiplicative effects of provocative and protective agents across the individual's life course". Thus, there is an obvious consensus that the development or not of psychosis, and more specifically of schizophrenia, depends upon the interaction between genetic and environmental factors during the development of the brain.

I will attempt to frame the contribution of the different risk factors within one model that considers schizophrenia as a disorder of brain maturation. For this, I would like to review first the concepts of synaptogenesis and synapse elimination, which are both crucial phenomena during the maturation of the brain. These data were brilliantly investigated by PR Huttenlocher and his collaborators [2–5] and will be summarized below.

Synaptogenesis in human neocortex occurs during the third trimester of gestation and during the two postnatal years. This period of intensive synaptic proliferation occurs concurrently with dendritic and axonal growth. It is then followed by a period of synapse elimination, during which synaptic density and number decrease to about 60 % of the maximum. In humans, synaptogenesis and synapse elimination are heterochronous in different cortical regions. For instance maximum synaptic density in the auditory cortex is reached at age 3 months, while in the middle frontal gyrus at age 15 months. The end of synapse elimination in the auditory cortex is reached by age 12 years, but in the prefrontal cortex at midadolescence.

One decisive factor for the development and maintenance of synaptic connections is synaptic activity, which determines the competition for neurotrophic factors. As a simple rule, synapses that work tend to remain, those that do not, are eliminated. Thus, the input of environmental stimuli may influence the rates of synapse formation and elimination. The human brain is a product of genetic instructions, cellular interactions and influences of innate activity and external stimulation [7].

The effect of external stimulation upon activity-dependent synaptic modification has been investigated in animal experiments. O'Kusky [9] reported that visually deprived (dark-reared) cats showed a twofold increase in synaptic elimination in the visual cortex compared to normally reared cats. Similarly Meisami & Firoozi [8] found that rats submitted to odor deprivation during the neonatal period showed in the olfactory bulb neuronal loss and permanent reduction of growth, total cell number and enzymes related to the metabolism of neurotransmitters.

These data show the profound modifications that environmental stimuli exert upon brain maturation. It is not unlikely that the interaction of the different environmental factors with the individual genetic constitution may increase the risk of schizophrenia through a disruption of the physiological process of synapse modification. Thus, the propositions of the three prior authors would very nicely fit into a model (Fig. 1), in which the risk of psychosis would depend upon the interaction of the different factors (H. Verdoux) acting continuously ... rather

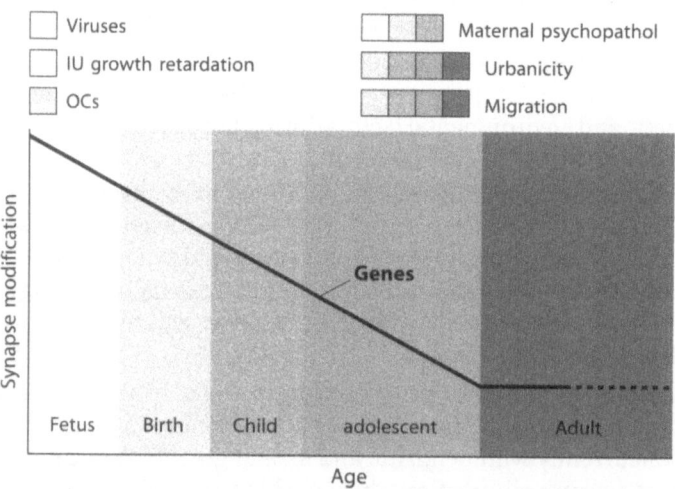

Fig. 1. Timing of environmental influences against the degree of synapse modification during the maturation of the brain. The result of the interaction between both is modulated by the genetic factors (*IU* intra-uterine; *Ocs* obstetric complications).

than at some specific vulnerable period (P. Mortensen), involving multiplicative effects of provocative and protective agents across the individual's life course (G. Harrison).

▪ Childhood meningitis and adult schizophreia

I would like to present now a preliminary evaluation of our data showing that a meningitis infection during childhood may increase the risk of psychosis in general, and of schizophrenia in especial during adulthood. The basis for our study was a meningitis epidemic that affected the population of São Paulo from 1971 until 1974, in which the infection rates increased from 2 cases to 170 cases per 100,000 inhabitants. Ninety percent of the infected individuals were committed to the Hospital Emilio Ribas, a 400 bed academic hospital linked to our Faculty of Medicine of the University of São Paulo.

The objectives of our study were to evaluate the lifetime psychiatric morbidity in adults infected by meningitis at age 0–4 years and to compare this morbidity to a control group matched by genetic and environmental (cultural, socioeconomic, etc.) backgrounds. For this purpose, we chose as a control group the siblings of our subjects who had not been infected by meningitis.

Our database was the microfilmed medical records from Hospital Emílio Ribas, which provided us with the individual data: name, birth date, name of the parents, age at meningitis, CSF exam and duration of hospitalization. With these data a team of psychiatrists and psychologists tried to localize the individuals or their relatives through an Internet telephone directory (www.telefonica.net.br) (mean 150 calls to localize one subject).

When the subjects were localized, the following script was said to them: "Here is Dr. X, from the University of São Paulo. We are doing a research about meningitis. We would like to interview personally you and one of your siblings, with the closest age to yours. Your collaboration will be important for our study. You will receive for this interview an honorarium of R$100 to cover part of your costs."

If patients accepted, then we would give him the address at the *Institute of Psychiatry*. This script was made to avoid the pre-selection of a sample with an

Table 1. Sample description of adults infected by meningitis at age 4 years or less and their siblings without childhood meningitis infection (* p < 0.05)

	Meningitis (n = 173)	Siblings (n = 141)
Male	77 (44 %)	50 (36 %)
Female	96 (56 %)	91 (64 %)
Age (years)	29.1 ± 1.6	30.0 ± 5.9
Years at school	11.6 ± 3.6	11.4 ± 4.0
IQ (estimated)	89.1 ± 10.4	88.8 ± 12.6
Income (R$/month)	938 ± 953	734 ± 806 *

overrepresentation of psychiatric morbidity, interested in receiving priority in psychiatric care at the University Department. This bias could be expected in a city like São Paulo, in which there is a shortage of psychiatric facilities as compared to the existent need.

We found 4951 records of individuals who had a meningitis at age 4 or less. From these, we searched up to now (October 2001) for 1745 individuals, and we found and contacted 331; from these, 173 (52%) came to the interview, bringing with them 141 siblings without childhood meningitis. The samples were well matched regarding age, sex distribution, educational performance and IQ. The only significant difference was a higher income in the meningitis group (!) as compared to their siblings (Table 1).

All individuals underwent a semi-structured interview based on the ICD-10 Checklist [6], followed by a neurological exam and a neuropsychological test battery evaluating IQ, frontal function and logical memory (neuropsychological data will not be presented here).

In general, we found a similar prevalence of psychiatric disorders in the meningitis (62.2%) and the siblings (58.2%, n.s.) groups. This prevalence is higher then that observed in a representative sample of the population from São Paulo [1]. In general, individuals with childhood meningitis had a 5-fold higher prevalence of psychotic disorders than their siblings (20.8% vs. 4.3%, p < 0.001). This difference was observed for each of the diagnoses schizophrenia, mood disorder with psychotic symptoms and 'other psychoses' (Fig. 2). No differences were found between both groups in the prevalence of the other psychiatric disorders (anxiety, personality disorder, alcohol and drugs abuse, mood disorder without psychotic symptoms).

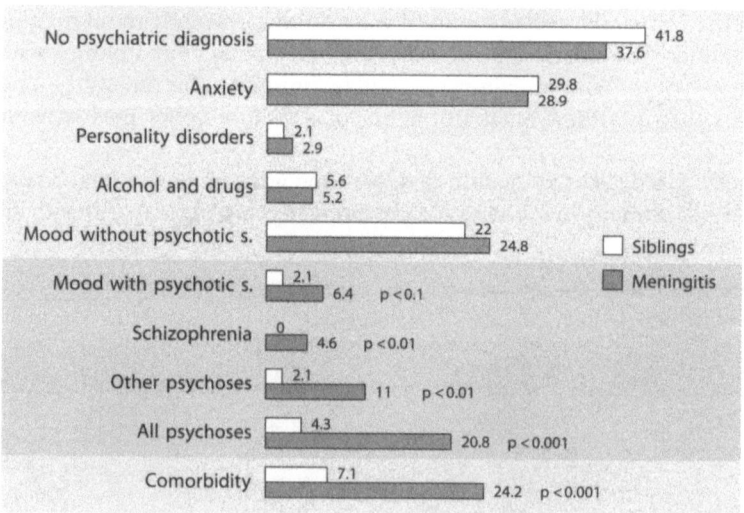

Fig. 2. Lifetime prevalence (%) of psychiatric disorders in adults infected by meningitis at age 4 years or less (n = 173) and their siblings without meningitis infection (n = 141).

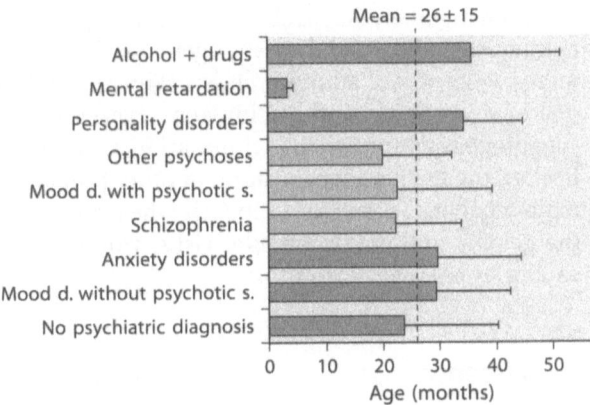

Fig. 3. Mean age at meningitis infection (in months) by diagnosis.

As expected, individuals with childhood meningitis had a higher prevalence of neurological disorders (24.8% vs. 5.6% in their siblings, p < 0.001), being the most frequent deafness (10.4%). Because there are some studies suggesting an association between deafness and psychoses, we analyzed the data separately in individuals with and without deafness. The increased prevalence of psychoses remained in the individuals with childhood meningitis (p < 0.001), whereas no other difference regarding the remaining diagnoses arose. Moreover, the association between meningitis and psychoses remained significant (p < 0.001) when we excluded from the sample all individuals with neurological diagnoses.

The mean age at the time of the meningitis infection was 26 ± 15 months. No difference was found in the timing of the meningitis between individuals with psychosis and those without a psychiatric diagnosis (Fig. 3).

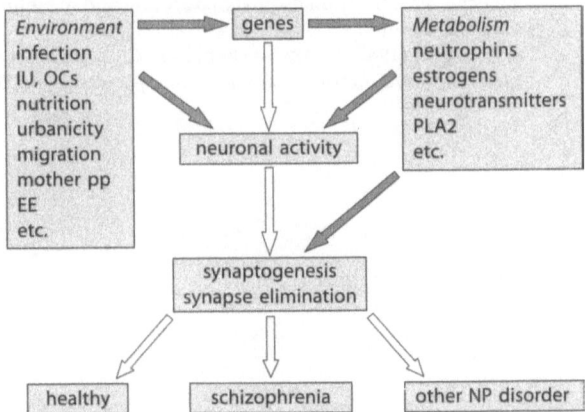

Fig. 4. Model for the effects of genetic and environmental factors on synapse modification during the maturation of the brain. Environmental factors may influence gene expression or directly neuronal activity disrupting synapse modification. Genes affect directly programmed neuronal activity or determine metabolic changes which, in turn, affect neuronal activity or synapse modification. Depending upon the degree (and probably localization) of synapse changes, an individual can develop schizophrenia or other neuropsychiatric disorders. Conversely, the interaction of these factors can have a protective effect in an individual prone to develop psychosis.

Taken together, the results from our prospective study suggest that childhood meningitis could enter the heterogeneous list of environmental factors that may increase the risk of adult psychosis (Fig. 4). All these factors may be operant at one or more levels, influencing gene expression, neuronal activity or directly synaptogenesis and synapse elimination, ending in some cases in schizophrenia. Besides the further identification of other potential risk factors, I think that our major challenge would be to identify the protective agents which, counteracting the genetic and environmental risks, would avoid or attenuate the suffering caused by a psychotic outburst.

▒ References

1. Andrade LHSG, Lólio CA, Gentil V, Laurenti R (1999) Epidemiologia dos transtornos mentais em uma área definida de captação da cidade de São Paulo, Brasil. Rev Psiq Clin 26: 257–261. Also available in http://www.hcnet.usp.br/ipq/revista/r265/artigo(257).htm
2. Huttenlocher PR (1984) Synapse elimination and plasticity in developing human cerebral cortex. Am J Ment Defic 88: 488–496
3. Huttenlocher PR, de Courten C (1987) The development of synapses in striate cortex of man. Hum Neurobiol 6: 1–9
4. Huttenlocher PR, Dabholkar AS (1997) Regional differences in synaptogenesis in human cerebral cortex. J Comp Neurol 387: 167–178
5. Huttenlocher PR, de Courten C, Garey LJ, Van der Loos H (1982) Synaptogenesis in human visual cortex – evidence for synapse elimination during normal development. Neurosci Lett 33: 247–252
6. Janca A, Hiller W (1996) ICD-10 Checklists – A tool for clinicians use of the ICD-10 classification of mental and behavio0ral disorders. Comprehensive Psychiatry 37: 180–187
7. Lagercrantz H, Ringstedt T (2001) Organization of the neuronal circuits in the central nervous system during development. Acta Paediatr 90: 707–715
8. Meisami E, Firoozi M (1996) Acetylcholinesterase activity in the developing olfactory bulb: a biochemical study on normal maturation and the influence of peripheral and central connections. Brain Res 353: 115–124
9. O'Kusky JR (1985) Postnatal changes in the numerical density and total number of asymmetric and symmetric synapses in the hypoglossal nucleus of the rat. Brain Res Dev Brain Res 108: 179–191

Indicators of Schizophrenia in Childhood and Adolescence

Risk factors for schizophrenia in childhood and youth

P. B. JONES

Department of Psychiatry, University of Cambridge, U.K.

■ Why look in youth and childhood for the causes of the schizophrenia syndrome?

The syndrome we call schizophrenia usually always appears in early to mid-adult life [24, 51, 52]. However, there is ample evidence that those who will develop it are a little different from their peers long before this, at a much earlier stage of the life course. These differences may be the manifestations of the same causes that later lead to schizophrenia, they may be distinct from these effects, or they may be the age-related, non-psychotic manifestations of schizophrenia itself; we don't know.

A far-reaching, longitudinal view of disease causation is transforming our understanding of a number of chronic physical disorders [6–9, 76, 86]. The same is happening for schizophrenia [74], although the life course or developmental approach has, we should acknowledge, been prevalent in research regarding psychological illness for much longer than physical disease [115, 116]. These longitudinal formulations raise the prospects of understanding psychosis causation [117–119] and could underpin early intervention.

■ What do we see in childhood and youth before schizophrenia?

Evidence of developmental differences between those who will later become psychotic and those who will not is difficult to refine. Kraepelin [75] and Bleuler [10, 11] both noticed that a considerable proportion of people who developed the psychotic syndrome of schizophrenia had been different, in terms of character and behaviour, during childhood and youth.

Their astute clinical observations were possible because they were, in large part, informally observing their patients' children before some developed illnesses similar to their parents. Thus, they made opportunistic use of genetic high-risk and cohort designs. However, the inference that the remainder of those who would develop schizophrenia had entirely *normal* development may not be justified.

Much of the evidence for abnormal development prior to psychosis, such as from studies of minor physical anomalies and neuropathology (see Falkai, this volume), is best (but not, necessarily, completely) explained in terms of developmental processes having gone wrong [152]. However, these processes are not observed directly. Genetic high-risk studies have shown subtle differences in neurological development in high-risk children [39, 42, 43, 147].

Parnas (this volume) considers these genetic high-risk studies. Here, evidence from general population samples is discussed. The evidence is convergent between the two research paradigms, each having its advantages and disadvantages. General population cohorts can be considered as another type of high-risk paradigm where the children who will develop schizophrenia are at 100% risk, and are compared with their peers at zero risk.

Early milestones and motor development

There is direct evidence of neuro-developmental differences. One source is the remarkable research by Walker and colleagues [147, 148] who studied "home movies" of families in which one child later developed schizophrenia. They rated emotion and motor function blind to that child's identity amongst their siblings. The pre-schizophrenic children were distinguished on both accounts, with some fairly gross, but transitory motor differences. Similar developmental differences have now been demonstrated in several general population samples from around the world.

Jones and colleagues [64] studied the British 1946 birth cohort (the Medical Research Council National Survey of Health and Development; NSHD; 145, 146), the first of the long-term, birth cohort studies that now support much life course research. The NSHD began as a survey of all children born in one week in March 1946, with a stratified, random sample of 5362 being followed to date. There were 11 data collection points before the age of 16 years. Information was collected from multiple sources, and in many domains including socio-economic status, development, educational attainment and behaviour. Those survey members who developed psychosis between 16 and 43 years of age were identified from the survey records and from the Mental Health Enquiry; until 1987 this was, in effect, a national, psychiatric hospital discharge register. DSM-III-R criteria [3] were applied to clinical case notes of those with serious mental illness. This identified 30 of them as fulfilling these narrow criteria for schizophrenia. This group was compared with the remaining population alive in the UK at age 16 years.

Milestones were assessed by maternal recall at age 24 months. All those recorded, sitting, standing, walking and talking, were delayed [64]. Teething was, if anything, a little early indicating that these results were not the result of information bias inherent in the recall at two years.

There were other indications that language development was different in these children. Health visitors were more likely to notice no speech by 2 years in the children who developed schizophrenia as adults, and school doctors noted speech delays and problems throughout childhood.

The delay in walking unsupported was only about six weeks, not anything that would concern a parent. Similarly, delayed speech would not have been prominent in most of these children; both milestones have great variability in normal children. This demonstrates one of the important advantages of prospective data. Not only do they guard against distortion of information on the basis of outcome, these unbiased data may also reveal subtle effects that would simply be beyond the resolution of memory over a decade or two. The recall only of gross events or differences, with the remainder classified as normal or unaffected may have led to the assumption that only sub-groups of cases with very different early life exposures constituted a special, or distinct group – the neurodevelopmental group. This is explored again later.

These developmental differences have been replicated in other cohorts. The British 1958 cohort (the National Child Development Study; NCDS) is the second of the three British birth cohorts and involves all children born in the same week as the NSHD, but twelve years later. The third of these cohorts involves the same methods in 1970. All babies born in the week have been followed in the NCDS. Crow, Done, Johnstone and colleagues applied similar case-finding methods as were used in the NSHD to identify subjects with schizophrenia [38]. They showed [33] that pre-schizophrenic children at age 7 had been slower to develop continence, and had poor co-ordination and vision. At age 16 they were rated clumsy.

Cannon [20] assembled a large case-control study of schizophrenia nested within a cohort of births in Helsinki between 1951 and 1960. Birth and school records are available on all those who appear on the Finnish Hospital Discharge Register with a diagnosis of schizophrenia and a group of controls sampled from the birth records. Cases of schizophrenia were rated at school as having problems with sports and handicrafts. This may be a manifestation of the same unco-ordinated motor characteristics as Crow [33] demonstrated, and of the delayed milestones noted in the earlier British cohort [64].

The North Finland 1966 birth cohort involves all the issue from all pregnancies of women in northern Finland (Oulu and Lapland provinces) due to deliver during 1966 [111]; there were 12,058 live births. The study was planned to investigate pre- and perinatal causes of mental retardation and cerebral palsy [112]. It arose from Rantakallio's consideration of the National Collaborative Perinatal Project in the United States (see 102 for description and references), and is now becoming a resource for longitudinal research in schizophrenia [59, 60, 67].

Isohanni and colleagues [61] have indicated that the developmental differences are present even earlier than was shown in the NSHD. In this cohort, delayed motor development as assessed at age 1 year distinguished babies who would develop adult schizophrenia, with the effect most marked in males. Once again the effect was subtle, though stronger in boys. There was evidence of a dose-response relationship between the age at which a boy could stand or walk without support, and his risk of subsequent schizophrenia; the later he walked, the more likely he was to develop schizophrenia.

Requiring support to walk at age one is by no means abnormal, the absolute size of these effects is small, and schizophrenia is not solely a disorder of motor development. However, a dose-response relationship is a very potent finding in epidemiology, and the important thing about this one is that it operates within the normal range. Subjects who would later develop schizophrenia may have been walking just a little later than they might have been had they not have been subject to some pathological process that increased the risk of schizophrenia. It is not helpful to consider those who were late walkers in terms of being well below the mean as being at particular, or different risk compared with the rest of the children who developed schizophrenia.

The latest results regarding early maturational effects before schizophrenia comes from the Dunedin birth cohort study in which continuity between self-reported psychotic experiences in childhood and a fairly broad concept of schizophreniform disorder arising by the early twenties has been reported recently [109]. Cannon and her colleagues [21] have demonstrated similarly widespread developmental delays in several modalities before schizophreniform disorder, these being rather specific to this disease category.

These subtle effects have become one of the most replicated findings in the developmental epidemiology of schizophrenia over the past decade. Each of the remarkable studies that have been investigated brings a slightly different view of the phenomenon. Regardless of their small size, these developmental differences are likely to betray biologically significant processes relevant to the development of schizophrenia. They also indicate that causal processes were already active in very early life. As in Walker's studies (see above) and in some of the high risk work [43], it seems that the differences were most apparent "on the cusp" of developmental processes. Grown-up, the children did not have gross motor or speech problems, although psychosis and the motoric aspects of the schizophrenia syndrome [46] may be the later manifestations of the same mechanism(s), with the study by Poulton and colleagues [109] indicating hitherto unrecognised continuity of psychopathology.

Behavioural development

Studies of behaviour have also evolved from early clinical accounts, through retrospective research methodologies to cohort designs. Sophisticated rating scales for the retrospective assessment of behaviour and personality demonstrate differences prior to psychosis, with the most common being characteristics of a rather shy, schizoid habit [2, 22, 44, 48].

Robins [115] carried out a pioneering, historical cohort study in which she followed a group of boys who had been referred to a child guidance clinic. Antisocial behaviour was associated with later schizophrenia in this sample. Watt & Lubensky [150, 151] traced the school records of cases of schizophrenia (chart diagnosis) from a geographically defined neighbourhood in Massachusetts, thus reconstructing a school-based cohort. Ratings on a variety dimensions were constructed from the teachers' unstructured comments, and compared with controls from the same schools. Girls who were to develop schizophrenia were introverted throughout kindergarten into adolescence. Boys in the same predicament were "disagreeable", but only in the later school grades (7-12); Done and colleagues [37] have identified a remarkably similar behavioural pattern in the British 1958 birth cohort, including the changes over time.

The differences between the cohorts in the behavioural predictors of schizophrenia may be a result of several things (see 68 for discussion). The behavioural rating scales are different in their design, with different items and foci. Asking teachers to make free or semi-structured comments may result in very different responses from questionnaires demanding a forced choice on all children. Naughty behaviours are much more likely to be noted in the former, and "shy" behaviour may not seem so odd in girls as it may in boys. The role of chance and sampling variation should not be forgotten. Just because a cohort is a remarkable sample does not mean that it will inevitably give a true result; there will be a range of variation when these samples are compared, just as with any review of samples.

Two cohort studies that have used forced-choice scales yielding continuous scores tell us more than individual behavioural items. In the 1946 birth cohort (the NSHD; see above), Jones and colleagues [64, 66] investigated the differences in behaviour between children who were to develop schizophrenia and their peers. They used the children's own ratings of their behaviour at age 13 years, and teachers' ratings two years later, at age 15 years. There was no evidence of antisocial traits in the pre-schizophrenia group, but a strong association with shy, "schizoid" behaviours at both ages; the two views gave a very similar picture. Moreover, when the continuous behavioural scores were analysed there was a highly significant trend in this association such that the more asocial a teenage was, the greater the likelihood of later schizophrenia. Just as for the milestone findings from the North Finland cohort [61] there was a dose response relationship, rather than a subgroup of very socially awkward individuals accounting for the association.

The findings have been replicated in both the dose-response relationship and regarding the content. Malmberg and colleagues [85] studied a cohort of some 50,000 late adolescent male conscripts in Sweden. At age 17-20 years, the age of conscription into the army, these men had undergone a range of tests and assessments. Record linkage identified those 192 who had later had hospital contact for ICD-8 schizophrenia. It was in this cohort that Andreasson and colleagues [4] demonstrated a dose-response relationship between cannabis consumption at conscription and later schizophrenia.

Four behavioural variables at age 18 were particularly associated with later schizophrenia: having fewer than two close friends, preferring to socialise in small groups, feeling more sensitive than others and not having a steady girlfriend [85]. Accumulation of exposure to these variables was associated with a linear increase in the risk of developing schizophrenia; a dose-response relationship, just as in the British 1946 birth cohort [64] but with much greater statistical precision. Cannon et al. [19] also noted the same relationship in a case-control design. This study used retrospective maternal accounts of behaviour, but had much higher statistical power.

Another remarkable conscript study from Israel is now providing important information about late adolescent characteristics that pre-date adult schizophrenia [2, 36]. Mark Weiser describes the results in detail elsewhere in this volume.

Briefly, Davidson and his colleagues linked the Israeli draft board registry with the national psychiatric hospitalisation case registry. The draft board tests measured intelligence, social functioning, organisational ability, interest in physical activity, and individual autonomy. Over 500 cases with schizophrenia were compared with controls, some 9000 adolescents who did not appear in the registry (N = 9,215), matched to patients by age, gender, and school attended at time of testing. One of the strongest predictors for schizophrenia were deficits in social functioning. As in other studies, there was a dose-response relationship.

Given current views (again re-learning what Kraepelin and Bleuler already thought) concerning the cognitive disturbances that accompany, and may underpin psychosis, it seems a reasonable and parsimonious hypothesis that the early developmental and behavioural effects may be linked through cognition. The motor and language findings betray a disturbance or difference in developmental processes. This is manifest in behavioural terms because the same processes affect cognitive development, particularly in the realm of social cognition. Any difference in behaviour and interaction with others may well, itself, lead to attenuation of social environment and further deviance in development through perturbation of the normal genetic, social-environmental and neurodevelopmental interactions that are involved in brain growth.

This suggestion of a "self-perpetuating cascade" arising from the results from the 1946 cohort [64] is discussed later. However, before being too carried away with conjecture, we should first review evidence to suggest that cognition really is different prior to psychosis.

Cognitive function and IQ

Studies of pre-psychotic personality have largely confirmed the earliest clinical accounts, investigation of pre-psychotic has IQ challenged the initial notion of a deteriorating, dementing course after onset of psychosis; the field remains controversial. By the mid part of the century poorer performance on standardised measures of intellectual function by people with schizophrenia was established, in line with Kraepelin's idea of dementia praecox. However, the questions were unanswered as to whether this really was deterioration in function, whether there was a pre-psychotic deficit, and when such a deficit might occur [56, 57, 83, 87, 114].

Albee and colleagues [1, 79] compared childhood Stanford-Binet scores with Wechsler-Bellevue scores during adult schizophrenic psychosis in 112 people. The scores at the two time points were very similar on a number of statistical parameters. Their longitudinal perspective allowed the authors to conclude that their results *"seriously challenge the belief that intellectual loss occurs as a consequence of adult schizophrenia"*. Russell and colleagues [120] have provided confirmatory evidence for this, but the effect remains controversial. In fact, the argument as to whether there is a developmental or degenerative process is probably a debate over a spurious dichotomy, given that a single, life-course process may be affected by a pathological process.

Aylward, Walker and Bettes [5] have provided a comprehensive review of intelligence in schizophrenia. They concluded that performance on standardised measures of intellectual function is lower in pre-psychotic individuals than in age-matched controls. Linking the pre-psychotic deficit to outcome, they raise the question as to whether IQ may be an independent factor that can protect otherwise vulnerable individuals, or whether the deficits are part of that vulnerability. The conclusion that there may be a causal sub-type of schizophrenia characterised by intellectual deficits has guided many searches for such causes. Developments in cohort studies have shed some new light on this issue; just as for milestones and behaviour the evidence does not support a sub-group effect.

In the 1946 British birth cohort (see above) several measures of educational achievement were collected on all children at ages 8, 11 and 15 years [107, 108]. Jones and colleagues [64] compared the first principal component of these measures (analogous to a standardised IQ score) in children who developed schizophrenia and the remainder who did not. The data and results are summarised by Jones [63, 64].

Statistical analysis of these data confirmed that the mean values in the case data were lower than in age-matched controls, with the greatest effect at age 15 years. There was a trend in the association between childhood IQ and risk of later schizophrenia such that the lower the IQ the higher the risk, although that risk remained small. A trend operated throughout the distribution; there was no evidence of a sub-group of very low scores that account for the finding. The data were compatible with all children who would later develop schizophrenia having scored somewhat less than expected, with a consequent shift downwards for the whole at-risk group.

The finding was replicated in the Swedish and Israeli conscript studies, mentioned above. The ability measures were from later in life than from the birth cohorts. The benefits from the larger numbers of cases were only slightly diluted by the measurement error that arose from the case notes and other clinical material not being scrutinised. With this greater statistical power, David et al. [35] used the Swedish conscript cohort study to confirm a linear trend in the association between pre-psychotic IQ and risk of later schizophrenia: the lower the IQ the greater the risk. Further replication and extension came from the Israeli conscripts [36] described above. Lower organisational ability and lower IQ showed strong associations with IQ, both with a dose-response relationship (see Weiser in this volume). Thus, there was no evidence of a threshold effect below or above which this relationship did not hold. Very bright individuals did develop schizophrenia but they were much less likely to than those who are less able. Put another way, any individual is more likely to develop schizophrenia than someone who is more able in terms of IQ, although the effect is small.

This formulation, possible only with the general population controls available in the large birth cohort and conscript studies, argues against Aylward and colleagues' [5] notion of a sub-group, though their hypotheses about sex differences and risk versus protection remain un-tested. Current interest in the cognitive aspects of schizophrenia [34, 50] suggests a parsimonious conclusion that pre-psychotic IQ deficits (and perhaps social characteristics) may, indeed, be manifestations of the same abnormal cognitive processes that later result in psychosis, just as was suggested earlier.

■ Longitudinal approaches to investigations of causes

Earlier on, the notion was considered that some of the developmental, cognitive and behavioural effects seen before psychosis may, *themselves*, act as causal factors by attenuating further CNS development in a non-linear manner by altering the immediate environment [62, 64]. In general, though, causes are often considered as the first or most distal external effect that might begin or trigger such a cascade effect, as well as having a predisposing action in some cases. Several environmental effects are candidates as parts of causes of the pre-psychotic manifestations that have been reviewed here.

Early infections

A link between severe psychiatric disorder and date of birth was noted by Tramer [142]. The proportion of people with schizophrenia born in the colder, winter and spring months of the year is slightly (5–15%) higher than the general population [13, 55]. It is also higher than those with other psychiatric disorder, particularly neurosis [12, 53, 110]. The pursuit of the explanation of this "season of birth effect" is a fair model to trace the development of longitudinal studies of early causes.

The controversial season of birth effect [80, 81, 139, 141, 149] has had a huge impact on developmental epidemiological research in schizophrenia. The season of birth effect is robust, rather than an artefact (see for varying views and evidence: 54, 71, 72, 80, 81, 125, 139). It also survives rigorous statistical techniques for time trends [72], and behaves in a biologically plausible manner, being reversed in the southern hemisphere and absent at the equator [91, 99, 104, 105]. Differential fertility and breeding patterns have been excluded by elegant series of family studies [54].

An environmental factor that changes with the season and has its effects around the time of birth has been posited. Perhaps the most exciting, new explanatory idea has come from John McGrath [89, 90]. He has suggested that varying levels of vitamin D in early life, caused by seasonal meteorological and solar rhythms, may be the causal factor, operating through low levels impinging upon CNS development. This would be consistent with, and perhaps explain (wholly or partially) much of the descriptive epidemiology of the disease [67].

Infections were originally considered as causes of schizophrenia only in adult life [23, 25, 29, 30, 97, 138]. Until McGrath's idea, they have more recently been the most consistent candidate out of a range of other possible explanations [126, 127, 140] prevalent before McGrath's new ideas. Many infectious agents have been investigated [155]; influenza is implicated in congenital [27, 28] and other central nervous system disorders [88], and has been the key target of investigation in schizophrenia.

A great deal the evidence regarding the role of these early infections has come ecological, or population-association studies. Regarding influenza, Mednick and colleagues [94] demonstrated an association between mid-trimester fetal life during the 1957/58 influenza A_2 pandemic and schizophrenia in adult life. This exciting and important finding spawned many studies well reviewed by McGrath et al. [92] and Morgan et al. [99].

Attempts at direct replication have yielded contradictory results (e.g., 40, 71, 72, 95, 103, 123, 131). Generally, positive results have come from studies of longer-term trends in the association between the timing of influenza epidemics over the century and the birth dates of people with schizophrenia [77, 99, 124, 134].

The relative risk associated with season of birth is somewhere between 1.05 and 1.15; small effects. This indicates that the association is some distance from being directly causal, although the situation in individuals may be quite different; McGrath et al. [92] review this carefully. Ecological designs have limitations, particularly regarding confounding with other factors explaining the association. If a true causal factor were linked with fetal influenza exposure – exposure to maternal fever, antipyretic drugs are possibilities [94] – then these studies are vital signposts. The notion of fetal exposure to a possible cause leads to a major limitation of the design. We cannot be certain that the (fetal) individuals in the population who were exposed to influenza in utero, if any, are the same (adult) individuals who get the schizophrenia as adults.

These caveats point towards the need for other methodologies where more details of the individual histories are documented. Cohort and case control designs fulfil this need in different ways. The main problems for the latter design in developmental epidemiology are the long period over which early, subtle (perhaps even un-noticed) exposures have to be recalled, and the ever-present difficulty of finding appropriate controls. For cohort studies, opportunistic use has to be made of others' judicious recording of appropriate material (including biological samples) in early life, several decades before the period of risk for schizophrenia begins. This collection is usually without any thought of a future psychiatric use for the data. The relative rarity of schizophrenia also means that large numbers of individuals must be studied, and their outcome traced in terms of a disorder that is notoriously difficult to define. Nevertheless, such samples are available. They are having a major impact on developmental formulations of causation and are likely to have a huge impact as ever larger and more comprehensive (particularly in terms of collection of genetic data) samples are studied. Some are reviewed below.

Mednick and colleagues [96] identified those people with schizophrenia who had been in utero during the 1957 influenza epidemic in Helsinki, and who had been the basis of the original, ecological report [94]. With narrative confirmation of maternal exposure to influenza, including some contemporary data, and comparison with a control group, an association with specific schizophrenia psychopathology was demonstrated.

Cohort studies have provided less support for the influenza-schizophrenia association. Cannon and her colleagues [18] followed a group in Dublin who had been exposed to the same 1957 influenza pandemic. Information on exposure was confirmed by an earlier report by Coffey and Jessop [27, 28] who had reported an increase in congenital defects in the same exposed group. Cannon found no evidence of an excess of schizophrenia in the exposed group during adult life, although a secondary analysis suggested a link with affective disorder.

The British 1958 birth cohort has relevant information (see above for details of the sample). About 6 weeks after they had given birth in the original survey, mothers were asked whether they had suffered influenza (the same A_2 pandemic, yet again) during pregnancy. Done and colleagues [38] identified those cohort members who suffered schizophrenia as adults, and showed no association between reported maternal influenza and schizophrenia in the offspring [31, 32]. Some critics indicated that the reported prevalence of maternal influenza was low given the pandemic through which they were pregnant, but it is difficult to conceive of sufficient, systematic bias to yield a spurious negative result.

The influenza hypothesis began the series of cohort studies of the effect of early infection, but other infections have been studied in other cohorts. In her North Finland 1966 cohort (see above) Rantakallio and colleagues [113] used record linkage to identify all cohort members who had been hospitalised during childhood for a central nervous system (CNS) infection (mainly encephalitis and meningitis). They identified those who had survived to age 16, the beginning of the period of risk for schizophrenia. They next used a similar record linkage technique to identify those members of the whole cohort who had been hospitalised for psychiatric illness. The investigators [59] applied DSM-III-R [3] criteria to the case notes of these people to make operational psychiatric diagnoses.

Children with serologically confirmed diagnosis and severe childhood CNS infections would have been the "tip of the iceberg" of CNS infection. Of 145 in this group, 4 (2.8% developed schizophrenia), compared with 0.7% of the unexposed majority. This 4-fold relative risk *may* underestimate the true risk because of the restriction to severe exposure [113]. If the relationship were causal, then an estimate of the population attributable fraction, the amount by which the population burden of schizophrenia may be reduced if the causal effect of the exposure were removed, is around 4%. This example shows the detailed conclusions that can be drawn from epidemiological samples where exposure and outcome are known precisely for individuals, although judgements on causality still have to made as carefully as ever. If this is a causal association, then only a minority of schizophrenia is explained.

It is biologically plausible for this association to be interpreted as being part of a cause. The CNS was known to have been affected in this group, something that is less clear for the studies of influenza, and similar findings have been shown in this sample for mental retardation and childhood epilepsy [112]. What was unexpected was the indication that the time window over which early toxic exposure may exert an effect extended beyond birth and into childhood. Only a minority of schizophrenia could be explained, the exposure was not a specific cause for schizophrenia, and the period over which it acted was not limited (if it were a cause at all). The caveat for these conclusions, as for any causal inference, is the danger of reverse causality. The CNS may have been already abnormal in the individuals that developed infection and schizophrenia, and such abnormalities may have made the individuals liable to CNS infection. Alternatively, tertiary factors (probably genetic) may have made the individuals vulnerable to a "schizophrenogenic" effect.

The idea of a continuum of outcomes of problems during pregnancy and delivery in terms of time and severity, from catastrophic CNS anomaly, through mental handicap to behavioural and psychiatric disorder is well known in neurology [106]. The early infections data applies these ideas to schizophrenia. The report by Gattaz (this volume) of a similar association between childhood meningitis and later schizophrenia is important evidence and develops these ideas, considerably.

A 50-year longitudinal study of a small cohort of people exposed to rubella in utero was assembled soon after the original reports from Australia of the congenital rubella syndrome. The long-term outcomes of this study provide further support for schizophrenia being part of the spectrum [93]. The causal mechanism of a higher expected incidence of schizophrenia is obscure given the excess of deafness in the group and the possibility that this may be the specific causal agent, with rubella exposure being but one possible antecedent. Brown and colleagues [14] are investigating a cohort of individuals exposed to rubella, first assembled by Chess [26]. They find evidence of schizophrenia phenomenology emerging in the teenage years, independent of hearing defects [15, 16]. Jones and colleagues [70] have followed a large group of individuals, the mothers of whom were identified during pregnancy as suffering from identified viral infections. Health outcomes have been compared with those of a group not known to have been so exposed (see 41 for explanation of the sample). Here, too, there appears to be some evidence linking neurotropic virus exposure with a range of adverse CNS outcomes including mental retardation, epilepsy and psychosis.

The development and testing of hypotheses about early infection are good examples of the development of thought and methodology over the century. They began with the season of birth observation, moved through ecological studies of infections, to general population cohorts and enriched samples where specific exposures are identified. The original prospect of single, specific infectious causes, possibly with specific time windows during which the developing brain was vulnerable to the putative "schizophrenogenic" effects have melted away. In their place has emerged an equally exciting but more complex set of findings. A variety of agents, acting over a variety of developmental epochs, may be linked to a variety of outcomes one of which is the syndrome of schizophrenia. New exposures, such as hypovitaminosis-D, have been added. The role of genetic diathesis remains unclear [100] but there are intriguing findings concerning HLA status and other putative susceptibility factors [47, 154]. The future almost certainly lies in the combination of molecular biological techniques to define exposure [155], molecular genetics to define susceptibility, and the opportunistic use of population-based samples. Such samples exist [17], and the work is ongoing.

Other putative pre-natal epigenetic risks

There are many other putative risk factors that act in early life. These have been reviewed elsewhere (e.g., 60, 62), and span an enormous range. They include pre-natal famine [129, 130, 132]; and indicators of psychosocial stress affecting the mother [58, 64, 66, 101, 144] or elicited from the child [64, 66].

These latter findings regarding behavioural interactions involved inter-personal conditions as well as genetics. The adoption paradigm is probably the design most suited to investigating these complex issues. This area is tackled by Tienari (this volume) with particular reference to his important Finnish Adoption Study [136, 137].

Pregnancy and delivery complications (PDCs) have been found more commonly in the histories of adults with schizophrenia than controls. Many studies have shown this [17, 69, 70, 82, 103], but not all [38]. The direction of causality is a matter of debate [49, 129]. Kendell et al. [73] have reviewed this field in detail, but a consideration of the role of cohort studies is of interest here; Geddes and Lawrie [45] undertook a meta-analysis. They found evidence of some publication bias in favour of small, positive, case-control studies. There were generally negative [38] or small effects [17] in general population birth cohort studies with unbiased assessments of exposure and outcome. Recent studies, such as that by Zornberg et al. [156, 157] and Jones et al. [69] indicate that specific exposures that actually damage the CNS, such as hypoxic-ischaemic insult, are strongly associated with later schizophrenia. This is further evidence for the continuum of casualty noted above. However, the true causal pathways are likely to be very complex, as reviewed and discussed by Verdoux in this volume; she also reviews all the relevant studies.

■ Conclusions from the study of childhood and youth

There is unlikely to be a single, early cause. This simple statement is based on a very complex set of propositions. Any putative cause may result in, or contribute to schizophrenia in a proportion of cases; this (small) proportion can be roughly estimated in some cohort studies. However, the large number of these possible causes suggests no single cause. Even if not all the results are valid, those that are, are very unlikely to be explained by one mechanism, or by a single confounding factor. It is much more likely that these individual putative causes can contribute to several complexes of causes and, depending on the other constituents of these causes, to several possible outcomes.

The most likely unifying mechanism would be a genetic one. Other factors are epi-genetic, always to be seen in a genetic context. In nature, interactions between genes and the environment are more likely to be the rule, even though the ability to model them in research is presently the exception. However, our notions of a genetic effect need to become sophisticated. The remarkable finding by Malaspina and colleagues [84] that paternal age is crucially related to risk for schizophrenia suggests the importance of non-Mendelian mechanisms, as may recent findings from functional genomic investigations (see Falkai, this volume; 98).

Are there causal sub-groups?

There may be many routes by which risk for schizophrenia may be increased. Indeed, many or perhaps *any* factors that can have a deleterious effect on the developing brain in early life may result in an increased risk of disorder. Precisely what might constitute a sufficient causal constellation will inevitably be much more complex. Small effect sizes for many of these individual factors suggest that on their own they are unlikely necessary and sufficient causes.

Regarding developmental effects, recent cohort studies have cast new light on the way some of these may be operating. There is evidence for dose-response relationships between risk for schizophrenia and hypoxia, timing of developmental milestones, pre-psychotic IQ and behaviour. This suggests that many children at 100 % risk for schizophrenia are showing small effects, not scoring as highly as they would have done if they had not been subject to some abnormal developmental mechanism. Thus, the whole population of children at 100 % risk is shifted relative to the population at zero risk. As noted in the previous paragraph, there may be a number of possible causes for such a shift. The notion of multiple genes of small effect (Quantitative Trait Loci; QTL) being involved in schizophrenia allows genetic effects to be involved in this way. So, too, precipitating factors such as drugs. Cannabis consumption has a dose-response relationship with later risk of schizophrenia [4]. The notion of stress occurring in discrete packets or "life events" suits research rather more than real life where there is not evidence of a threshold after which psycho-social stress becomes toxic.

As already mentioned, this shift may in itself be a part of a cause in that some of the effects have arrows impinging on development as causes. Once a child suffers a developmental perturbation in any domain, then its micro- or social environment is changed and the development of brain and mind will also be affected. This might further impinge upon the environment, setting-up what has been termed a self-perpetuating cascade of abnormal development [64]. Under this form of dynamic model, no two routes to schizophrenia would be alike, and many children at risk would not develop the disorder.

However, linear trends in associations may still hide sub-groups. These may not be apparent in terms of single variables such as IQ, but may exist in multivariate domains. Sets of many risk factors may combine in discrete ways that are not apparent when individual factors are looked at in isolation. If this were the case then any one multivariate subgroup would likely account for only a very small proportion of schizophrenia. They would also be beyond the statistical resolution of current cohort studies. The prevalence of some individual risk factors is low so the numbers of cases with certain combinations is too low for analysis.

In addition, it may be that only a small proportion of cases has been affected, say in terms of a slightly lower IQ. If only 10 % of children at risk of schizophrenia have an equal decrement in their IQ, but this decrement occurs regardless of what would have been their IQ then the whole group will appear to have shifted.

The same argument could be mounted for behaviour if a sub-group were a little more anxious in social situations than they might have been, for instance. However, huge effects in this sub-group would be necessary to shift the mean value.

It is necessary to judge abnormality in terms of what the value would have been, not in terms of some arbitrary cut-off defined by population norms. Take the example of mental handicap. This may be defined as scoring below 70 points on an IQ test. A decrement of 10 points is a large effect that may betray an important neurobiological process. It would be missed in a bright child with a score of 130 if judged against an arbitrary definition of abnormality.

In this way, binary definitions of normal versus abnormal, and of causes being present or absent are inadequate to describe the patterns arising from this kind of analysis where the greater the dose of a cause, the greater the likelihood of disorder. Susser [133] picks up this theme familiar to the epidemiology of other chronic diseases. Similarly, genetic research now acknowledges that the presence or absence of a single gene is unlikely to explain genetic liability to schizophrenia. Multiple genes of small effect acting in distributed or dose-response fashion are more likely to be involved.

The analysis of general population cohorts allows these effects to be demonstrated, but it does not allow the distinction between a widespread effect in children who go on to develop schizophrenia and a small group being affected relative to their expected characteristics. Analysis of monozygotic twin pairs discordant for schizophrenia suggests the effects are widespread. Suddath and colleagues [128] demonstrated that affected twins had a predictably increased cerebral ventricle system volume, and smaller temporal lobes than their unaffected twin, regardless of the absolute dimensions. This effect in cerebral structures was mirrored in an epidemiological analysis of a case-control study of ventricle dimensions [65]. The predictable decrement in affected twins has also been demonstrated in other domains such as cognitive function [141, 153]. Lane et al. [78] has shown a shift towards greater numbers of dysmorphic facial features in schizophrenia; the same notion of a dose-response relationship with a physical, developmental risk factor.

These effects are unlikely to be specific for schizophrenia [135], though Cannon et al. [21] suggest contrary findings for a broad outcome category where lack of specificity may have different implications compared with studies using narrow criteria. In general, research has concentrated on schizophrenia in its various definitions over the century, rather than on other disorders. Much more evidence is required. In the British 1958 birth cohort Done and colleagues [37] demonstrated differences in the behaviour of children who developed affective and other disorders in adult life; these were different from the effects seen in schizophrenia. In the 1946 cohort, van Os and colleagues [143] demonstrated similar developmental precursors in affective disorder as those that had been shown for schizophrenia. Behaviour was different, and the magnitude of developmental effects somewhat smaller. Cannon and colleagues [9] showed a similar pattern, with developmental effects prior to affective psychosis intermediate between the histories of normal controls and subjects with schizophrenia, at odds with the New Zealand data [21].

Lack of specificity for developmental effects in schizophrenia is, in some senses, disappointing because we value distinctions in classification systems more than similarities. However, the developmental variables in even the best epidemiological studies are relatively crude. There may be a variety of reasons why a milestone may be delayed or school achievement poor. Early psycho-social risk factors are accepted in the case of affective disorder [122]. In both physical and psycho-social risk factors, similar manifest effects may be the result of quite distinct neurobiological (or psychological) mechanisms in different disorders. In terms of prevention, (see Klosterkötter, this volume) lack of specificity may be an advantage.

In conclusion, causal models of schizophrenia need to include early life, childhood and youth, the periods of the life-course when psychotic syndromes are rare or absent. Epidemiological research is now able to exploit remarkable longitudinal samples that suggest a rich variety of causal factors may antedate the pre-psychotic manifestations of schizophrenia. Those antecedents may, themselves, become part of the genesis of the syndrome, and may betray abnormal or different cognitive developmental processes that lead to vulnerability to psychosis, and determine functional outcome. We know that genetic factors will be part of these developmental processes, but the details remain obscure and a challenge for schizophrenia research. Study of the early stages of the life course will reveal the answers to causes, mechanisms and prevention of this enigmatic condition.

Acknowledgment The author gratefully acknowledges support from the Stanley Foundation.

■ References

1. Albee GW, Lane EA, Corcoran C, Werneke A (1963) Childhood and inter-current intellectual performance of adult schizophrenics. J Consult Psychology 27 (4): 364–366
2. Ambelas A (1992) Preschizophrenics: adding to the evidence, sharpening the focus. Br J Psychiatry 160: 401–404
3. American Psychiatric Association (1987) Diagnostic and Statistical Manual of Mental Disorders. Third Edn – Revised. Washington, DC: American Psychiatric Association
4. Andreasson S, Allebeck P, Engstrom A, Rydberg U (1987) Cannabis and schizophrenia. A longitudinal study of Swedish conscripts. Lancet ii:1483–1486
5. Aylward E, Walker E, Bettes B (1984) Intelligence in schizophrenia: meta-analysis of the research. Schizophrenia Bull 10: 430–459
6. Barker DJP (1992) (ed) Fetal & Infant Origins of Adult Disease. Papers written by the Medical Research Council Environmental Epidemiology Unit London: Br Med J
7. Barker DJP, Osmond C (1986) Childhood respiratory infection and chronic bronchitis in England and Wales. Br Med J 293: 1271–1275
8. Barker DJP, Winter PD, Osmond C, Margetts B, Simmonds SJ (1989) Weight in infancy and death from ischaemic heart disease. Lancet ii: 577–580
9. Barker DJP, Bull AR, Osmond C, Simmonds SJ (1990) Fetal and placental size and risk of hypertension in adult life. Br Med J 301: 259–262
10. Bleuler E (1908) Die Prognose der Dementia Praecox – Schizophreniegruppe. Allgemeine Zeitschrift fur Psychiatrie 65: 436–464. Translated in: Cutting J, Shepherd M (eds) The Clinical Roots of the Schizophrenia Concept (1987). Cambridge CUP pp 59–74
11. Bleuler E (1911) Dementia praecox oder Gruppe der Schizophrenien. Deuticke, Leipzig, Vienna

12. Boyd JH, Pulver AE, Stewart W (1986) Season of birth: schizophrenia and bipolar disorder. Schizophrenia Bull 12: 173–185
13. Bradbury TN, Miller GA (1985) Season of birth in schizophrenia: a review of evidence, methodology, and etiology. Psychological Bulletin 98: 569–594
14. Brown AS, Susser E, Cohen P (1997) Psychosis after prenatal exposure to rubella. Schizophr Res 24 (1,2): 247
15. Brown AS, Cohen P, Greenwald S, Susser E (2000) Non-affective psychosis after prenatal exposure to rubella. Am J Psychiatry 157 (3): 438–443
16. Brown AS, Cohen P, Harkavy-Friedman J, Babulas V, Malaspina D, Gorman JM, Susser ES (2001) Bennett Research Award. Prenatal rubella, premorbid abnormalities, and adult schizophrenia. Biol Psychiatry 49 (6): 473–486
17. Buka SL, Tsuang MT, Lipsitt LP (1993) Pregnancy/delivery complications and psychiatric diagnosis. A prospective study. Arch Gen Psychiatry 50: 151–156
18. Cannon M, Cotter D, Sham PC, Larkin C, Murray RM, Coffey VP, O'Callaghan E (1996) Schizophrenia in an Irish sample following prenatal exposure to the 1957 influenza epidemic: a case-controlled, prospective follow-up study. Abstr Schizophr Res 11: 95
19. Cannon M, Jones P, Gilvarry C, Rifkin L, McKenzie K, Foerster A, Murray R (1997) Premorbid social functioning in schizophrenia and Bipolar disorder. Similarities and differences. Am J Psychiatry 154 (11): 1544–1550
20. Cannon M, Jones P, Huttunen M, Tanskanen A, Huttunen T, Rabe-Hesketh S, Murray RM (1999) School performance in Finnish children and the latter development of schizophrenia: a population-based longitudinal study. Arch Gen Psychiatry 56: 457–463
21. Cannon M, Caspi A, Moffitt T, Harrington H-L, Taylor A, Murray RM, Poulton R (2001) Evidence for early, pan-developmental impairment specific to schizophreniform disorder. Results from a longitudinal birth cohort. Arch Gen Psychiatry 59 (5): 449–456
22. Cannon-Spoor HE, Potkin SG, Wyatt RJ (1982) Measurement of premorbid adjustment in chronic schizophrenia. Schizophr Bulletin 8 (3): 470–484
23. Castillo SM, Cabrera JS (1979) Estudio de las particulas semejantes a virus observadas en la esquizofrenia. Rev Hosp Psiquiatr Habana 10: 725–736
24. Castle D, Wessley S, Der G, Murray RM (1991) The incidence of operationally-defined schizophrenia in Camberwell 1965–84. Br J Psychiatry 159: 790–794
25. Chacon C, Monro M, Harper I (1975) Viral infection and psychiatric disorders. Acta Psychiatr Scand 51: 101–103
26. Chess S, Korn SJ, Fernandez PB (1971) Psychiatric Disorders of Children with Congenital Rubella. Butterworths, London
27. Coffey VP, Jessop WJE (1959) Maternal influenza and congenital deformities: a prospective study. Lancet ii: 935–938
28. Coffey VP, Jessop WJE (1963). Maternal influenza and congenital deformities. A follow-up study. Lancet i: 748–751
29. Cooper SJ, King DJ (1987) Can psychiatric nurses 'catch' schizophrenia? Br J Psychiatr 151: 546–548
30. Crow TJ, Done J (1986) Age of onset of schizophrenia in siblings: a test of contagion hypothesis. Psychiatr Res 18: 107–117
31. Crow TJ, Done J (1992) Prenatal exposure to influenza does not cause schizophrenia. Br J Psychiatry 161: 390–393
32. Crow TJ, Done DJ, Johnstone EC (1991) Schizophrenia and influenza. Lancet 338: 116–117
33. Crow TJ, Done DJ, Sacker A (1995) Childhood precursors of psychosis as clues to its evolutionary origins. Eur Arch Psychiatry & Clin Neurosci 245 (2): 61–69
34. David AS, Cutting J (1994) (eds) The Neuropsychology of Schizophrenia. Lawrence Erlbaum, Hove
35. David AS, Malmberg A, Brandt L, Allebeck P, Lewis G (1997) IQ and risk for schizophrenia: a population-based cohort study. Psychol Medicine 27: 1311–1323
36. Davidson M, Reichenberg A, Rabinowitz J, Weiser M, Kaplan Z, Mark M (1999) Behavioral and intellectual markers for schizophrenia in apparently healthy male adolescents. Am J Psychiatry 156 (9): 1328–1335

37. Done DJ, Crow TJ, Johnstone EC, Sacker A (1994) Childhood antecedents of schizophrenia and affective illness: social adjustment at ages 7 and 11. Br Med J 309: 699–703
38. Done J, Johnstone EC, Frith CD, Golding J, Shepard PM, Crow TJ (1991) Complications of pregnancy and delivery in relation to psychosis in adult life: data from the British Perinatal Mortality Survey. Br Med J 302: 1576–1580
39. Erlenmeyer-Kimling L, Cornblatt B, Friedman D et al. (1982) Neurological, electro-physiological and attentional deviations in children at risk of schizophrenia. In: Henn FA, Nasrallah H (eds) Schizophrenia as a Brain Disease. OUP, New York, pp 61–98
40. Erlenmeyer-Kimling L, Folnegovic Z, Hrabak-Zerjavic V, Borcic B, Folnegovic-Smalc V, Susser E (1994) Schizophrenia and prenatal exposure to the 1957 A2 influenza epidemic in Croatia. Am J Psychiatry 151 (10): 1496–1498
41. Fine PEM, Adelstein AM, Snowman J, Clarkson JA, Evans SM (1985) Long term effects of exposure to viral infections in utero. Br Med J 290: 509–511
42. Fish B (1977) Neurobiological antecedents of schizophrenia in children. Arch Gen Psychiatry 34: 1297–1313
43. Fish B, Marcus J, Hans SL, Auerbach JG, Perdue S (1992) Infants at risk for schizophrenia: sequelae of a genetic neurointegrative defect. Arch Gen Psychiatry 49: 221–235
44. Foerster A, Lewis SW, Owen MJ, Murray RM (1991) Pre-morbid adjustment and personality in psychosis. Effects of sex and diagnosis. Br J Psychiatry 158: 171–176
45. Geddes JR, Lawrie SM (1995) Obstetric events in schizophrenia: a meta-analysis. Br J Psychiatry 167: 786–793
46. Gervin M, Browne S, Lane A, Clarke M, Waddington JL, Larkin C, O'Callaghan E (1998) Spontaneous abnormal involuntary movements in first episode schizophrenia and schizophreniform disorder: baseline rate in a group of patients from an Irish catchment area. Am J Psychiatry 155: 1202–1206
47. Gilvarry CM, Sham PC, Jones PB, Cannon M, Wright P, Lewis SW, Bebbington P, Toone BK, Murray RM (1996) Autoimmune diseases and psychosis: a case control family study. Schizophr Res 19: 33–40
48. Gittleman-Klein R, Klein DF (1969) Premorbid social adjustment and prognosis in schizophrenia. J Psych Research 7: 35–53
49. Goodman R (1988) Obstetric complications and schizophrenia. Br J Psychiatry 153: 850
50. Green MF (1998) Schizophrenia from a Neurocognitive Perspective. Probing the Impenetrable Darkness. Allyn & Bacon, Needham Heights, MA
51. Hafner H, Riecher A, Maurer K, Loffler W (1989) How does gender influence age at first hospitalisation for schizophrenia? A transnational case register study. Psychol Med 19: 903–918.
52. Hafner H, Maurer K, Loffler W, Riecher-Rossler A (1993) The influence of age and sex on the onset and early course of schizophrenia. Br J Psychiatry 162: 80–86
53. Hare EH (1975) Season of birth in schizophrenia and neurosis. Am J Psychiatry 132: 1168–1171
54. Hare EH (1976) The season of birth of siblings of psychiatric patients. Br J Psychiatry 129: 49–54
55. Hare EH, Price JS, Slater ETO (1974) Mental disorder and season of birth: a national sample compared with the general population. Br J Psychiatry 124: 81–86
56. Hunt H (1952) Testing for psychological deficit. In: Brower D, Abt LE (eds) Progress in Clinical Psychology. Vol I Ronald Press, New York
57. Hunt JMcV, Cofer C (1944) Psychological deficit. In: Hunt JMcV (ed) Personality and the Behavior Disorders. Ronald Press, New York.
58. Huttunen M, Niskanen P (1978) Prenatal loss of father and psychiatric disorders. Arch Gen Psychiatry 35: 427–431
59. Isohanni M, Mäkikyrö T, Moring J, Rasanen P, Hakko H, Partanen U, Koiranen M, Jones PB (1997) A comparison of clinical and research DSM-III-R diagnoses of schizophrenia in a Finnish national birth cohort. Soc Psychiatry Psychiatric Epidemiol 32: 303–308

60. Isohanni M, Jones PB, Kemppainen L, Croudace T, Isohanni I, Veijola J, Rasanen S, Wahlberg KE, Tienari P, Rantakallio P (2000) Childhood and adolescent predictors of schizophrenia in the Northern Finland 1966 birth cohort – a descriptive life-span model. Eur Arch Psychiatry Clin Neurosci 250 (6): 311–319

61. Isohanni M, Jones P B, Moilanen K, Rantakallio P, Veijola J, Oja H, Koiranen M, Jokelainen J, Croudace T, Jarvelin MR (2001) Early developmental milestones in adult schizophrenia and other psychoses. A 31-year follow-up of the North Finland 1966 birth cohort. Schizophr Res 52: 1–19

62. Jones PB (1999) Longitudinal approaches to the search for the causes of schizophrenia: past, present and future. In: Hafner H, Gattaz WF (eds) Search for the Causes of Schizophrenia, Vol. IV. Darmstadt: Steinkopff (Springer), Berlin, pp 91–119

63. Jones PB (1996) Childhood motor milestones and IQ prior to adult schizophrenia: results from a 43-year-old British birth cohort. Psychiatria Fennica 26: 63–80

64. Jones PB, Rodgers B, Murray RM, Marmot MG (1994) Child developmental risk factors for adult schizophrenia in the British 1946 birth cohort. Lancet 344: 1398–1402

65. Jones PB, Guth CW, Lewis SW, Murray RM (1994) Low intelligence and poor educational achievement precede early onset schizophrenic psychosis. In: David AS, Cutting J (eds) The Neuropsychology of Schizophrenia Lawrence Erlbaum, Hove, pp 131–144

66. Jones PB, Murray RM, Rodgers B (1995) Childhood risk factors for schizophrenia in a general population birth cohort at age 43 years. In: Mednick SA, Hollister JM (eds) Neural Development in Schizophrenia: Theory and Practice. Plenum Press, New York, pp 151–176

67. Jones PB, Cannon M (1998) The new epidemiology of schizophrenia: common methods for genetics and environment. Psychiatric Clinics of North America 21 (1): 1–25

68. Jones PB, Done DJ (1997) From birth to onset: a developmental perspective of schizophrenia in two national birth cohorts. In: Keshavan MS, Murray RM (eds) Neurodevelopment and Adult Psychopathology. Chapter 9 CUP: Cambridge, pp 119–136

69. Jones PB, Rantakallio P, Hartikainen AL, Isohanni M, Sipila P (1998) Schizophrenia as a long-term outcome of pregnancy, delivery and perinatal complications: a 28-year follow-up of the 1966 North Finland general population birth cohort. Am J Psychiatry 155: 355–364

70. Jones PB, Pang D, Piracha S, Fine PEM (1998) The long-term effects of viral infections in utero: a 35 year follow-up study. Presentation at the Stanley Foundation symposium on bipolar disorder. Royal Society, London, September 1998

71. Kendell RE, Kemp IW (1989) Maternal influenza in the etiology of schizophrenia. Arch Gen Psychiatry 46: 878–882

72. Kendell RE, Adams W (1991) Unexplained fluctuations in the risk for schizophrenia by month and year of birth. Br J Psychiatry 158: 758–763

73. Kendell RE, McInneny K, Juszczak E, Bain M (2000) Obstetric complications and schizophrenia. Two case-control studies based on structured obstetric records. Br J Psychiatry 176: 516–522

74. Keshavan MS, Murray RM (eds) (1997) Neurodevelopment and Adult Psychopathology. CUP, Cambridge

75. Kraepelin E (1896) Dementia Praecox. Psychiatrie 5th Edition. pp 426–441. Barth: Leipzig. Translated in: Cutting J, Shepherd M (eds) The Clinical Roots of the Schizophrenia Concept (1987). CUP Cambridge, pp 13–24

76. Kuh D, Ben-Shlomo Y (eds) (1997) A Life-Course Approach to Chronic Disease Epidemiology. OUP, Oxford

77 Kunugi H, Nanko S, Takei N, Saito K, Hayashi N, Kazamatsuri H (1995) Schizophrenia following in utero exposure to the 1957 influenza epidemics in Japan. Am J Psychiatry 152: 450–452

78. Lane A, Kinsella A, Murphy P, Byrne M, Keenan J, Colgan K, Cassidy B, Sheppard N, Horgan R, Waddington JL, Larkin C, O'Callaghan E (1997) The anthropometric assessment of dysmorphic features in schizophrenia as an index of its developmental origins. Psychol Med 27: 1155–1164

79. Lane EA, Albee GW (1963) Childhood intellectual development of adult schizophrenics. J Abnorm Soc Psychol 67: 186–189

80. Lewis MS, Griffin PA (1981) An explanation for the season of birth effect in schizophrenia and certain other diseases. Psychol Bull 89: 589–596
81. Lewis MS (1989) Age incidence and schizophrenia: Part 1. The season of birth controversy. Schizophr Bull 15: 59–73
82. Lewis SW, Owen MJ, Murray RM (1989) Obstetric complications and schizophrenia: methodology and mechanisms. In: Schulz SC, Tamminga CA (eds) Schizophrenia – A Scientific Focus. Oxford University Press, New York, pp 56–68
83. Lubin A, Gieseking CF, Williams HL (1962) Direct measurement of cognitive deficit in schizophrenia. J Consult Psychol 26: 139–143
84. Malaspina D, Harlap S, Fennig S, Heiman D, Nahon D, Feldman D, Susser ES (2001) Advancing paternal age and the risk of schizophrenia. Arch Gen Psychiatry 58 (4): 361–367
85. Malmberg A, Lewis G, David A, Allebeck P (1998) Premorbid adjustment and personality in people with schizophrenia. Br J Psychiatry 172: 308–313
86. Marmott M, Wadsworth MEJ (eds) (1997) Fetal and early childhood environment: long-term health implications. Br Med Bull 53 (1): 126–146
87. Mason CF (1956) Pre-illness intelligence of mental hospital patients. J Consult Psychol 20: 297–300
88. Mattock C, Marmot M, Stern G (1988) Could Parkinson's disease follow intra-uterine influenza? a speculative hypothesis. J Neurol. Neurosurg Psychiatry 51: 753–756
89. McGrath J (1999) Hypothesis: is low prenatal vitamin D a risk-modifying factor for schizophrenia? Schizophr Res 40 (3): 173–177
90. McGrath J (2001) Does 'imprinting' with low prenatal vitamin D contribute to the risk of various adult disorders? Med Hypoth 56 (3): 367–371
91. McGrath JJ, Pemberton MR, Welham JL, Murray RM (1994) Schizophrenia and the influenza epidemics of 1954, 1957 and 1959 : a southern hemisphere study. Schizophr. Res 14: 1–8
92. McGrath JJ, Castle D, Murray RM (1995) How can we judge whether or not prenatal exposure to influenza causes schizophrenia. In: Mednick SA, Hollister JM (eds) Neural Development and Schizophrenia. Theory and Research. Plenum Press, New York
93. McIntosh ED, Menser MA (1992) A fifty-year follow-up of congenital rubella. Lancet 340: 414–415
94. Mednick SA, Machon RA, Huttunen MO, Bonett D (1988) Adult schizophrenia following prenatal exposure to an influenza epidemic. Arch Gen Psychiatry 45: 189–192
95. Mednick SA, Machon RA, Huttunen MO (1990) An update on the Helsinki influenza project. Letter to Editor. Arch Gen Psychiatry 47: 292
96. Mednick SA, Huttunen MO, Machon RA (1994) Prenatal influenza infections and adult schizophrenia. Schizophr Bull 20: 263–267
97. Menninger KA (1926) Influenza and schizophrenia. Am J Psychiatry 5: 469–529
98. Mimmack ML, Ryan M, Baba H, Navarro-Ruiz J, Iritani S, Faull RLM, McKenna PJ, Jones PB, Arai H, Starkey M, Emson PC, Bahn S (2002) Gene expression analysis in schizophrenia: reproducible upregulation of several members of the apolipoprotein L family located in a high susceptibility locus for schizophrenia on chromosome 22. Proc Natl Acad Sci 99 (7): 4680–4685
99. Morgan V, Castle D, Page A, Fazio S, Gurrin L, Burton P, Montgomery P, Jablensky A (1997) Influenza epidemics and incidence of schizophrenia, affective disorders and mental retardation in Western Australia: no evidence of a major effect. Schizophr Res 26: 25–39
100. Murray RM, Jones PB, O'Callaghan E, Takei N, Sham PC (1992) Genes, Viruses and Neurodevelopmental Schizophrenia. J Psychiatric Res 26 (4): 225–235
101. Myhrman A, Rantakallio P, Isohanni M, Jones PB, Partanen U (1996) Does unwantedness of a pregnancy predict schizophrenia? Br J Psychiatry 169: 637–640
102. Nelson KB, Ellenberg JH (1986) Antecedents of cerebral palsy: multivariate analysis of risk. New Eng J Med 315: 81–86
103. O'Callaghan E, Sham P, Takei N, Glover G, Murray RM (1991) Schizophrenia after prenatal exposure to 1957 A2 influenza epidemic. Lancet 337: 1248–1250
104. Parker G (1978) Schizophrenia and season of birth: further southern hemisphere studies. Aus NZ J Psychiatr 12: 65–67

105. Parker G, Neilson M (1976) Mental disorder and season of birth – a southern hemisphere study. Br J Psychiatry 129: 355–361
106. Pasamanick B, Rodgers ME, Lilienfield AM (1956) Pregnancy experience and behaviour disorder in children. Am J Psychiatry 112: 613–618
107. Pidgeon DA (1964) Tests used in the 1954 and 1957 surveys. In: Douglas JWB (ed) The Home and the School. MacGibbon & Kee, London, pp 129–132
108. Pidgeon DA (1968) Appendix: details of the fifteen year tests. In: Douglas JWB, Ross JM, Simpson HR (eds) All Our Futures. Peter Davies, London, pp 194–197
109. Poulton R, Caspi A, Moffitt TE, Cannon M, Murray R, Harrington H (2000) Children's self-reported psychotic symptoms and adult schizophreniform disorder: a 15-year longitudinal study. Arch Gen Psychiatry 57 (11): 1053–1058
110. Price JS, Hare EH (1969) Birth Order Studies: some sources of bias. Br J Psychiatry 115: 633–646
111. Rantakallio P (1969) Groups at risk in low birth weight infants and perinatal mortality. Acta Paediatrica Scandinavia Supplement 193: 1–71
112. Rantakallio P, von Wendt L (1986) A prospective comparative study of the etiology of cerebral palsy and epilepsy in a one-year birth cohort from Northern Finland. Acta Paediatr Scand 75: 586–592
113. Rantakallio P, Jones P, Moring J, Von Wendt L (1997) Association between central nervous system infections during childhood and adult onset schizophrenia and other psychoses: a 28-year follow- up. Int J Epidemiol 26: 837–843
114. Rappaport SR, Webb WB (1950) An attempt to study intellectual deterioration by pre-morbid testing. J Consult Psychol 14: 95–98
115. Robins LN (1966) Deviant Children Grown Up. A Sociological and Psychiatric Study of Sociopathic Personality. Williams and Wilkins, Baltimore
116. Robins LN, Rutter M (eds) (1990) Straight and Devious Pathways from Childhood to Adulthood. Cambridge University Press, Cambridge 1991, c1990
117. Rothman KJ (1976) Causes. Am J Epidemiol 104: 587–592
118. Rothman KJ (1977) Causes and risks. In: Clark MA (ed) Pulmonary Disease: Defense Mechanisms and Populations at Risk. Tobacco and Health Research Institute, Lexington, KY
119. Rothman KJ (ed) (1988) Causal Inference. Epidemiology Resources, Chestnut Hill, MA
120. Russell AJ, Munro JC, Jones PB, Hemsley DR, Murray RM (1997) Schizophrenia and the myth of intellectual decline. Am J Psychiatry 154 (5): 635–639
121. Sacker A, Done DJ, Crow TJ, Golding J (1995) Antecedents of schizophrenia and affective illness. Obstetric complications. Br J Psychiatry 166 (6): 734–741
122. Sadowski H, Ugarte B, Kolvin I, Kaplan C, Barnes J (1999) Early life family disadvantages and major depression in adulthood. Br J Psychiatry 174: 112–120
123. Sèlten JPCJ, Slaets JPJ (1994) Second-trimester exposure to 1957 A2 influenza epidemic is not a risk factor for schizophrenia. Abstr Schizophr Res 11: 95
124. Sham PC, O'Callaghan E, Takei N, Murray GK, Hare EH, Murray RM (1992) Schizophrenia following pre-natal exposure to influenza epidemics between 1939 and 1960. Br J Psychiatry 160: 461–466
125. Schur E, Hare EH (1983) Age prevalence and the season of birth effect in schizophrenia: a response to Lewis and Griffin. Psychol Bull 93: 373–377
126. Stevens JR, Hallick LM (1992) Viruses and schizophrenia. In: Specter S, Bendinelli M, Friedman H (eds) Neuropathogenic Viruses and Immunity. Plenum, New York, pp 27–53
127. Stevens JR, Albrecht P, Godfrey L, Krauthammer E (1983) Viral antigen in the brain of schizophrenic patients? In: Morozov PV (ed) Research on the Viral Hypothesis of Mental Disorders. Karger, Basel, pp 76–96
128. Suddath RL, Christison GW, Torrey EF, Casanova MF, Weinberger DR (1990) Anatomical abnormalities in the brains of monozygotic twins discordant for schizophrenia. New Eng J Med 322: 789–794
129. Susser E, Lin SP (1992) Schizophrenia after prenatal exposure to the Dutch hunger winter of 1944–1945. Arch Gen Psychiatry 49: 983–988

130. Susser E, Lin SP (1994) Schizophrenia after prenatal exposure to the Dutch hunger winter of 1944–1945. Arch Gen Psychiatry 51: 333–334
131. Susser ES, Lin SP, Brown AS, Lumey LH, Erlenmeyer-Kimling L (1994) No relation between risk of schizophrenia and prenatal exposure to influenza in Holland. Am J Psychiatry 151: 922–924
132. Susser E, Neugebauer R, Hoek HW, Brown AS, Lin S, Labovitz D, Gorman JM (1996) Schizophrenia after prenatal famine. Arch Gen Psychiatry 53: 25–31
133. Susser E, Brown AS, Gorman JM (eds) (1999) Prenatal Exposures in Schizophrenia. American Psychiatric Association Press: Washington DC
134. Takei N, Sham P, O'Callaghan E, Murray GK, Glover G, Murray RM (1994) Prenatal exposure to influenza and the development of schizophrenia: is the effect confined to females? Am J Psychiatry 151: 117–119
135. Tarrant J, Jones PB (1999) Precursors to schizophrenia: do biological markers for schizophrenia have specificity? Can J Psychiatry 44: 176–195
136. Tienari P, Sorri A, Lahti I, Naarala M, Wahlberg K, Moring J, Pohjola J, Wynne LC (1987) Genetic and psychosocial factors in schizophrenia: The Finnish Adoptive Family Study. Schizophr Bull 13 (3): 477–484
137. Tienari P, Wynne LC, Moring J, Laksy K, Nieminen P, Sorri A, Lahti I, Wahlberg K-E, Naarala M, Kurki-Suonio K, Saarento O, Koistinen P, Tarvainen T, Hakko H, Miettunen J (2000) Finnish adoptive family study: sample selection and adoptee DSM-III-R diagnoses. Acta Psychiatr Scand 101 (6): 433–443
138. Torrey EF, Peterson MR (1973) Slow and latent viruses in schizophrenia. Lancet 2: 22–24
139. Torrey EF, Bowler AE (1990) The seasonality of schizophrenic births: a reply to Marc S Lewis. Schizophr Bull 16 (1): 1–3
140. Torrey EF, Bowler A (1990) Geographical distribution of insanity in America: evidence for an urban factor. Schizophr Bull 16: 591–604
141. Torrey EF, Bowler AE, Rawlings R, Terrazas A (1993) Seasonality of schizophrenia and stillbirths. Schizophr Bull 19: 557–562
142. Tramer T (1929) Uber die biologische Bedeutung des Geburtesmonnates fur die Psychogerkrankung. Schweizer. Archiv fur Neurologie und Psychiatrie 24: 17–24
143. van Os J, Jones PB, Lewis G, Wadsworth M, Murray R (1997) Developmental precursors of affective illness in a general population birth cohort. Arch Gen Psychiatry 54: 625–631
144. van Os J, Selten J-P (1998) Prenatal exposure to maternal stress and later schizophrenia: the May 1940 invasion of the Netherlands. Br J Psychiatry 172: 324–326
145. Wadsworth MEJ (1987) Follow-up of the first national birth cohort: findings from the Medical Research Council National Survey of Health and Development. Paediatric and Perinatal Epidemiology 1: 95–117
146. Wadsworth MEJ (1991) The Imprint of Time. Childhood history and adult life. Clarendon Press, Oxford
147. Walker E, Lewine RJ (1990) Prediction of adult-onset schizophrenia from childhood home movies of the patients. Am J Psychiatry 147: 1052–1056
148. Walker EF, Grimes KE, Davis DM, Smith AJ (1993) Childhood precursors of schizophrenia: facial expressions of emotion. Am J Psychiatry 150: 1654–1660
149. Watson CG, Kucala T, Angulski G, Brunn C (1982) Season of birth and schizophrenia: a response to the Lewis and Griffin critique. J Abnorm Psychol 91: 120–125
150. Watt NF (1978) Patterns of childhood social development in adult schizophrenics. Arch Gen Psychiatry 35: 160–165
151. Watt N, Lubensky A (1976) Childhood roots of schizophrenia. J Consult Clin Psychol 44: 363–375
152. Weinberger DR (1995) From neuropathology to neurodevelopment. Lancet 346: 552–557
153. Weinberger DR, Berman KF Suddath R, Torrey EF (1992) Evidence for a prefrontal-limbic network in schizophrenia: a magnetic resonance and regional cerebral blood flow study of discordant monozygotic twins. Am J Psychiatry 149: 890–897
154. Wright P, Sham PC, Gilvarry C, Jones PB, Cannon M, Sharma T, Murray RM (1996) Autoimmune disorders in the pedigrees of schizophrenic and control subjects. Schizophr Res 20: 261–267

155. Yolken RH, Torrey EF (1995) Viruses, schizophrenia and bipolar disorder. Clin Microbiol Rev 8: 131–145
156. Zornberg GL, Buka SL, Tsuang MT (2000) Hypoxic-ischemia-related fetal/neonatal complications and risk of schizophrenic and other nonaffective psychoses: a 19-year longitudinal study. Am J Psychiatry 157 (2): 196–202
157. Zornberg GL, Buka SL, Tsuang MT (2000) The problem of obstetrical complications and schizophrenia. Schizophr Bull 26 (2) 249–256

Association between cognitive and behavioral functioning, non-psychotic psychiatric diagnoses, and drug abuse in adolescence, with later hospitalization for schizophrenia

M. Weiser
Sheba Medical Center, Tel Hashomer, Israel

Many efforts are being made to identify factors which increase the risk of later schizophrenia. This is important both in the hope that these markers will shed light on the pathophysiology of the illness, and might enable identification of persons very early in the course of the illness. This chapter will briefly review the main risk factors which have been identified for schizophrenia and will focus on risk factors for schizophrenia in adolescence.

▪ Risk factors for schizophrenia

Having a family history of schizophrenia is the strongest risk factor of future schizophrenia, studies indicating that approximately 12% of children with one parent with schizophrenia, up to 40% of children with two parents with schizophrenia, and up to 50% of identical twins are later diagnosed with the disease [1, 2]. However, although genetic factors significantly increase the risk for future illness, 90% of persons with schizophrenia will have neither parent ill with schizophrenia [3]. Other risk factors include maternal exposure to infection [4], and obstetric complications, including low birth weight [5], asphyxia at birth [6–8], preterm birth [9] and preeclampsia [10]. Delayed childhood development has been shown to be associated with future schizophrenia: delays in ages at learning to stand [11], walk [11, 12] and becoming potty-trained [11]. In addition, poor social functioning, including solitary play preferences even at age 4 [12], and fewer expressions of joy and more negative affects as children [13] have been associated with future schizophrenia. Below-normal intellectual functioning and school marks at ages 4, 10, and other ages [12], have also been associated with later onset of schizophrenia.

The purpose of this chapter is to present a series of studies on risk factors for schizophrenia which are present in adolescents aged 16–17. The studies presented here are a follow-back or historical prospective study. This has the advantage that is drawn from an epidemiological population, not from a sample, and that it captures a very large population of cases; hence it can examine markers predicting vulnerability to the illness with high statistical power. This was done by merging the Israeli National Psychiatric Hospitalization Case Registry with the Draft Board Registry, which contains the scores of cognitive and behavioral assessments, psychiatric diagnoses obtained at age 16–17 for the entire population, and records self-reported drug abuse for males identified as having behavioral problems.

The following is a summary of cognitive and behavioral functioning [14], non-psychotic psychiatric diagnoses [15], and drug abuse [16] that were identified as risk factors for schizophrenia in adolescence identified using this study design. Because the in-depth Draft Board assessment is applied only to males, these risk factors are relevant for male adolescents only.

▪ Method

Draft Board assessment

Israeli law requires that all adolescents between the ages of 16 and 17 undergo pre-induction assessment to determine their intellectual, medical and psychiatric eligibility for military service. This assessment is compulsory and is administered to the entire, unselected, population of Israeli adolescents. It includes individuals who will be eligible for military service, as well as those who will be excused from service based on medical, psychiatric or social reasons. The initial Draft Board assessment consists of a cognitive test battery and an interview assessing personality and behavioral traits conducted by a psychometrician, which are administrated to all male adolescents. Those adolescents identified as problematic and are referred for an in-depth psycho-social assessment, including screening for drug abuse. If a psychiatric diagnosis is likely, the adolescent is referred to a psychiatrist who assigns a psychiatric diagnosis where deemed appropriate. The draft board assessment is described in detail elsewhere [15, 17, 18].

The *cognitive test battery* yields a total score which is a highly valid measure of general intelligence equivalent to a normally distributed IQ score. The cognitive assessment is comprised of four sub-tests which assess arithmetic ability (Arithmetic-R); verbal abstraction and concept formation (Similarities-R); visiospatial abilities (RPM-R), and the ability to understand written instructions (OTIS-R).

The *behavioral assessment* is done by a trained psychometrician who administers a structured interview evaluating:
a) *social functioning* which assess social potency (e.g., likes to take charge, likes to be noticed at social events), and social closeness (e.g., sociable, have close interpersonal ties),
b) *individual autonomy* which assesses personal autonomy, maturity and self-directed behavior (e.g., ability to function and make decisions independently),
c) *organizational ability* which assesses compliance to time tables, self-mastery and self-care (e.g., ability to adhere to a schedule and tidiness responsibility), and
d) *physical activity* which assesses the involvement in extracurricular activities concentrating in health-related physical activities (e.g., interest in sports and hiking).

The behavior is rated on a 1 (worst) to 5 (best) scale based on predetermined reliable and validated instructions. Examples of questions in the interview are: how many good friends do you have? do you tend to be the center of attention at parties?, how often are you late for school?, do you consider yourself organized?, and who cleans your room? After this initial screening interview, those adolescents who are suspected of having significant behavioral problems are referred for an in-depth psychosocial assessment.

Screening for drug abuse: all adolescents who meet the criteria for referral for the in-depth psychosocial assessment are first asked a general screening question: "Have you ever used drugs?". Those who respond affirmatively are then questioned in detail regarding the kind of drugs used, the frequency of drug use, and the psychological and physical effects of the drug. The interviewer assesses if the subject is addicted to drugs, if the use of drugs is daily and/or is a significant part of his life style or social life, and if these criteria are met, he is reported as a drug user in a yes/no format. Sporadic users are classified as non-users. Although the types of drugs used are not specified, data from several door-to-door studies on drug use between ages 12–18, carried out by the Israeli health authorities in 1989, 1992 and again in 1995, the time period that the data reported here were collected, indicate that the majority of drug users in this age group principally used marijuana.

The *mental health assessment* is a comprehensive psycho-social examination performed by a clinical social worker or psychologist, who inquires about personal and family history, previous psychological and psychiatric treatments, interpersonal relationships, self-esteem, self-injurious and anti-social acts, and functioning within the family and in school. If the clinician suspects that the adolescent suffers from psychopathology, a provisional diagnosis is suggested, and the adolescent is then referred for evaluation to a board certified psychiatrist experienced in treating adolescents. Adolescents who had previously been treated by mental health professionals, or who had been hospitalized, are required to present treatment summaries and/or discharge letters. Diagnoses during the time covered by this study were based on ICD-9 criteria. In cases of co-morbidity, the examining psychiatrist decides which diagnosis is most clinically significant, and only that diagnosis is recorded, without the co-morbid condition. For the sake of simplicity, personality disorders were divided into three groups: schizophrenia spectrum personality disorders (schizotypal and paranoid personality disorders), anti-social personality disorder, and other personality disorders (avoidant, dependent, histrionic, obsessive-compulsive, narcissistic, borderline or schizoid personality disorders). Because the ICD-9 code for affective disorders includes affective disorder with or without psychotic features, and because we were interested in future schizophrenia in adolescents with non-psychotic psychiatric diagnoses, adolescents diagnosed with affective disorders in the draft board were not included in the analysis, as some of the adolescents with affective disorders had psychotic as well as affective symptoms.

The National Psychiatric Hospitalization Case Registry is a complete listing of all psychiatric hospitalizations in the country, including the diagnosis assigned and coded upon admission and discharge by a board-certified psychiatrist at the facility. During the time covered by this study, ICD 9 diagnoses were used by the registry. All inpatient psychiatric facilities in the country, including psychiatric hospitals, day hospitals and psychiatric units in general hospitals, are required by law to report all admissions and discharges to the registry.

Study populations

Due to periodic changes in Draft Board procedure, each of the three research questions addressed utilized the assessments of adolescents examined by the draft board during slightly different time periods and therefore examined slightly different, but overlapping populations assessed by the draft board during the 1980s and 1990s. Follow-up periods ranged from 4–15 years, and the risk for schizophrenia in this population was 0.46 – 0.52%, which is compatible with the age-adjusted incidence of schizophrenia in other studies carried out in Israel [11], and the United States [12]. In order to limit this analysis to apparently healthy individuals with no obvious signs of disease, draftees who presented clinically detectable signs or symptoms of any mental illness or of mental retardation for which they were exempted from the draft, were excluded from further analysis. Also, in order to lessen the chance of including patients in the prodrome or initial stages of their disease, individuals who had a psychiatric hospitalization prior to the Draft Board assessment or within one year from the date of Draft Board assessment were excluded. The scores of the cases were compared to the mean scores of a control group made up of all individuals tested at the same age and attending the same high school who were found eligible for military service and did not appear in the Psychiatric Hospitalization Registry. Matching cases to non-cases by high school attended at the time of testing was an attempt to control for educational and social opportunities.

Results

The analysis of behavioral and cognitive scores focused on examining the extent to which test scores could be used to correctly classify draftees as cases or controls. The 509 cases were compared to their matched control schoolmates using a paired samples t-test. As a group, individuals destined to develop schizophrenia (n = 509) obtained statistically significant lower (worse) scores on all measures as compared to matched non-cases (n = 9,215) and to the entire population (all p values were lower than 0.0001). The differences between future cases and controls ranged from 0.3 – 0.5 standard deviations. To examine the extent to which the behavioral and cognitive measures discriminated between the cases and matched controls, Table 1 displays the distribution of the scores in these two groups. For these analyses the mean score of the non-case matched comparisons was used. As can be seen, there are large and statistically significant differences on all behavioral measures. The most pronounced differences were in social functioning, where 8.3% of cases had the lowest score and 35.1% had the second to lowest score, whereas only 0.8% and 6.2% of non-cases respectively had scores

Table 1. Contingency table comparing cases and non-cases on behavioral measures (**A**) and on intellectual functioning (cases and the mean scores of controls; row percentages)

A.	1-Low	2	3	4	5-High	Significance	
Social Functioning						$\chi^2 = 214.7$, $p < 0.000$	df = 4,
Cases	8.3 %	35.1 %	46.6 %	9.6 %	0.4 %		
Comparisons	0.8 %	6.2 %	85.6 %	7.4 %	0.0 %		
Organizational ability						$\chi^2 = 96.0$, $p < 0.000$	df = 4,
Cases	11.6 %	16.6 %	59.3 %	11.0 %	1.5 %		
Comparisons	0.8 %	13.4 %	81.0 %	4.8 %	0.0 %		
Physical activity						$\chi^2 = 78.5$, $p < 0.000$	df = 4,
Cases	17.1 %	25.0 %	44.3 %	12.3 %	1.2 %		
Comparisons	2.6 %	22.8 %	66.0 %	7.6 %	1.0 %		
Individual autonomy						$\chi^2 = 173.8$, $p < 0.000$	df = 4,
Cases	3.3 %	22.2 %	54.7 %	16.0 %	3.9 %		
Comparisons	0.4 %	2.2 %	87.2 %	9.6 %	0.6 %		

B.	1-Low	2	3	4	5	6	7	8	9-High	Significance
Intellectual Functioning										$\chi^2 = 79.3$, df = 8, $p < 0.000$
Cases	0.2%	0.8 %	0.8 %	24.2 %	32.6 %	24.4 %	11.2 %	2.9 %	2.9 %	
Comparisons	0.0%	0.0 %	0.0 %	8.3 %	37.5 %	34.4 %	18.1 %	1.2 %	0.6 %	

in these categories. Table 1 indicates that although a high proportion of cases perform below the range of *their* comparisons, as a group, future schizophrenics perform over the entire range of possible normal performance (i.e., comparing the distribution of all cases to the distribution of all controls).

The follow-up of adolescents with non-psychotic psychiatric diagnoses found that having any non-psychotic psychiatric disorder in adolescence increased the risk of future hospitalization for schizophrenia, compared with the risk for schizophrenia in the entire cohort of adolescents. Table 2 displays the number of adolescents who were assigned each of the non-psychotic psychiatric diagnoses by Draft Board psychiatrists, and the rate of later hospitalization for schizophrenia. The prevalence of non-psychotic psychiatric disorders in future schizophrenia patients was 26.8%, as compared to 7.4% of non-psychotic, non-major affective psychiatric disorders in the general population of adolescents (OR = 4.5, 95% CI = 3.6 – 5.6).

An association was found between the different disorders in adolescence, and schizophrenia. The magnitude of this association differed between the different diagnostic groups. For example, patients with a registry diagnosis of schizophrenia were about 21.5 times more likely to have had a pre-morbid diagnosis of schizophrenia-spectrum personality disorder in adolescence, compared with the prevalence of schizophrenia-spectrum personality disorder in the general

Table 2. Association between non-psychotic psychiatric diagnoses and later hospitalization for schizophrenia in a population of 17 year old male adolescents

Diagnosis	Prevalence in total population	Prevalence in future schizophrenia patients	Number hospitalized for schizo-phrenia *	OR	95 % CI	OR con-trolled for IQ	95 % CI
Schizophrenia spectrum personality disorders [A]	0.11	1.95	4.7	21.5	12.6–36.6	14.4	5.9–29.4
Adjustment disorder	0.03	0.28	2.6	11.8	2.5–55.2	12.2	0.7–58.7
Antisocial personality disorder and impulse control disorder	0.15	1.11	2.0	8.9	3.9–20.3	4.8	1.4–11.4
Mental retardation	0.49	2.79	1.6	7.1	4.1–12.1	3.2	1.5– 6.1
Alcohol and Drug abuse	0.05	0.27	1.5	6.8	1.2–37.4	5.3	0.3–24.9
Other personality disorders [B]	5.43	17.03	0.9	3.9	3.0– 5.1	2.7	2.0– 3.6
Neurosis [C]	1.17	3.35	0.8	3.6	2.1– 6.2	2.5	1.3– 4.4
Total non-psychotic diagnoses	7.43	<16> 26.82					

OR odds ratios; CI confidence interval

* Number of adolescents later diagnosed for schizophrenia/number of adolescents assigned non-psychotic psychiatric diagnosis

[A] paranoid personality disorder or schizotypal personality disorder

[B] obsessive-compulsive personality disorder, avoidant personality disorder, dependent personality disorder, narcissistic personality disorder, schizoid personality disorder, borderline personality disorder or histrionic personality disorder

[C] anxiety, phobias, OCD, reactive depression or PTSD

[D] Entire population, including adolescents hospitalized within a year of draft board assessment and adolescents diagnosed with psychotic or affective disorders in draft board

population of adolescents. On the other hand, patients with a registry diagnosis of schizophrenia were only about 3.6 times more likely to have had a pre-morbid diagnosis of neurosis in adolescence, compared with the prevalence of neurosis in the general population of adolescents.

Sub-normal intellectual functioning is present in some persons with non-psychotic psychiatric disorders [21, 22], and is also associated with future schizophrenia in this population of adolescents (OR 2.16, 95 % CI = 2.004 – 3.430), and in other similar populations [23]. We therefore asked if sub-normal intellectual performance is a confounder for the risk for schizophrenia in adolescents with non-psychotic psychiatric disorders. The association between each psychiatric diagnosis and later hospitalization for schizophrenia was re-calculated while controlling for intellectual performance. In this analysis we applied separate hierarchical logistic regression models for each of the psychiatric diagnoses. In each regression model intellectual performance was entered first, and the psychiatric diagnosis was entered in the second step. Controlling for intellectual functioning decreased the association with future schizophrenia for most of the non-psychotic disorders, the decreases in OR reaching 65 % across the different diagnoses (Table 2).

Among the adolescents who were identified by the Draft Board screening process as having behavioral disturbances and were systematically asked about drug abuse, subjects with baseline drug abuse were two times more likely (12.4%, vs. 5.9%, adjusted RR = 2.033, 95% CI = 1.322 – 3.126) to be later hospitalized for schizophrenia, in comparison to adolescents who did not report drug use. This effect was specific for schizophrenia, as the rate of drug abuse in patients later hospitalized for affective disorders was not different than the rate of drug abuse in the entire cohort: 5.1% of the adolescents later hospitalized for affective disorder reported using drugs in the Draft Board, vs. the 5.9% rate of drug abuse in the cohort, RR = 0.9075, 95% CI = 0.2813 – 2.9272. The observed association between drug abuse and later hospitalization with schizophrenia was maintained after controlling for the presence of below-normal cognitive functioning, below-normal social functioning, and/or the presence of a non-psychotic psychiatric disorder in the Draft Board assessment (Wald Chi-square = 6.53, df = 1, p = 0.0106, RR = 1.70, 95% CI: 1.13 – 2.56).

The observed overall increase in drug use before the onset of illness might be explained by self-medication of the non-psychotic symptoms often preceding psychosis in schizophrenia patients. Consistent with this, it would be expected that the prevalence of drug abuse would increase as the first psychotic episode draws closer. To investigate this assumption, we evaluated the association between drug abuse and risk for future schizophrenia in the years preceding the first psychiatric admission. Table 3 shows the number of future schizophrenia patients who abused drugs/total number of patients in the cohort hospitalized for each year following the Draft Board assessment. The Kaplan-Meier survival analysis showed that those individuals who abused drugs were hospitalized later after the Draft Board assessment, rather than closer to it (Log rank = 8.54, df = 1, p = 0.0035). The finding that adolescents who abuse drugs were hospitalized later, rather than closer to hospitalization does not support the hypothesis that pre-morbid drug abuse reflects self-medication of non-psychotic symptoms preceding the onset of psychosis. This interpretation was also supported by finding

Table 3. Percentage of future schizophrenia patients who abused drugs relative to the total number of future schizophrenia patients, for each year elapsed between the Draft Board assessment and hospitalization*

Years between Draft Board assessment and hospitalization	Drug abusers/ all future patients (%)
1	0
2	13.3
3	8.3
4	12
5	11.4
6	10.7
7	10.7
8	0
9	42.9
10 – 11	25

that patients who abused drugs had a later mean age of first hospitalization, compared to those who did not report abusing drugs (23.48 ± 2.23 years vs. 21.98 ± 2.6 years, respectively; $t = 2.79$, $df = 261$, $p = 0.006$).

The comparison of social functioning in future schizophrenia patients with social functioning of those male adolescents in this cohort who were not later hospitalized found that future schizophrenia patients who abused drugs had non-significantly better social functioning compared with future schizophrenia patients who did not abuse drugs (2.65 ± 1.06 vs. 2.36 ± 0.80, $t = 1.69$, $p = 0.092$), a finding which does not support the hypothesis that drug abuse reflects self-medication of pre-morbid social withdrawal.

▦ Discussion

These data confirm and extend existing reports indicating that as a group, individuals destined to develop schizophrenia manifest subtle cognitive and behavioral abnormalities before the symptoms essential to diagnose schizophrenia manifest. In addition, 26.8 % of the males hospitalized for schizophrenia suffered from non-psychotic psychiatric disorders in adolescence, in comparison to 7.4 % prevalence of non-psychotic psychiatric disorders in the general population of adolescents. These findings are consistent with and extend previous studies [24, 25] which found that persons with schizophrenia often suffer from behavioral and emotional disturbances years before the manifestation of psychosis. More unique are the findings of the follow-up, which found that adolescents with non-psychotic psychiatric disorders had an increased risk for future schizophrenia (1.03 %), as compared with the risk for schizophrenia in the entire population (0.46 %). Taken together, these may indicate that although many patients with schizophrenia have behavioral deviations in adolescence, these behavioral deviations alone lack the specificity necessary to predict future schizophrenia, because the vast majority of adolescents (approximately 99 %) who have non-psychotic psychiatric disorders do *not* later suffer from schizophrenia.

Another singular finding of this report is the gradient of association between the various psychiatric disorders and future schizophrenia. While the OR of persons with other personality disorders and neuroses were 3.6 – 3.9, adolescents with anti-social personality disorder, mental retardation or drug abuse had OR in the range of 7 – 9. Moreover, adolescents with schizophrenia spectrum personality disorders (SSPD's) had an OR of 21.5. It could be hypothesized that those non-psychotic psychiatric disorders with higher ORs share more genetic or environmental factors in common with schizophrenia. This makes sense particularly for the SSPDs, which are phenomenologically more similar to schizophrenia [26].

The data presented here are consistent with high-risk studies [27, 28] of children and siblings of persons with schizophrenia that found increased prevalence of non-psychotic symptoms and diagnoses in these persons, and increased prevalence of schizophrenia at follow-up. Furthermore, the finding that adolescents with SSPDs have increased chances of future schizophrenia replicates and expands other studies, which found that magical thinking [29, 30] and schizo-typal symptoms [31] increase the risk of future schizophrenia. The findings in this report replicate very closely a recently published paper with a similar design [33], which followed conscripts screened by the Swedish draft board for future hospitalization for schizophrenia. That study reported that 38% of the future patients had a diagnosis of non-psychotic psychiatric disorder at age 18, with OR of 4.6 for neurosis, 8.2 for personality disorder, 5.5 for alcohol abuse, and 14.0 for substance abuse. The great similarity of the findings in that paper with the present report support the reliability of the data reported here.

Drug abuse, mainly marijuana, was also found to be a risk factor for schizo-phrenia. In a cohort of 50,413 male adolescents who were suspected of having behavioral problems, those adolescents who self-reported abuse of drugs at age 16 – 17 were 2.0 times more likely to be later hospitalized for schizophrenia. These data are compatible with the previous, longitudinal study on Swedish army conscripts which utilized a similar study design, and found that over a 15 year follow-up, the relative risk of hospitalization for schizophrenia in heavy cannabis users (more than fifty occasions) was 6.0, compared to non-users [32]. Similarly, a retrospective study in which patients with schizophrenia were asked about the use of cannabis before the onset of the illness reported higher rates of cannabis use in patients compared with controls [34]. Taken together, these findings indi-cate that use of drugs might interact with other risk factors contributing to the manifestations of schizophrenic symptoms in vulnerable individuals. Support for this idea is drawn from a basic science report which found that the density of canabinoid receptors was increased in the dorsolateral prefrontal cortex in sub-jects with schizophrenia, compared with controls [35]. This increased density of canabinoid receptors might be an example of an underlying brain pathology which increases vulnerability, and when the vulnerable brain is exposed to the trigger (illicit drugs), this may increase the risk of later symptom manifestation. Yet another view [36] of the association between schizophrenia and drug abuse before the onset of overt psychosis is based on evidence that developmental neu-ropathology in hippocampal and pre-frontal cortical pathways contributes both to symptoms of schizophrenia and to vulnerability to addictive behavior, via dys-functional interactions with the nucleus accumbens.

The finding that drug use is more prevalent among adolescents who develop schizophrenia farther from, rather than closer to the questioning about drug use is not consistent with the explanation that illicit drugs are used to ameliorate the anxiety, depression, and confusion that characterize prodromal schizophrenia.

Limitations

The diagnoses assigned by Draft Board psychiatrists are not research but clini-cal diagnoses, raising concerns about their accuracy. However all the psychia-trists working for the Draft Board are board-certified, received their postgradu-ate education after the introduction of DSM III, and are instructed and super-vised on a regular basis for quality and consistency. The three-stage screening procedure used by the Draft Board dictates that even before the adolescent is referred to the psychiatrist, both the interviewer assessing personality and behavioral traits, and the clinical social worker or clinical psychologist identify him as having significant behavioral problems. In addition, the clinical social worker or clinical psychologist assigns a tentative diagnosis, so that the psychiatric diagnosis assigned reflects the consensus diagnosis between them and the psychiatrist. Disagreements between the two are resolved by consensus with the help of another, senior psychiatrist. A related concern is the fact that the case registry diagnoses are clinical, not research diagnoses. However, these diagnoses are also assigned by board-certified psychiatrists who have had the benefit of observing the patient throughout one or more hospitalizations, and had been trained and re-trained in the use of the diagnostic criteria of the ICD 9. Moreover, studies which have compared clinical diagnoses of schizophrenia assigned in state hospitals [37] with research diagnoses have shown a high degree of concordance. The results are limited to males since the Draft Board administers behavioral tests only to males (females only undergo cognitive assessment). Since male patients are more likely than female patients to be hospitalized for schizophrenia [38], and since male patients may suffer from a more severe form of illness [39], the more severely ill schizophrenic patients might be over represented in this study.

The prevalence of non-psychotic psychiatric diagnoses made by the Draft Board in the population of adolescents, approximately 7.4%, is lower than the prevalence of psychiatric disorders found in some, but not all, other studies [40]. One reason for the relatively low prevalence rates observed may be that the Draft Board screening procedure sets a high threshold for diagnosis of minor psychiatric disturbances, compared with screening instruments used in epidemiological surveys. For example, diagnoses such as specific phobias (included here in the "anxiety" category), which are relatively common in epidemiological surveys, are less common in the present sample.

The Draft Board assessment is intended to screen adolescents before military service, and not specifically to detect recruits who will manifest schizophrenia, and the instruments used reflect this. It is clear that the optimal design of a study assessing the association between cognitive and behavioral functioning, non-psychotic psychiatric diagnoses, and drug abuse in adolescence with later hospitalization for schizophrenia would screen subjects using structured research instruments which specifically assess cognitive and behavioral functioning known to be impaired in patients with schizophrenia, and to ascertain diagnoses both of the non-psychotic psychiatric disorders at baseline and of schizophrenia using the SCID or similar instruments. However, the incidence of schizophrenia in the population is between 0.5 – 1%, and not all patients have abnormal cognitive and behavioral functioning, non-psychotic psychiatric disorders, or abuse drugs before manifesting psychosis. In order to yield significant results, this hypothetical protocol would therefore necessitate screening of hundreds of thousands of adolescents and then following them for years, a project which is probably not feasible in the near future.

▪ Conclusions

The results of this study, based on the screening of an entire population of 16 – 17 year old males, indicate that years before the onset of illness, future schizophrenia patients have subtle impairments in cognitive and behavioral functioning, and that non-psychotic psychiatric disorders in adolescence are associated with future schizophrenia. Drug abuse is also associated with future schizophrenia, and is probably not due to self-medication of pre-morbid symptoms. Unfortunately, the predictive power of cognitive and behavioral impairments, non-psychotic psychiatric diagnoses and drug abuse are not strong enough to recommend prophylactic treatment with antipsychotic or other medications. Hence, these data advocate for intensive research in this area, rather than suggesting immediate clinical implications. Additional studies combining information about genetic, obstetric and intellectual risk factors, together with behavioral disturbances in adolescence, may enable more accurate identification of persons who will later suffer from schizophrenia.

▪ References

1. Kendler KS, Diehl SR (1993) The genetics of schizophrenia: a current, genetic-epidemiologic perspective. Schizophr Bull 19 (2): 261–285
2. Tsuang MT, Gilbertson MW, Faraone SV (1991) The genetics of schizophrenia. Current knowledge and future directions. Schizophr Res 4 (2): 157–171
3. Gottesman, II, Erlenmeyer-Kimling L (2001) Family and twin strategies as a head start in defining prodromes and endophenotypes for hypothetical early-interventions in schizophrenia. Schizophr Res 51 (1): 93–102
4. Brown AS, Cohen P, Harkavy-Friedman J, Babulas V, Malaspina D, Gorman JM, Susser ES (2001) A.E. Bennett Research Award. Prenatal rubella, premorbid abnormalities, and adult schizophrenia. Biol Psychiatry 49 (6): 473–486
5. Kunugi H, Nanko S, Murray RM (2001) Obstetric complications and schizophrenia: prenatal underdevelopment and subsequent neurodevelopmental impairment. Br J Psychiatry 178 (Suppl 40): S 25–29
6. Dalman C, Thomas HV, David AS, Gentz J, Lewis G, Allebeck P (2001) Signs of asphyxia at birth and risk of schizophrenia: population-based case-control study. Br J Psychiatry 179 (5): 403–408
7. Cannon TD, Rosso IM, Hollister JM, Bearden CE, Sanchez LE, Hadley T (2000) A prospective cohort study of genetic and perinatal influences in the etiology of schizophrenia. Schizophr Bull 26 (2): 351–366
8. Zornberg GL, Buka SL, Tsuang MT (2000) Hypoxic-ischemia-related fetal/neonatal complications and risk of schizophrenia and other nonaffective psychoses: a 19-year longitudinal study. Am J Psychiatry 157 (2): 196-202
9. Ichiki M, Kunugi H, Takei N, Murray RM, Baba H, Arai H, Oshima I, Okagami K, Sato T, Hirose T, Nanko S (2000) Intra-uterine physical growth in schizophrenia: evidence confirming excess of premature birth. Psychol Med 30 (3): 597–604
10. Dalman C, Allebeck P, Cullberg J, Grunewald C, Koster M (1999) Obstetric complications and the risk of schizophrenia: a longitudinal study of a national birth cohort. Arch Gen Psychiatry 56 (3): 234–240
11. Isohanni M, Jones PB, Moilanen K, Rantakallio P, Veijola J, Oja H, Koiranen M, Jokelainen J, Croudace T, Jarvelin M (2001) Early developmental milestones in adult schizophrenia and other psychoses. A 31-year follow-up of the Northern Finland 1966 Birth Cohort. Schizophr Res 52 (1–2): 1–19

12. Jones P, Rodgers B, Murray R, Marmot M (1994) Child development risk factors for adult schizophrenia in the British 1946 birth cohort. Lancet 344 (8934): 1398–1402

13. Walker EF, Grimes KE, Davis DM, Smith AJ (1993) Childhood precursors of schizophrenia: facial expressions of emotion. Am J Psychiatry 150 (11): 1654–1660

14. Davidson M, Reichenberg A, Rabinowitz J, Weiser M, Kaplan Z, Mark M (1999) Behavioral and intellectual markers for schizophrenia in apparently healthy male adolescents [In Process Citation]. Am J Psychiatry 156 (9): 1328–1335

15. Weiser M, Reichenberg A, Rabinowitz J, Kaplan Z, Mark M, Bodner E, Nahon D, Davidson M (2001) Association between nonpsychotic psychiatric diagnoses in adolescent males and subsequent onset of schizophrenia. Arch Gen Psychiatry 58 (10): 959–964

16. Weiser M, Reichenberg A, Rabinowitz J, Kaplan Z, Caspi A, Yazvitsky R, Mark M, Nahon D, Davidson M (2002) Self-reported drug abuse in male adolescents with behavioural disturbances, and follow-up for future schizophrenia. (Submitted)

17. Rabinowitz J, Reichenberg A, Weiser M, Mark M, Kaplan Z, Davidson M (2000) Cognitive and behavioural functioning in men with schizophrenia both before and shortly after first admission to hospital. Cross-sectional analysis. Br J Psychiatry 177: 26–32

18. Gal R (1986) The selection, classification and placement process. In: Westport CT (eds) A Portrait of the Israeli Soldier. Greenwood Press, p 77

19. Levav I, Kohn R, Dohrenwend BP, Shrout PE, Skodol AE, Schwartz S, Link BG, Naveh G (1993) An epidemiological study of mental disorders in a 10-year cohort of young adults in Israel Psychol Med 23 (3): 691–707

20. Bromet EJ DM, Eaton W (1995) Epidemiology of psychosis with special reference to schizophrenia. In: Tsuang MT, Tohen M, Zahner GEP (eds). Psychiatric Epidemiology. John Wiley & Sons, pp 283–300

21. Asmundson GJ, Stein MB, Larsen DK, Walker JR (1994) Neurocognitive function in panic disorder and social phobia patients. Anxiety 1 (5): 201–207

22. Burgess JW (1992) Neurocognitive impairment in dramatic personalities: histrionic, narcissistic, borderline, and antisocial disorders. Psychiatry Res 42 (3): 283–290

23. David AS, Malmberg A, Brandt L, Allebeck P, Lewis G (1997) IQ and risk for schizophrenia: a population-based cohort study. Psychol Med 27 (6): 1311–1323

24. Done DJ, Crow TJ, Johnstone EC, Sacker A (1994) Childhood antecedents of schizophrenia and affective illness: social adjustment at ages 7 and 11 [see comments]. BMJ 309 (6956): 699–703

25. Jones PB, Bebbington P, Foerster A, Lewis SW, Murray RM, Russell A, Sham PC, Toone BK, Wilkins S (1993) Premorbid social underachievement in schizophrenia. Results from the Camberwell Collaborative Psychosis Study. Br J Psychiatry 162: 65–71

26. Siever LJ, Kalus OF, Keefe RS (1993) The boundaries of schizophrenia. Psychiatr Clin North Am 16 (2): 217–244

27. Parnas J, Cannon TD, Jacobsen B, Schulsinger H, Schulsinger F, Mednick SA (1993) Lifetime DSM-III-R diagnostic outcomes in the offspring of schizophrenic mothers. Results from the Copenhagen High-Risk Study. Arch Gen Psychiatry 50 (9): 707–714

28. Erlenmeyer-Kimling L (2000) Neurobehavioral deficits in offspring of schizophrenic parents: liability indicators and predictors of illness. Am J Med Genet 97 (1): 65–71

29. Chapman LJ, Chapman JP, Kwapil TR, Eckblad M, Zinser MC (1994) Putatively psychosis-prone subjects 10 years later. J Abnorm Psychol 103 (2): 171–183

30. Kwapil TR, Miller MB, Zinser MC, Chapman J, Chapman LJ (1997) Magical ideation and social anhedonia as predictors of psychosis proneness: a partial replication. J Abnorm Psychol 106 (3): 491–495

31. Fenton WS, McGlashan TH (1989) Risk of schizophrenia in character disordered patients. Am J Psychiatry 146 (10): 1280–1284

32. Andreasson S, Allebeck P, Engstrom A, Rydberg U (1987) Cannabis and schizophrenia. A longitudinal study of Swedish conscripts. Lancet 2 (8574): 1483–1486

33. Lewis G, David AS, Malmberg A, Allebeck P (2000) Non-psychotic psychiatric disorder and subsequent risk of schizophrenia: cohort study [In Process Citation]. Br J Psychiatry 177: 416–420

34. Hambrecht M, Hafner H (2000) Cannabis, vulnerability, and the onset of schizophrenia: an epidemiological perspective. Aust N Z J Psychiatry 34 (3): 468–475
35. Dean B, Sundram S, Bradbury R, Scarr E, Copolov D (2001) Studies on [3H]CP-55940 binding in the human central nervous system: regional specific changes in density of cannabinoid-1 receptors associated with schizophrenia and cannabis use. Neuroscience 103 (1): 9–15
36. Chambers RA, Krystal JH, Self DW (2001) A neurobiological basis for substance abuse comorbidity in schizophrenia. Biol Psychiatry 50 (2): 71–83
37. Pulver AE, Carpenter WT, Adler L, McGrath J (1988) Accuracy of the diagnoses of affective disorders and schizophrenia in public hospitals. Am J Psychiatry 145 (2): 218–220
38. Munk-Jorgensen P (1985) The schizophrenia diagnosis in Denmark. A register-based investigation. Acta Psychiatr Scand 72 (3): 266–273
39. Meltzer HY, Rabinowitz J, Lee MA, Cola PA, Ranjan R, Findling RL, Thompson PA (1997) Age at onset and gender of schizophrenic patients in relation to neuroleptic resistance. Am J Psychiatry 154 (4): 475–482
40. Roberts RE, Attkisson CC, Rosenblatt A (1998) Prevalence of psychopathology among children and adolescents. Am J Psychiatry: 715–725

Specificity of basic symptoms in early onset schizophrenia

F. Resch[1], P. Parzer[1], L. Poustka[1], E. Koch[1], H. Meng[2], D. Bürgin[2]
[1]Dept. of Child and Adolescent Psychiatry, University of Heidelberg, Germany
[2]Dept. of Child and Adolescent Psychiatry, University of Basel, Switzerland

■ Introduction

Developmental psychopathology addresses several important questions of the pathogenesis of psychotic disorders proposing a conceptual framework, which includes developmental psychology, neurobiology and clinical psychopathology. The first question to be raised is the contribution of normal developmental processes to the pathogenesis of psychotic symptoms, ending up with the second question, what impacts psychopathology itself may exert on normal development concerning defects, vulnerabilities and disturbances of age-dependent adaptive processes [11]. Normal cognitive and emotional development seems to be a prerequisite for symptom formation. These assumptions may help us in the interpretation of different psychotic and prodromal phenomena in children and adolescents. Looking at the table of ages, we find overlapping disturbances in various age groups. First manifestations of pervasive developmental disorders – Kanner-Autism [7] – can be detected in the age group from birth to six years. Asperger syndrome [2] may be particularly detected in the age group between six and nine years. In this age group also very early onset psychosis can be elucidated, which shows predominantly formal thought disorder and inappropriate affect. Very early onset psychoses presenting with hallucinations and delusions rather seem to start off in the age group between nine and twelve years. Of these patients, 60 % show developmental disorders of speech and language, and about one third present with pervasive developmental disorders in prodromal stages [1]. Early onset psychoses with a lifetime prevalence of about 0.23 % begin in the age group between twelve and eighteen [3]. Adult psychosis presents with prodromal features that reach back into ages around and before puberty [5]. From an epidemiological point of view all these groups of disorders may be found during the adolescent age.

In schizophrenia research, the main focus is set on early detection of the disorder [9]. Especially psychosis with early onset before the age of eighteen present with a very poor outcome, which seems to be related to features of the prodromal period and the duration of untreated psychosis [10]. Yung and McGorry [13] widened the scope on prodromal symptoms at first manifestations. They reported the following disturbances in a ranking of descending significance, beginning with disturbances of concentration and attention, disturbances of drive and motivation, sleeping disorders, anxiety spells, social withdrawal, suspiciousness, loss of performance in school or work and irritability. So in summary, these prodromal features include phenomena of a decline of social functioning. According to the literature, prodromal symptomatology is known to be nonspecific for schizophrenia and may be found in the initial phase of other psychiatric illnesses as well. The most important aspect of Yung and McGorry's metaanalysis was that the subjective experiences of prodromal and early psychotic signs clearly preceded the behavioral changes recognizable by the social environment. So it can be stated that patients realize their deficits and changes of experiences particularly earlier before they change their overt behavior! In this respect it seems quite reasonable to refer to subjective complaints in the clinical context of early recognition. The basic symptom concept [6] as an integrative clinical approach in accordance with a vulnerability stress cope model may shed light on the pathogenesis of schizophrenia. The concept of basic symptoms relies on subjective experiences of cognitive, affective and neurobehavioral deficits that are interpreted as dysfunctional processes in neuroadaptive regulation. Such basic symptoms may reflect the underlying pathogenetic process from vulnerability to overt psychosis [8]. Basic symptoms can be assessed in a semistructured clinical interview called the Bonn Scale for the Assessment of Basic Symptoms [4]. The assessment consists of retrospective questions that are rated in a qualitative way. The basic symptom concept is of clinical use in adult and adolescent patients as it has been assessed earlier [12].

The Bonn Scale Instrument (BSABS) in the short version consists of fifty items that are distributed in four categories. Category A consists of direct minus symptoms (6 items), e.g., changes in basic mood and emotional reactivity. Category B consists of indirect minus symptoms (7 items), e.g., increased impressionability due to everyday events and other irritation symptoms. Category C consists of cognitive symptoms (26 items). The subgroup C 1 comprises thought disturbances, e.g., thought blocking. C 2 consists of perception disturbances, e.g., micropsia and macropsia. And C 3 relates to motor disturbances, e.g., the loss of automatic skills. Category D consists of coenesthetic complaints (11 items), e.g., electric sensations.

▨ Cross-sectional study

In our study we try to address the question of specificity in a cross-sectional approach with retrospective assessment procedures. Sample 1 consisted of 75 consecutive non-psychotic inpatients referred to the ward of the Heidelberg Clinic in the years 1995 and 1996: 44% were males, 56% females, the mean age was 14.2, standard deviation 2.0. One patient had a disorder due to substance abuse, five patients suffered from affective disorders, nineteen patients had neurotic and stress-related disorders, nine patients suffered from eating disorders, four patients had borderline personality disorder, four patients had pervasive developmental disorder and 33 patients suffered from behavioral and emotional disorders of childhood. Diagnosis was made according to the ICD-10 research criteria.

Sample 2 consisted of 66 schizophrenic inpatients of the early onset type. Of these patients, 36 were examined in Heidelberg and Vienna by our own group of developmental psychopathologists. Thirty patients were examined by different co-workers of our VESPA Network in childhood schizophrenia (Verbundstudie Psychosen der Adoleszenz) and consisted of schizophrenic patients recruited in Basel, Hamburg, Tübingen and several other clinics in Austria and Switzerland. 55% were males, 54% females, mean of age was 16.5, standard deviation 1.2. We administered the Bonn Scale for the Assessment of Basic Symptoms in retrospection. In those 36 patients examined by our group, the long version of the BSABS was administered. In the 30 patients examined within the Network, the short version was administered. For this analysis we used only the fifty items of the BSABS, which represent a subgroup of the long version and define the short version of the BSABS. Schizophrenia diagnosis was certified according to both the DSM-IV and ICD-10 research criteria.

The first question to be raised was whether there exists any specificity in the occurrence of basic symptoms in adolescent patients. We addressed this question by looking at the percentage of patients with at least one basic symptom in each of the different categories. In category A (direct minus symptoms) 81.8% of schizophrenics, compared to 57.3% of adolescent patients with other diagnoses had at least one symptom (Fisher's exact test: $p = 0.002$). In the indirect minus symptom group, 83.3% of the schizophrenics showed symptoms of irritations compared to 50.7% of adolescents with other diagnoses (Fisher's exact test: $p < 0.001$). In the cognitive symptom category (C) 97% of schizophrenics scored positively in at least one basic symptom compared to 64% of patients with other diagnoses (Fisher's exact test: $p < 0.001$). Coenesthetic complaints (Category D) were reported by 56.1% schizophrenics compared to 38.7% of patients

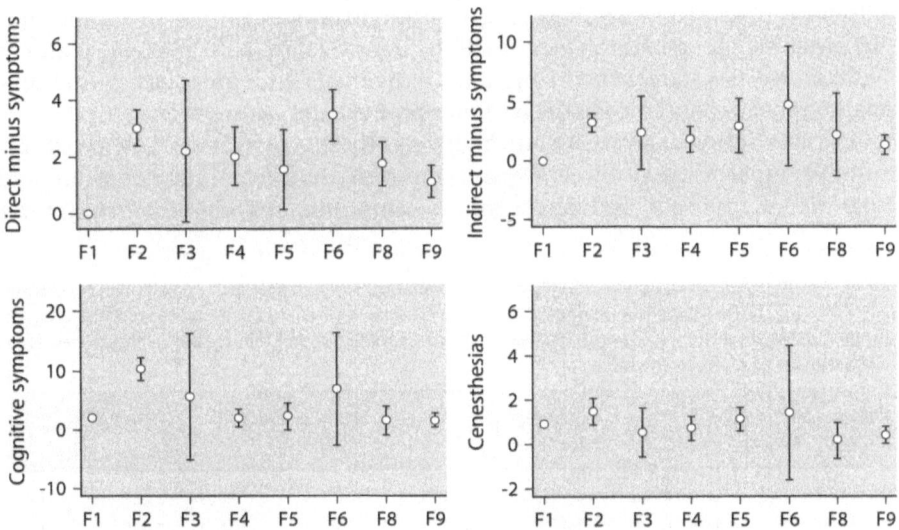

Fig. 1. Means and 95% confidence intervals of the number of basic symptoms in the ICD-10 diagnostic groups.

Table 1. Means, results from t-tests and effect sizes for the number of basic symptoms in schizophrenic and non-schizophrenic adolescent patients

BSABS category	Mean (SD) of the number of symptoms schizophrenic	other diagnoses	t-test p	Effect size
Direct minus symptoms	2.6 (1.8)	1.6 (1.8)	0.001	0.54
Indirect minus symptoms	3.1 (2.3)	1.9 (2.5)	0.005	0.47
Cognitive symptoms	9.3 (5.5)	2.4 (3.8)	< 0.001	1.18
Coenesthesias	1.4 (1.7)	0.7 (1.1)	0.003	0.50

with other diagnoses (Fisher's exact test: p = 0.044). Although schizophrenic patients in all the categories differ significantly from non-schizophrenics, concerning the occurrence of at least one basic symptom within the basic symptom category, there is no specificity in having basic symptoms in this rather qualitative approach. It is noteworthy that at least 2/3 of patients with non-schizophrenic diagnoses had at least one cognitive complaint and about one half suffered from subjective minus symptoms.

In a more dimensional approach, we first looked at the number of basic symptoms within different diagnostic groups (Fig. 1). Direct and indirect minus symptoms do occur rather often in schizophrenics, but direct minus symptoms are equally found in affective and borderline patients, irritation symptomatology may be found quite more often in borderline patients compared to schizophrenics. Coenesthesias are quite rare in all diagnostic groups. In cognitive symptomatology schizophrenics show the highest scores, only borderline patients presenting with similar amounts of cognitive basic symptomatology. Taken together the comparison of schizophrenics and non-schizophrenics shows that the number of basic symptoms is significantly increased in schizophrenics compared to a non-psychotic group of adolescent patients. This finding holds true for all four categories of the Bonn Scale (Table 1). At this point of analysis, we may state that schizophrenic individuals show more basic symptoms than non-schizophrenics in the last few months before admission.

In a correlation analysis, we find highly significant correlations between direct minus symptoms and indirect minus symptoms, indirect minus symptoms and cognitive symptoms, and direct minus symptoms and cognitive symptoms

Table 2. Regression coefficients between the number of BSABS minus symptoms (minuss.) and the number of BSABS cognitive symptoms in schizophrenics and patients with other diagnoses. The p-values next to the coefficients test the hypothesis that the coefficient is zero, the p-values in the column 'difference' test the hypothesis that the regression coefficients are equal in both groups

Regression	Schizophrenic coefficient	p	Other diagnoses coefficient	p	Difference p	R^2
Indirect minuss. → direct minuss.	0.48	< 0.001	0.52	< 0.001	0.657	0.48
Indirect minuss. → cogn. sympt.	1.45	< 0.001	0.86	< 0.001	0.038	0.57
Direct minuss. → cogn. sympt.	1.85	< 0.001	1.13	< 0.001	0.054	0.56

Table 3. Partial correlation coefficients between minus symptoms (minuss.) and cognitive symptoms in schizophrenics and patients with other diagnoses

	Schizophrenic direct minuss.	indirect minuss.	Other diagnoses direct minuss.	indirect minuss.
Indirect minuss.	0.40		0.60	
Cognitive sympt.	0.36	0.36	0.23	0.30

(Table 2). More direct minus symptoms are accompanied by more indirect minus symptoms. In schizophrenics and other disorders the same effect can be detected. The more indirect minus symptoms a patient has, the more cognitive disturbances of thought, speech and motor activity are to be found. In addition the regression line of schizophrenics is steeper, thus, representing the fact that with increasing indirect minus symptoms, the cognitive symptoms show higher increase rates in schizophrenics than in other diagnostic groups. Even with less irritation symptoms schizophrenics present with high scores of cognitive disturbances. This could reflect a vulnerability for the schizophrenic disorder. More direct minus symptoms lead to more cognitive symptoms. And again, schizophrenics show a tendency to have more cognitive symptoms with increasing direct minus symptoms reflecting apathy and affective blunting compared to other patients. Partial correlations between minus symptoms and cognitive symptoms do not significantly differ from each other in different patient groups. But as a tendency, partial correlations reflect a slightly different pattern in patients with schizophrenia compared to patients with other diagnoses (Table 3). Whereas in non-schizophrenics direct minus symptoms and indirect minus symptoms show the strongest partial correlation, leaving only weaker correlations of each with cognitive disturbances, in schizophrenic patients the partial correlations are equally strong between the three symptom categories. This may again reflect a stronger relative contribution of cognitive complaints to the clinical picture of schizophrenic prodrome.

In the next step, we looked at the contribution of the BSABS categories on the discrimination of schizophrenia and other diagnoses. We used a method of a stepwise logistic regression to prove which variable remains significant in the context of the others. As a dependent variable, the schizophrenia diagnosis (yes/no) was added. The independent variables consisted of the number of basic symptoms in the four categories of the BSABS. Results showed a model of prediction, including indirect minus symptoms and cognitive symptoms (Table 4).

Table 4. Result of stepwise logistic regression using backward elimination ($p > 0.05$) with schizophrenia (yes/no) as independent variable and the number of symptoms in the BSABS-categories A, B, C, D and E as predictors

Predictor	Odds ratio	p	95 % Confidence interval	
Number of indirect minus symptoms	0.79	0.042	0.63	0.99
Number of cognitive symptoms	1.51	< 0.001	1.31	1.74

The classification table has a sensitivity of 75.8 % and the specificity of 89.3 %, so that 83 % could be classified correctly. On the basis of basic symptomatology, the prediction of psychotic risks can be tried in this patient sample with 75 % sensitivity and nearly 90 % specificity, which does not seem satisfying. Although this psychopathological model may serve as a clinical tool for the detection of early risk in adolescent samples, a methodological problem of early diagnosis has to be raised, if we take into account that the prevalence of adolescent schizophrenia is 0.23 %. This means that in an epidemiological sample 23 out of 10,000 present with schizophrenic symptomatology. If our test presents with a sensitivity of 75 % and a specificity of 90 %, we may detect seven out of 23 schizophrenics, but we will detect 998 false positives. So only 1.7 % of the real schizophrenics in an epidemiological group can be classified correctly. Even if we optimize the psychopathological model and get a screening instrument with a sensitivity of 99 % and a specificity of 99 %, we may detect all 23 schizophrenics, but we already have 100 false positives. So, only 18 % real schizophrenics in an epidemiological group may be classified correctly.

If the prevalence of the disorder is so low, the screening for primary prevention will be difficult, concerning the therapeutic intervention. If one should try therapy before the onset of psychotic symptomatology, a false positive group has to be taken into account! Therapy with neuroleptics or intensive specific psychotherapy may be burdened with a high risk of treating people who actually do not need it. For ethical reasons, in unselected samples, only symptom-guided psychosocial intervention should be provided for adolescents! The psychopathological screening model only seems to be fruitful for clinical samples with high prevalence rates of schizophrenic symptomatology; in addition, screening instruments should include biological data and family history data, and not only rely on psychopathology.

▓ Follow-up study

On 90 consecutive patients of the Heidelberg sample (1995/1996, 75 non-psychotics and 15 psychotics) a follow-up study was done. Preliminary data analysis shows that until now 46 of 90 patients participated. The mean follow-up interval is 4.3 years, minimum 2.7 years and a maximum of 5.7 years. As instruments served the KIDDY-SADS and the BSABS. We could not detect significant differences between participants and non-participants in gender, age, diagnosis and BSABS scores at the first assessment. What could be found was that 22 of the non-psychotic patients presented with no psychiatric diagnosis at all at the follow-up term. None of the non-schizophrenic patients had diagnosis changed to schizophrenia! And none of the schizophrenic patients had his diagnosis changed to another nosological entity. The stability of the BSABS scores are shown in Table 5. The correlation coefficients seem to be rather low. There exists a weak tendency toward stability exhibited by single individuals, while others change their scores dramatically. Basic symptoms in adolescents do not seem to represent trait parameters. They are more prone to subjective complaints, which seem to

Table 5. Correlation coefficients between the number of basic symptoms at admission and at follow-up

BSABS category	r	p
Direct minus symptoms	0.34	0.021
Indirect minus symptoms	0.43	0.003
Cognitive symptoms	0.44	0.003
Coenesthesias	0.27	0.081
Central vegetative symptoms	0.26	0.091

be related to developmental tasks and emotional turmoil without any specificity for schizophrenia in this age group.

Conclusions

Thus, the occurrence of any single basic symptom in adolescent samples does not show schizophrenic specificity. The number of basic symptoms in the BSABS categories is significantly increased in schizophrenics compared to other diagnoses. The correlation between minus symptoms and cognitive symptoms slightly differ between schizophrenics and other diagnoses. The follow-up study reveals low stability of basic symptoms over four years in adolescents, so the subjective complaints concerning the psychotic process present with the qualities more of a state than a trait marker. There may be an intensification of underlying trait deficits in trigger situations, but adolescence itself may serve developmental demands that cause emotional turmoil, identity diffusion or cognitive disturbances, which as single complaints do not show any specificity in the direction of schizophrenia proneness. But in a quantitative approach, schizophrenia-prone individuals seem to present with high scores of minus symptoms and cognitive symptoms in the last few months before the onset of psychotic symptomatology.

References

1. Asarnow JR, Karatekin C (2001) Neurobehavioral perspective. In: Remschmidt H (ed) Schizophrenia in Children and Adolescents. Cambridge: Cambridge University Press, pp 135–167
2. Asperger H (1944) Die "autistischen Psychopathen" im Kindesalter. Archiv für Psychiatrie und Nervenkrankheiten 117: 76–136
3. Gillberg C (2001) Epidemiology of early onset schizophrenia. In: Remschmidt H (ed) Schizophrenia in Children and Adolescents. Cambridge: Cambridge University Press, pp 43–59
4. Gross G, Huber G, Klosterkötter J, Linz M (1987) BSABS. Bonner Skala für die Beurteilung von Basissymptomen. Heidelberg: Springer.
5. Häfner H, an der Heiden W (1997) Epidemiology of schizophrenia. Canadian Journal of Psychiatry 42: 139–151
6. Huber G (1983) Das Konzept substratnaher Basissymptome und seine Bedeutung für Theorie und Therapie schizophrener Erkrankungen. Nervenarzt 54: 23–32

7. Kanner L (1944) Child psychiatry: early infantile autism. Journal of Pediatrics 25: 211–217
8. Klosterkötter J, Hellmich M, Steinmeyer EM, Schultze-Lutter F (2001) Diagnosing schizophrenia in the initial prodromal phase. Archives of General Psychiatry 58 (2): 158–164
9. McGorry P, Jackson HJ (eds) (1999) The Recognition and Management of Early Psychosis. A Preventive Approach. Cambridge: University Press
10. Resch F (1992) Therapie der Adoleszentenpsychosen: psychopathologische, psychobiologische und entwicklungspsychologische Aspekte aus therapeutischer Sicht. Stuttgart: Thieme
11. Resch F, Parzer P, Brunner M, Haffner J, Koch E, Oelkers R, Schuch B, Strewlow U (1999) Entwicklungspsychopathologie des Kindes- und Jugendalters. Ein Lehrbuch. (2 ed). Weinheim: Psychologie Verlags Union
12. Resch F, Schuch B, Amminger GP (1993) Investigation of basic symptoms in children and adolescents. Neurology, Psychiatry and Brain Research 1: 201–203
13. Yung AR, McGorry PD (1996) The initial prodrome in psychosis: descriptive and qualitative aspects. Australian and New Zealand Journal of Psychiatry 30: 587–599

Discussion: indicators of schizophrenia in childhood and adolescence

D. J. DONE

Department of Psychology, University of Hertfordshire, Hatfield, UK

The first two papers in this chapter were concerned with childhood (Jones) or adolescent (Weiser) premorbid antecedents of adult onset schizophrenia, whereas the third (Resch) was focused on prepsychotic signs in adolescent onset schizophrenia. What are the themes common to these three papers? Firstly the underlying research questions are similar. Whereas the research questions in the late 1960s and 1970s centred around using premorbid status to identify the sub-types of schizophrenia (e.g., paranoid-nonparanoid; process-reactive), and predicting outcome [14, 32], these three presentations highlight the contemporary research questions. These can be summarised as:

■ What is the neurodevelopmental pathway of schizophrenia?
■ Can we identify the endophenotype [31]?
■ Can the evidence available allow us to develop effective intervention programmes for children at risk of developing schizophrenia?

Answers to all of these research questions requires piecing together a jigsaw from a diverse range of studies, principally because high quality evidence is very difficult to find. Research on the birth (Jones) and conscript (Weiser) cohorts provide some pieces, but these depend on data collected from studies not principally designed for research into the antecedents of schizophrenia. Over the last decade, research on childhood-onset schizophrenia has added a new dimension to understanding the neurodevelopmental pathway of this disorder. Comparisons of the premorbid neurodevelopmental pathways of childhood and adult onset schizophrenia are now possible. With the premorbid deficits being more common and the duration of premorbid and prodromal phases much shortened in the former [13, 26] it is a method that is contributing much toward answering these research questions. From the diversity of evidence then, on what issues is there agreement, and where are there disagreements? Firstly we need to separate studies into those which follow back (i.e. retrospective) from adulthood to childhood and those which follow-up (i.e. prospective) groups of children (i.e. typically those deemed to be at risk of schizophrenia for various reasons).

◼ Agreements across studies

Follow-back studies

The largest reported effect sizes are found in the area of social functioning. A variety of abnormalities of social behaviour have been reported from birth and conscription cohort studies [8, 10, 16, 36], or retrospective recall studies [3, 23]. This has also been characterised as schizoid or schizotypal personality disorder [24, 35], and Mark Weiser reported that a substantial number meet criteria for a diagnosis of adjustment or personality disorder [21]. Rejection by peers has also been reported [15]. Peter Jones noted that studies typically report Pre-S children to be more anxious, neurotic, or depressed [10, 16, 21]. IQ is reduced by about 0.5 standard deviation [7, 8, 16] but perhaps more interestingly is the point that Peter Jones raised, namely the 'dose- response' relationship between reduced IQ and risk of schizophrenia, rather than a specific group of low IQ children at increased risk. Motor/neurological soft signs and delayed milestones are reported especially in the birth cohort studies [19, 31]. And again, Peter Jones noted the a dose-response relationship between one soft sign (delay in learning to stand without support) and risk of schizophrenia. Later in childhood/adolescence a small number of Pre-S children appear to have an uncommon disorder of communication perhaps unintelligible language but not dysarticulation [7, 16]. This pattern of premorbid deficits and dysfunctions has also been reported in childhood onset schizophrenia, although the language disorder seems more marked [13, 26]. This broad picture was summed up by Peter Jones as reflecting the different fragments of a complex constellation of causes. Finally, these constellations do not qualitatively distinguish Pre-S children from those who develop other types of adult onset psychopathology. Instead we find a dose-response relationship again, i.e. Pre-S children differ by virtue of an increase in both severity and frequency, but not type, of early abnormalities [10, 20, 24, 33]. Resch reported the same finding in his sample of adolescents, which replicates recent findings from other studies of childhood onset schizophrenia [26].

Follow-up studies

There are really only two important findings that come from the follow-up studies from populations at risk such as children with marked antisocial behaviour [28], juvenile delinquents [12], children referred to children's clinics [25, 34], or shy children [17, 18]. Firstly the probability of developing schizophrenia in such children is extremely low for a putative endophenotype, and secondly the consequences for adult psychopathology are diverse.

◼ Disagreements across follow-back studies

Given the variety of interpersonal behaviour problems in children, it is not unreasonable to expect some to be better predictors than others, but current evidence provides marked disagreements. Peter Jones reminded us that Bleuler noted early withdrawal and irritability, which have also been noted in other recent studies [16, 24, 35]. Other evidence characterises Pre-S boys as exhibiting excess degrees of externalising behaviour with little sign of withdrawal [10, 28, 36]. Mark Weiser's presentation raises the question of whether there are any characteristic behaviours, since these boys had various forms of dysfunctional social behaviour. Perhaps then risk is conferred by degree of disordered social behaviour rather than type, but we need more evidence before we can resolve this question. We are also unclear about whether there is stability, gradual deterioration [10, 28], or precipitate decline at critical periods [35] in cognitive, social or affective functioning. Resch reported instability, even over a short period of time. Peter Jones raised the challenging view that change across the life span can be regarded as either developmental or degenerative; the distinction is arbitrary. Also, recent studies have contributed little to the debate on gender differences in premorbid functioning. Some studies have reported large, qualitative gender differences in trajectories [10, 36] whereas others report no differences [1, 16]. Finally, is the positive predictive value (PPV) from this constellation of indicators high enough to warrant intervention? Some studies have reported models with good 'predictive power' [4, 8] but Weiser and Jones cautioned that PPVs are too low. But even if we could develop screening programmes with, say, 95% specificity and sensitivity then the PPV would only be 16% (i.e. only 16% of test positives will be true positives) because of the 1% population prevalence of adult onset schizophrenia. And although this might appear to be low, it is in actuality quite high compared with other screening programmes [2] .

■ Methodological considerations

Many of the disagreements and unresolved issues on childhood/adolescent indicators probably arise from use of less than satisfactory evidence obtained opportunistically, i.e. an opportunity to link prospective childhood data with case registers. Data has often been collected in different eras (e.g. 1960s through to 1990s) and with different procedures (e.g. teachers vs parental vs self report). Definitions (e.g. problem/withdrawn behaviour) can change over time and reliability can be low when comparing different reporting procedures for problem behaviour and anxiety [11, 17]. Time series data is required to identify the longitudinal phenotype suggested by Peter Jones, and as I shall note later resilience research requires such data. But this sort of data is limited to birth cohorts; conscript studies being cross sectional rather than longitudinal. Also current attempts to identify the endophenotype have not appreciated marked transitions between childhood and adolescence. The assessments reported in Weiser's presentation were completed in 16 – 17 year olds but it would be unwise to extrapolate back into childhood. The very different needs of children and adolescents has been embodied in most educational systems [30]; gender differences in susceptibility to depression only appear in adolescence [27], and externalising behaviour increases exponentially in males during mid adolescence [30].

■ Resilience and intervention research

Given the expectation of PPVs not exceeding 16%, we can expect that many endophenotype positive cases will not go on to develop schizophrenia per se, although if a positive case is defined as any adult psychiatric disorder then the PPV will inevitably be substantially higher. Coupled with the findings from the follow-up studies this would suggest that many 'at risk' individuals are resilient or there is a 'self righting tendency' [6]. Either way we should be able to identify protective factors, i.e. factors that reduce risk, but to date we have practically no evidence on what protects children at risk of schizophrenia. It is therefore worthwhile considering some lessons that arise from the literature on resilience where primary outcomes in adulthood have not included schizophrenia. Firstly the majority of putative high risk children show what Clarke and Clarke called the 'self righting tendency' rather than 'behaviour constancy' across the life span. This is true for extremely shy children [18], conduct disordered children [29], children with psychiatric disorders [34], mild/moderate birth complications [34], low IQ resulting from head injury [5], and those who have suffered severe adversity [6]. Surely then there is a strong case to assume self righting rather than constancy for cases meeting criteria for the neurodevelopmental endophenotype for schizophrenia?

Secondly resilience considered as a fixed trait, or constellation of factors at a particular point in development has been heuristically infertile [22]. Social behaviour, for example, is constantly being shaped and so self righting in children with dysfunctional social behaviour develops over time [18] and depends on multiple levels of influence, e.g. attributional style of the child, peer acceptance, school, and family [22]. Fostering resilience requires focusing on resilient trajectories not traits [22]. Interestingly probability of a good (or poor) adult outcome increases exponentially with the accumulation of protective (or risk) factors [22]. Evidence is emerging that a similar exponential function relates probability of schizophrenia with number of risk factors [1, 24]. Glyn Harrison (this publication) also reported that the risk for schizophrenia in Afro-Carribean English people increased exponentially with linear increase of need. Perhaps then, resilience to schizophrenia, just like other adverse adult outcomes, accord with a non-linear perhaps dynamic model of self righting. Protective factors reported in the resilience literature are not dissimilar to those we might expect in schizophrenia, such as high IQ, sociability, planning ability and a pro-social peer group. But whether these do act as protective factors for schizophrenia has yet to be evaluated. For this to be the case, high values on one or more factors would need to mitigate low scores on the other know risk factors. The protective effect of healthy (i.e. non-deviant) patterns of communication, reported (in this publication) by Tienari, may for example protect against the risk of schizophrenia in children with problem behaviour [9].

Finally it is interesting to see what lessons can be learnt from intervention studies. Peter Jones alluded to the potential for intervention. Early psycho-social interventions may well look premature given the limited evidence for protective factors and the low positive predictive value. However, if one accepts that the neurodevelopmental endophenotype increases the risk for a range of poor outcomes then the public health case for intervention strengthens. Furthermore intervention studies are not implemented purely on the back of a sound scientific base; political expediency also plays its hand (a good example is the School Violence Prevention programme in the USA) leading Zigler to coin the term 'disorder du Jour' [22]. And although the immediate cost may be prohibitive, the longer-term benefits can be substantial as demonstrated in the Perry Preschool Project. In this 1–2 year intensive preschool intervention with disadvantaged African-American children, the estimated cost saving was up to $90K/child by the time the cohort reached 27 years of age [6].

■ References

1. Bearden CE, Rosso IM, Hollister JM, Sanchez LE et al. (2000) A prospective cohort study of childhood behavioral deviance and language abnormalities as predictors of adult schizophrenia. Schiz Bull 26: 395–410
2. Bland M (1995) An Introduction to Medical Statistics. Oxford Medical Pubs
3. Cannon M, Jones P, Gilvarry C, Rifkin L et al. (1997) Premoorbid social functioning in schizophrenia and bipolar disorder: similarities and differences. Am J Psychiat 154: 1544–1550
4. Cannon M, Walsh E, Hollis C, Kargin M et al. (2001) Predictors of later schizophrenia and affective psychosis among attendees at a child psychiatry department. Brit J Psychiat 178: 420–426
5. Chadwick O, Rutter M, Shaffer D, Shrout PE (1981) A prospective study of children with head injuries: IV. Specific cognitive deficits. J Clin neuropsychol 3: 101–120
6. Clarke A, Clarke A (2000) Early Experience and the Life Path. Jessica Kingslet, London
7. David AS, Malmberg A, Brandt L, Allebeck P, Lewis G (1997) IQ and risk for schizophrenia: a population based cohort study. Psych Med 27: 1311–1323
8. Davidson M, Reichenberg A, Rabinowitz J, Weiser M et al. (1999) behavioral and intellectual markers for schizophrenia in apparently healthy male adolescents. Am J Psychiatry 156: 1328–1335
9. Doane JA, West KL, Goldstein MJ, Rodnick EH, Jones JE (1981) Parental communication deviance and affective style. Arch Gen Psychiat 38: 679–685
10. Done DJ, Crow TJ, Johnstone EC, Sacker A (1994) Childhood antecedents of schizophrenia and affective illness: social adjustment at ages 7 and 11. BMJ 309: 699–703
11. Elander J, Rutter M (1996) An update on the status of the Rutter parents' and Teachers' Scales. Child Psychol Psychiat rev 1: 31–35
12. Hartman E, Milofsky E, Vaillant G, Oldfield M et al. (1984) Vulnerability to schizopohrenia: prediction of adult schizophrenia using childhood information. Arch Gen Psychiat 41: 1050–1056
13. Hollis C (1995) Child and adolescent (juvenile onset) schizophrenia. A case control study of premorbid developmental impairments. Brit J Psychiat 166: 489–495
14. Houlihan JP (1977) Heterogeneity among schizophrenic patients: selective review of recent findings (1970–75). Schiz Bull 3: 246–261
15. John RS Mednick SA Schulsinger F (1982) Teacher reports as a predictor of schizophrenia and borderline schizophrenia: a bayseian decision analysis. J Abn Psychol 91: 399–413
16. Jones P, Rodgers B, Murray R, Marmot M (1994) Child development risk factors for adult schizophrenia in the British 1946 birth cohort. Lancet 344: 1398–1401
17. Kagan J (1992) Yesterday's premises, tomorrow's promises. Developmental Psychology 28: 990–997
18. Kerr M, Lambert WW, Bem DJ (1996) Life course sequelae of childhood shyness in Sweden: comparison with the United States. Dev Psychol 32: 1100–1105

19. Leask SJ, Done DJ, Crow TJ (in press) Adult psychosis in a national birth cohort; associatinos with meningitis and neurological soft signs, but not with common infectious illnesses. Brit J Psychiat
20. Lewine RRJ, Watt NF, Prentky RA, Fryer JH (1980) Childhood social competence in functionally disordered psychiatric patients and in normals. J Abn Psychol 89: 132–138
21. Lewis G, David A, Malmberg A, Allebeck P (2000) Non-psychotic disorder and subsequent risk of schizophrenia. Brit J Psychiat 177: 416–420
22. Luthar SS, Cicchetti D (2000) The construct of resilience: implications for interventions and social policies. Development and Psychopathology 12: 857–885
23. MacEwan TH, Athawes RWB (1997) The Nithsdale Schizophrenia Surveys. XV. Social adjustment in schizophrenia: associations with gender, symptoms and childhood antecedents. Acta Psychiat Scand 95: 254–258
24. Malmberg A, Lewis G, David A, Allebeck P (1998) Premorbid adjustment and personality in people with schizophrenia. Brit J Psychiat 172: 308–313
25. Michael CM, Morris DP, Soroker E (1957) Follow-up studies of shy withdrawn children: II. Relative incidence of schizophrenia. Am J Orthopsychiat 27: 331–337
26. Nicolson R, Lenane M, Singaracharlu S (2000) Premorbid speech and language impairments in childhood-onset schizophrenia: association with risk factors. Am J Psychiatry 157: 794–800
27. Nolen-Hoeksema S, Girgus JS (1994) The emergence of gender differences in depression during adolescence. Psychological Bulletin 115: 424–443
28. Robins LN (1966) Deviant Children Grow Up. Williams & Wilkins, Maryland
29. Robins LN, Ratcliff KS (1978) Risk factors in the continuation of childhood antisocial behavior into adulthood. Int J Ment Health 7: 96–116
30. Siegel AW, Scovill LC (2000) Problem behavior: the double symptom of adolescence. Development and Psychopathology 12: 763–793
31. Skuse DH (2001) Editorial: endophenotypes and child psychiatry. Brit J Psychiat 178: 395–396
32. Strauss JS, Klorman R, Kokes RF (1977) Part v. the implications of findings for understanding, research, and application. Schiz Bull 3: 240–244
33. Van Os J, Jones P, Lewis G, Wadsworth M, Muray R (1997) Developmental precursores of affective illness in a general population birth cohort. Archives of General Psychiatry 54: 625–631
34. Von Knorring A-L, Anderson O, Magnusson D (1987) Psychiatric care and course of psychiatric disorders from childhood to early adulthood in a representative sample. J Child Psychol Psychiat 28: 329–341
35. Walker EF, Walder DJ, Reynolds F (2001) Developmental changes in cortisol secretion in normal and at-risk youth. Development and Psychopathology 13: 721–732
36. Watt NF (1972) Longitudinal changes in the social behavior of children hospitalized for schizophrenia as adults. J Nerv Ment Dis 155: 42–54
37. Werner EE, Smith RS (1982) Vulnerable but Not Invincible: a Longitudinal Study of Resilient Children and Youth. New York, McGraw-Hill

■ Psychopathological Predictors of Onset and Course of Schizophrenia

Predicting the onset of schizophrenia

J. KLOSTERKÖTTER
Department of Psychiatry and Psychotherapy, University of Cologne, Germany

▓ Treatment and clinical course

Despite good progress in the treatment of schizophrenic psychoses in modern industrialized countries, in the majority of cases, the first diagnosis of and treatment for schizophrenia is still preceded by a succession of inadequate and, therefore, distressing contacts with counseling, medical and/or psychological services. Yet, as indicated by results from first episode research, the longer the start of an efficient therapy is delayed after the onset of first psychotic symptoms, i.e., the longer the 'Duration of Untreated Psychosis' (DUP), the more likely a negative clinical course becomes with regard to different outcome measures. A delayed begin of treatment correlates with:

- ▓ Delayed and incomplete remission of symptoms [27, 37, 6, 44, 38]
- ▓ Longer duration of hospitalization and higher risk for relapse [17]
- ▓ Less compliance, higher burden for the family and "expressed emotion" level [7, 48, 49]
- ▓ Weaker supportive social networks [35]
- ▓ Higher risk of depression and suicide [1, 2, 16, 29, 50]
- ▓ More stress in work and education-related situations [28, 34]
- ▓ More substance abuse and delinquent behavior [23]
- ▓ Possible cerebral pathophysiological changes [36, 52]
- ▓ Significantly higher treatment costs [45]

Studies showing a negative correlation between DUP and positive outcome have been assessed retrospectively and, albeit their number, are still far from being conclusive. First, they hold some methodological weaknesses. Second, some, though few, studies failed to show this correlation. A lack of association of the duration of untreated psychosis was found with:

- ▓ Severity of cognitive deficits or structural brain anomalies, i.e., lateral ventricular, temporal lobe and cerebral hemispheric volumes [20]
- ▓ Quality of life, symptom severity and time to remission of positive symptoms 6 months after first inpatient hospitalization – after controlling for the effects of age at onset (earlier onset associated with longer DUP) [19]
- ▓ 24-Month illness course, i.e., consensus rating of illness course, GAF score for worst week of last month before follow-up, affective and psychotic symptoms at 24-month follow-up [9]

Third, correlative findings in general do not allow for a causal interpretation, and – as Malla & Norman [39] pointed out – the negative correlation between DUP and outcome could as well be mediated by a third variable, e.g., the kind of onset – slow vs. acute. Future prospective studies will have to show the true nature of this relationship. Nevertheless, after a review of literature, Malla, Norman & Voruganti [40] concluded that already today "The arguments for early and optimal intervention are compelling" (p. 845).

Regarding the length of the DUP, which in most studies is defined as the time between occurrence of the first psychotic positive symptom and first hospitalization for schizophrenia, different data exists, but, in summary, a one to two years duration was specified most. A DUP of 1.1 year was also found in the most important epidemiological German retrospective study of the early course of schizophrenia, the Mannheim Age-Beginning-Course Study (ABC study), with a comprehensive assessment of first-episode patients in a circumscript area and time and a matched sample of healthy controls [14].

▪ Onset of illness and treatment

In most cases, the onset of first psychotic symptoms that meet diagnostic criteria of schizophrenia of ICD-10 or DSM-IV does not define the onset of the illness itself: Their occurrence is preceded by more or less unspecific disturbances of drive and affect, of thought, language, perception and motor action as well as by impaired bodily sensations, a reduced tolerance to normal stress and an increased emotional reactivity. These deficiencies do not meet the definition of negative symptoms by means of severity and, slightly varying in definition and differentiation, have been described as 'early symptoms' [8], 'early signs' [18, 5] or 'basic symptoms' [13, 21].

Basic symptoms can appear more or less continuously between two months and 35 years prior to their progression to the first psychotic symptoms. In the Bonn long-term study [22,], basic symptoms were found pre-psychotically in 37% of patients, and an additional 15% had shown an 'outpost syndrome' with the same kind of disturbances spontaneously remitting after their first occurrence, before transiting to a first episode after re-occurrence. Applying a more refined method, the Mannheim ABC study has meanwhile revealed even higher numbers with pre-psychotic deficiencies: On average five years before the first characteristic positive symptom, 75% of first-episode schizophrenic patients had reported negative and specially unspecific symptoms partly identical with basic symptoms (Fig. 1).

Thus, prodromal symptoms taken into account, the total delay of an adequate treatment is much longer than just one or two years: By the time of first inpatient treatment for schizophrenia, the true onset of illness dates back more than six years on average. And it was shown that the social deficits that are post-psychotically related to an incomplete recovery are not only a consequence of the acute psychosis itself but mainly develop and consolidate already very early in course, during the initial prodromal stage [41].

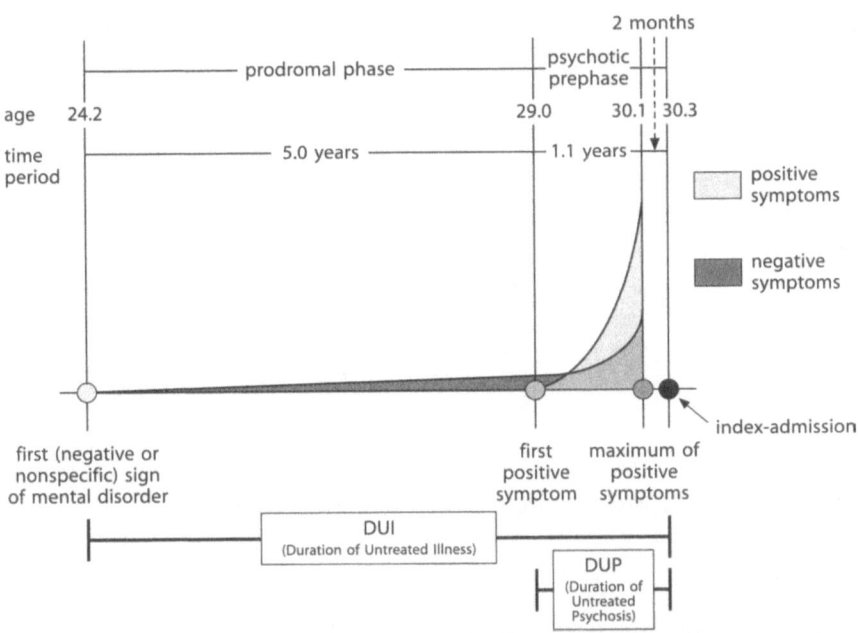

Fig. 1. The prephases of schizophrenia from first sign of mental disorder to first admission (modified from [41]).

▓ Shortening the duration of untreated illness

The conclusion to draw from these results is obviously the call for an early detection and intervention of schizophrenic psychoses. While only two German groups, the Bonn group of Gerd Huber and the Mannheim group of Heinz Häfner, have aimed for this in the past, this point of view is nowadays shared by an increasing number of researchers and clinicians world-wide. A preliminary peak of international interest in this topic was reached in 1996 with the edition of a whole volume of one of the most important special periodicals, the 'Schizophrenia Bulletin' (Vol. 22, No. 2), dedicated to "Early Detection and Intervention in Schizophrenia". Therein, McGlashan & Johannessen [42] deduced the rationale for this program and pointed out the different stages of schizophrenia (Fig. 2).

The first and most obvious therapeutic aim resulting from this phase model is the advancement of the onset of adequate treatment to the point of onset of psychotic symptoms, i.e., a shortening of the DUP. The second and probably more efficient aim representing a breakthrough in the treatment of schizophrenia is the advancement even beyond the onset of psychosis to the point of onset of prodromal symptoms, the onset of illness. Thereby, the acute psychotic symptomatology – as defined by ICD-10 and DSM-IV as schizophrenia – might be prevented or at least delayed and shortened. Such a prevention of frank psychosis would not be a primary but a secondary prevention like the prevention of pneu-

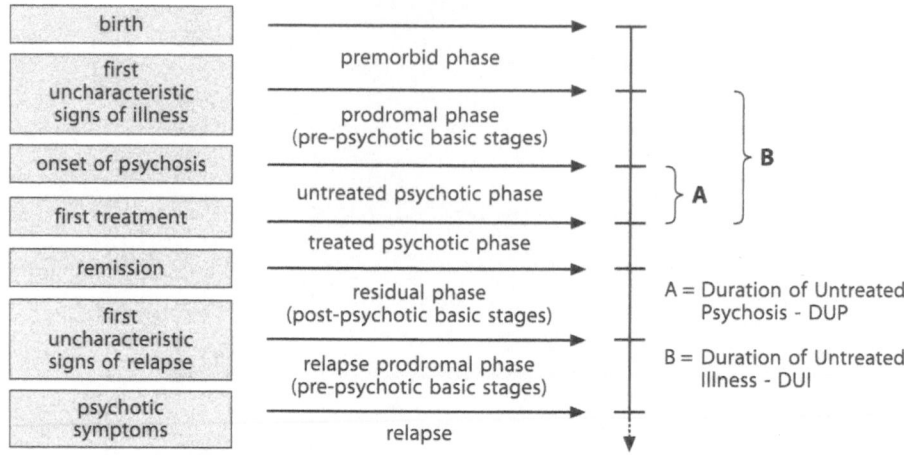

Fig. 2. Early course of schizophrenia – phases and definitions (modified from [42]).

monia by antibiotics in the pre-stage of cough. Yet as regards the requirements for early detection, such a shortening of the 'Duration of Untreated Illness' (DUI) is far more challenging than that of the DUP, because it has to be done by prodromal symptoms.

▪ Initial prodromal symptoms

Despite broad consensus on the presence of an initial prodromal stage in the majority of schizophrenic cases and on the necessity of an early detection and intervention that lead to the foundation of the 'International Early Psychosis Association' in 1996, there is less agreement as to what prodromal symptomatology predicts later schizophrenia with sufficient accuracy. Until recently, most groups focused on the DSM-III-R definition of all together nine prodromal (and residual) symptoms:

▪ Marked social isolation or withdrawal
▪ Marked impairment in role functioning as wage-earner, student, or home-marker
▪ Markedly peculiar behavior (e.g., collecting garbage, talking to self in public, hoarding food)
▪ Marked impairment in personal hygiene and grooming
▪ Blunted of inappropriate affect
▪ Digressive, vague, over-elaborate, or circumstantial speech, or poverty of speech, or poverty of content of speech
▪ Odd beliefs or magical thinking, influencing behavior and inconsistent with cultural norms, e.g., superstitiousness, belief in clairvoyance, telepathy, "sixth sense", "others can feel my feelings", over-valued ideas, ideas of reference

Table 1. Values for the predictive power of DSM-III-R prodromal symptoms

Prodromal symptom	Sensi-tivity	Speci-ficity	Positive predictive power	Negative predictive power	False positive predictions	False negative predictions
Social isolation or withdrawal	0.76	0.58	0.44	0.85	29.07 %	7.35 %
Marked impairment in role functioning	0.63	0.64	0.43	0.80	24.92 %	11.18 %
Markedly peculiar behavior	0.26	0.88	0.48	0.73	8.31 %	22.36 %
Marked impairment in personal hygiene	0.22	0.89	0.47	0.73	7.67 %	23.32 %
Blunted, flat or inappropriate affect	0.33	0.78	0.40	0.74	14.70 %	20.13 %
Digressive, vague or metaphoric speech	0.29	0.78	0.36	0.72	15.66 %	21.41 %
Odd or bizarre ideation	0.53	0.70	0.43	0.78	21.09 %	14.38 %
Unusual perceptual experiences	0.24	0.86	0.42	0.73	9.59 %	23.00 %
Marked lack of initiative, interests or energy	0.53	0.68	0.41	0.76	15.02 %	19.81 %

■ Unusual perceptual experiences, e.g., recurrent illusions, sensing the presence of a force or person not actually present
■ Marked lack of initiative, interest, or energy

No prospective study of the predictive accuracy of these symptoms has hitherto been published. Therefore, it cannot be decided whether the indices of diagnostic efficiency found in a thorough retrospective study of first-episode patients with different psychotic diagnoses [25] and given in Table 1 are an accurate estimation of their true value for an early detection. According to these results, the probability that no schizophrenic psychosis develops in the absence of any one of these symptoms (i.e., the negative predictive value, NPV) is between 0.72 and 0.85, whereas the opposite, the probability that a schizophrenia develops in the presence of any one symptoms (i.e., the positive predictive value, PPV) is at most 0.48 for 'markedly peculiar behavior'.

This as well as other studies of the prevalence, specificity and reliability of DSM-III-R-prodromal symptoms [24, 26, 43] could give no proof of the validity of these prodromal symptoms, but of an insufficient reliability of their assessment in first-episode schizophrenic patients and subsequently resulted in their removal from DSM-IV-diagnostic criteria of schizophrenia [26] with a subgroup of them subsumed among diagnostic criteria of schizotypal personality disorder. However, in a recently published, very subtle study with an improved statistical methodology, McGorry et al. [46] were indeed able to show that the diagnostic efficiency of these symptoms was definitely better in combination with a relatively prolonged functional deterioration. The failure to prove the validity of these symptoms themselves led to the conclusion that "... other symptoms, when taken in concert with one another, may have greater sensitivity and specificity, and more importantly, greater positive and negative predictive powers for psy-

Table 2. Number of patients with and without prodromal symptoms at first examination as regards outcome

	Transition to schizophrenia	No transition to schizophrenia	Σ
Basic symptoms present (at least one)	77	33	110
Basic symptoms absent	2	48	50
Σ	79	81	160

sensitivity: 0.98	positive predictive power: 0.70	% false positive predictions: 20.6%
specificity: 0.59	negative predictive power: 0.96	% false negative predictions: 1.3%
	correct predictions: 78.125%	
	(c^2 = 59.9; df = 1; p < 0.0001)	

chosis, but obviously more empirical work needs to be undertaken as regards such symptoms" [26]. And this was recently done with regard to basic symptoms, the most detailed conceptualization of prodromal symptoms in Germany.

In the 'Cologne Early Recognition (CER) study of schizophrenia' [32, 33], the first concluded prospective study on patients thought to be in the initial pro-dromal stage of a first-episode schizophrenia, 160 of 338 patients were followed up for the development of schizophrenia on average 9.6 years after their first examination. They had first been examined for prodromal symptoms with the Bonn Scale for the Assessment of Basic Symptoms (BSABS) [13] and for psy-chotic symptoms with the ninth version of the Present State Examination (PSE9) [51] before 1991 and had never shown any positive or negative symptoms of schizophrenia at this time. Yet, in the follow-up period, 79 patients developed schizophrenia according to DSM-IV criteria.

As shown in Table 2, the presence/absence of any one of the 66 BSABS-symp-toms at first examination ruled in/out the development of schizophrenia in the follow-up period with great accuracy: In the absence of any one BSABS-prodro-mal symptom, the probability of no schizophrenic psychosis was very high (NPV = 0.96; false-negatives: 1.3%), and regarding the sensitivity (0.98), specificity (0.59), positive predictive value (PPV = 0.70) and percentage of false-positive predictions (20.6%) of these symptoms in general, the resulting values are still, though little less satisfying. Thus BSABS-prodromal symptoms, when taken in concert with one another, correctly predicted the outcome in 78% of cases.

⬛ Subsyndromes of initial prodromes

Hierarchical cluster analysis of the 66 BSABS-prodromal symptoms on sample of 322 consecutively admitted inpatients and healthy controls had resulted in five subsyndromes explaining 53.25% of variance in the sample [30] "subsyndrome 1" with 35 thought, language, perception and motor disturbances, "subsyndrome 2" containing 13 impaired bodily sensations, "subsyndrome 3" subsuming five

Table 3. Prognostic accuracy of BSABS subsyndromes at a cut-point of 15 % symptoms present

BSABS subsyndrome	Sensi-tivity	Speci-ficity	Positive predictive power	Negative predictive power	False positive predictions	False negative predictions
Information processing disturbances (any 5 of 35)	0.56	0.84	0.77	0.66	8.1 %	21.9 %
Cenesthesias (any 2 of 13)	0.47	0.52	0.49	0.50	24.4 %	26.3 %
Vulnerability (any 1 of 5)	0.63	0.35	0.49	0.49	33.1 %	18.1 %
Adynamia (any 1 of 7)	0.92	0.16	0.52	0.68	42.5 %	3.8 %
Interpersonal irritation (any 1 of 6)	0.68	0.46	0.55	0.60	27.5 %	15.6 %

(The cut-point and number of symptoms included in the subsyndrome are given in parenthesis.)

symptoms describing an impaired tolerance to normal stress, "subsyndrome 4" consisting of seven disorders of emotion and affect including impaired thought energy, concentration and memory, and "subsyndrome 5" comprising six signs of increased emotional reactivity and impaired ability to maintain or initiate social contacts and disturbances in non-verbal expression.

In the CER study – as shown in Table 3 for a general cut-off of 15 % symptoms of subsyndrome present, BSABS symptoms of emotion and affect had the highest sensitivity for a transition schizophrenia (0.92) and a low percentage of false-negatives (3.8 %), but a low specificity (0.16) and PPV (0.52) along with the highest rate of false-positives (42.5 %). Disturbances of thought, language, perception and motor were also found frequently (sensitivity = 0.56), thereby satisfying the requirement for diagnostically relevant psychotic symptoms of sensitivity ≥ 0.30

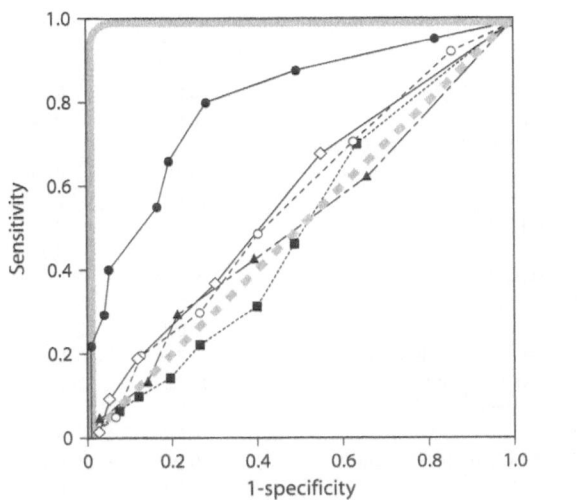

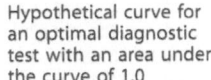

Hypothetical curve for an optimal diagnostic test with an area under the curve of 1.0

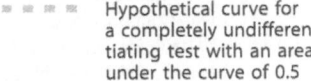

Hypothetical curve for a completely undifferen-tiating test with an area under the curve of 0.5

● Thought, language, perception and motor disturbances
■ Impaired bodily sensations
▲ Impaired stress tolerance
○ Disorders of emotion and affect
◇ Increased emotional reactivity

Fig. 3. ROC curves of BSABS subsyndromes (N = 160).

as given by Andreasen & Flaum [3], and, furthermore, had high specificity (0.84) and PPV (0.77) on top of the lowest percentage of false-positives of all subsyndromes (8.1%). Subsyndromes 2,3 and 5 held a mid-position between subsyndrome 4 and subsyndrome 1 regarding their values of indices of prognostic accuracy.

Analyses of the predictive accuracy of subsyndromes regardless of the cut-off carried out by analyses of the area under the Receiver Operating Characteristic (ROC) curve, c, DeLong, DeLong & Clarke-Pearson [11] confirmed the outstanding position of thought, language, perception and motor disturbances (see Fig. 3). With c = 0.8065 and a sensitivity of 0.80 at a specificity of 0.72, BIP discriminated significantly (p < 0.00) better between the outcome alternatives 'transition to schizophrenia' and 'no transition to schizophrenia' in nonparametric pairwise comparisons of c in related samples than any other subsyndrome. Their predictive discrimination was similar to "tossing a coin" (c = 0.5034 to 0.5810).

▓ Symptoms with the highest predictive accuracy

Table 4 shows all those 21 individual symptoms that were significantly more frequent among patients with a subsequent development of schizophrenia at the

Table 4. Prodromal symptoms significantly more frequent at first examination in the transited group

BSABS No.	Prodromal symptom	x^2 $(df = 1)$ p	p
A.8.4	Inability to divide attention	4.381	0.036
C.1.1	Thought interference	23.412	0.001
C.1.2	Thought perseveration	8.717	0.003
C.1.3	Thought pressure	28.692	0.001
C.1.4	Thought blockages	9.369	0.002
C.1.6	Disturbances of receptive language	20.677	0.001
C.1.7	Disturbances of expressive language	8.967	0.003
C.1.15	Decreased ability to discriminate between ideas and perception, fantasy and memories	14.211	0.001
C.1.17	Unstable ideas of reference	16.878	0.001
C.2.2s1	Hypersensitivity to light or certain optic stimuli	10.338	0.001
C.2.2s2	Photopsia	10.338	0.001
C.2.3s5	Changed perception of the face or body of others	9.778	0.002
C.2.3s6	Changed perception of the patient's own face	8.576	0.003
C.2.4s2	Acoasms	5.097	0.024
C.2.6	Disturbances of perception of olfactoric, gustatoric or sensible stimuli	4.703	0.030
C.2.8	Hyperdistractibility, feeling overwhelmed by stimuli	11.605	0.001
C.2.9	Captivation of attention by details of the visual field	7.506	0.006
C.2.11	Derealization	8.479	0.004
C.3.1	Motor interference exceeding simple lack of coordination	6.392	0.011
C.3.2	Motor blockages	4.670	0.031
C.3.3	Loss of automatic skills (psychomotor retardation)	10.467	0.001

Table 5. Prognostic accuracy of prodromal symptoms, which show a good predictive value and occur at least in a quarter of patients who later developed schizophrenia

Prodromal symptom	Sensitivity	Specificity	Likelihood ratio	Positive predictive value	Negative predictive value	False positive predictions	False negative predictions
Thought interference	0.42	0.91	4.66	0.83	0.62	4.4 %	28.8 %
Thought perseveration	0.32	0.88	2.66	0.71	0.57	6.3 %	33.8 %
Thought pressure	0.38	0.96	9.50	0.91	0.62	1.9 %	30.6 %
Thought blockages	0.34	0.86	2.42	0.71	0.57	6.9 %	32.5 %
Disturbances of receptive language	0.39	0.91	4.33	0.82	0.61	4.4 %	30.0 %
Decreased ability to discriminate between ideas and perception, fantasy and memories	0.27	0.95	5.40	0.84	0.57	2.5 %	36.3 %
Unstable ideas of reference	0.39	0.89	3.45	0.78	0.60	5.6 %	30.0 %
Derealization	0.28	0.90	2.80	0.73	0.56	5.0 %	35.6 %
Visual perception disturbances	0.46	0.85	3.06	0.75	0.62	7.5 %	26.9 %
Acoustic perception disturbances	0.29	0.89	2.63	0.72	0.53	5.6 %	35.0 %

index examination: these were disturbances of attention, thought, language, perception and motor.

To identify symptoms predicting the development of a first-episode schizophrenia best, two selection criteria were imposed: First, the symptom should have been present in at least a quarter of later schizophrenics at first examination, i.e., in the initial prodromal stage; this criterion equals a sensitivity ≥ 0.25 and thus is slightly more liberal than that of Andreasen & Flaum [3]. Second, at least 70 % of patients who had reported the symptom at first examination should have become schizophrenic during follow-up, i.e., PPV ≥ 0.70.

Alltogether 10 of the 66 BSABS-prodromal symptoms fulfilled these two selection criteria (see Table 5). Except 'unstable ideas of reference', these symptoms belong to thought, language, perception and motor disturbances, thereby underlining the outstanding predictive value of these self-experienced information processing disturbances. All other 56 symptoms had been present at first examination either too rarely or too frequently in both groups, thereby possessing a PPV below 0.70. Besides fulfilling selection criteria, the 10 chosen symptoms showed satisfying values for NPV and percentage of false-negatives and excellent values for specificity and percentage of false-positives. The latter measure plays an especially important role in early detection and intervention, because – as Bell [4] pointed out – those "... cases [falsely] considered at risk could suffer negative effects of intervention along with positive effects that they do not need" (p. 380). For each of the 10 selected symptoms, this percentage was clearly below 10 %.

▦ Consequences for future studies

Prodromal symptoms as defined by the BSABS have meanwhile been included in early detection instruments recently developed by two leading work groups in this field from Melbourne and New Haven, USA: the Comprehensive Assessment of At Risk Mental States (CAARMS) [53] and the Scale Of Prodromal Symptoms (SOPS) [47]; and, besides Attenuated Positive Symptoms (APS) and Brief Limited Intermitted Psychotic Symptoms (BLIPS), those BSABS-prodromal symptoms found to be highly predictive in the CER study have been added as inclusion criteria in the early intervention projects of these two groups. With a high PPV and a low rate of false-positives, they allow – for the first time – an intervention already very early in the prodromal phase when attenuated or transient psychotic symptoms have not yet been developed. In the past, early intervention mainly focused on the very late prodromal or early psychotic stage and a reduction of the DUP as identified APS and BLIPS, because reliable indicators of earlier stages had been missing (Fig. 4).

In Germany, a large Competence Network Schizophrenia was recently chosen for funding by the Ministry of Education and Research, and its first project unit Early Detection and Intervention (PU1) was given top priority. For this project unit, the Mannheim group of H. Häfner has developed an Early Recognition Inventory (ERIraos) that is based on findings with the Instrument for the Retrospective Assessment of the Onset of Schizophrenia (IRAOS) [15] and the BSABS as well as on other international conceptualizations of prodromal symptoms. Part of the ERIraos is a checklist that can be completed as a questionnaire by lay-

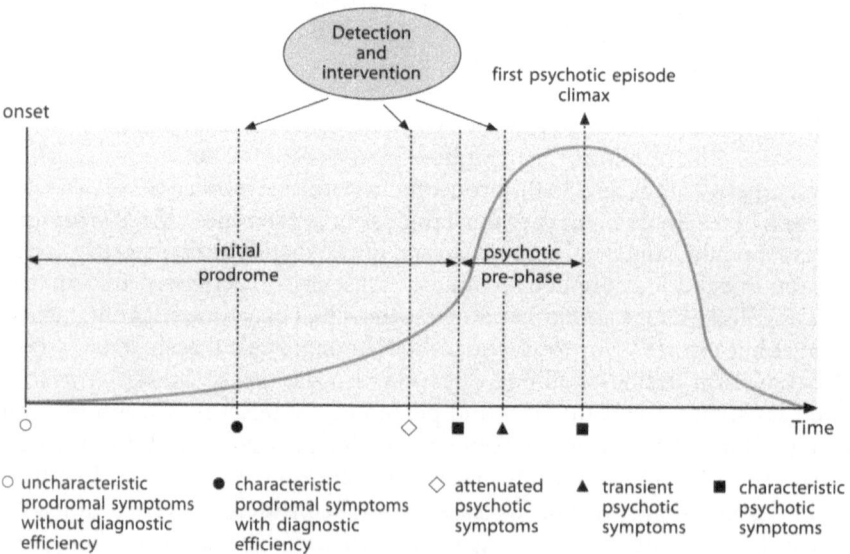

Fig. 4. Development of psychosis.

men and persons with mental problems or assessed by professionals in an interview. It serves a first risk-estimation and will be widely distributed among the addressees of the information campaigns of the Early Recognition and Intervention Center (ERIC) in Cologne and the other newly opened centers in Bonn, Düsseldorf and Munich participating in PU1. The checklist already includes some of the highly predictive BSABS-prodromal symptoms that, after the assessment of the comprehensive ERIraos, serve as one of the research criteria for the assumption of an 'early prodromal stage'.

First criterion: prodromal symptoms
a. ≥ 1 of the following symptoms with a severity ≥ 1 (ERIraos):
■ Thought interference
■ Thought perseveration
■ Thought pressure
■ Thought blockages
■ Disturbance of receptive language, either heard or read
■ Decreased ability to discriminate between ideas and perception or fantasy and true memories
■ Unstable ideas of reference
■ Derealization
■ Visual perception disturbances
■ Acoustic perception disturbances
b. multiple occurrence in ≥ 1 week

Second criterion: recent functional deterioration and risk factors
Loss of ≥ 30 GAF-M points (Global Assessment of Functioning according to DSM-IV) for ≥ 1 month plus
≥ 1 1st-degree relative with a life-time diagnosis of schizophrenia (ERIraos) or ante-/postnatal or obstetric complications (ERIraos).

■ Prospects

Albeit great and still growing international attention paid to the subject 'early detection and intervention in psychoses', just the first careful steps have been taken in practice. But as long as there is only one larger prospective early detection study concluded and only preliminary results from a pilot study of early intervention exist, it still remains unclear, if this approach will fulfill the high expectations. Early enthusiasm should also be avoided as one of the most cited arguments for an early detection and intervention, the negative effect of a long DUP on the clinical course of first psychotic episodes, is still not finally proven. However, even in the case that this assumption is proven wrong, one central aim of the approach will not be called into question: the gradual shift from curative treatment – that, at present, is still far from being successful in all cases – to preventive intervention [31]. Would it become possible to prevent a first psychotic exacerbation in a subgroup of patients, as indicated by the preliminary results from Melbourne, a breakthrough in the treatment of psychoses would have been reached that might as well bring along more positive effects than can be expected by a reduction of the DUP when frank psychosis is already present. And there is reason for cautious optimism now that psychosis predictive value was shown even for simple test parameters as applied by the Israeli draft board [10] and neuropsychological paradigms as assessed in the American high-risk project [12]. Such objective measures, when taken in concert with initial prodromal symptoms, might be able to optimize prediction of first-episode psychoses and to close the gap between the rather treatment oriented early detection and intervention approach and basic research, e.g., into the biological principles underlying the risk of psychoses. In an attempt towards closing this gap, patients participating in treatment studies of PU1 will be asked to additionally volunteer for neuropsychological, neurophysiological, imaging and molecular-genetic studies.

Regarding the growing number of early detection and intervention initiatives in different and the existing international co-operation between groups working in this field, it might not be overly optimistic to expect that the question of the efficacy of early detection and intervention can be answered in more detail in between the forthcoming 5 years.

■ References

1. Addington J, Addington D (1998) Effect of substance misuse in early psychosis. Br J Psychiatry 172 (Suppl 33): 134–136
2. Addington D, Addington J, Patten S (1998) Depression in people with first-episode schizophrenia. Br J Psychiatry 172 (Suppl 33): 90–92
3. Andreasen NC, Flaum M (1991) Schizophrenia: the characteristic symptoms. Schizophr Bull 17: 27–49
4. Bell RQ (1992) Multiple-risk cohorts and segmenting risk as solutions to the problem of false positives in risk for the major psychoses. Psychiatry 55: 370–381
5. Birchwood M, Smith J, McMillan JF (1989) Predicting relapse in schizophrenia: the development and implementation of an early signs monitoring system using patients and families as observers, a preliminary investigation. Psychol Med 19: 649–656
6. Birchwood M, McMillan JF (1993) Early intervention in schizophrenia. Aust N Z J Psychiatry 27: 374–378
7. Brown S, Birtwistle J (1998) People with schizophrenia and their families. Fifteen-year outcome. Br J Psychiatry (Aug) 173: 139–144
8. Chapman JP (1966) The early symptoms of schizophrenia. Br J Psychiatry 112: 225–251
9. Craig TJ, Bromet EJ, Fennig S, Tanenberg-Karant M, Lavelle J, Galambos N (2000) Is there an association between duration of untreated psychosis and 24-month clinical outcome in first-admission series. Am J Psychiatry 157: 60–67
10. Davidson M, Reichenberg A, Rabinowitz J, Weiser M, Kaplan Z, Mark M (1999) Behavioral and intellectual markers for schizophrenia in apparently healthy male adolescents. Am J Psychiatry 156: 1328–1335
11. DeLong ER, DeLong DM, Clarke-Pearson DL (1988) Comparing the areas under two or more correlated receiver operating characteristic curves: a nonparametric approach. Biometrics 44: 837–845
12. Erlenmeyer-Kimling L, Rock D, Roberts SA, Janal M, Kestenbaum C, Cornblatt B, Adamo UH, Gottesman II (2000) Attention, memory, and motor skills as childhood predictors of schizophrenia-related psychoses: the New York High-Risk Project. Am J Psychiatry 157 (9): 1416–1422

13. Gross G, Huber G, Klosterkötter J, Linz M (1987) Bonner Skala für die Beurteilung von Basissymptomen (BSABS: Bonn Scale for the Assessment of Basic Symptoms). Springer, Berlin, Heidelberg, New York

14. Häfner H, Maurer K, Löffler W, Riecher-Rössler A (1993) The influence of age and sex on the onset and early course of schizophrenia. Br J Psychiatry 162: 80–86

15. Häfner H, Riecher-Rössler A, Hambrecht M, Maurer K, Meissner S, Schmidtke A, Fätkenheuer B, Löffler W, van der Heiden W (1999) IRAOS: an instrument for the assessment of the onset and early course of schizophrenia. Schizophr Res 6: 209–223

16. Hambrecht M, Häfner H (1996) Substance abuse and the onset of schizophrenia. Biol Psychiatry 39: 1–9

17. Helgason L (1990) Twenty years' follow-up of first psychiatric presentation for schizophrenia: what could have been prevented? Acta Psychiatr Scand 81: 231–235

18. Herz MI, Szymanski MV, Simon JC (1982) Intermitted medication of stable schizophrenic outpatients: an alternative to maintenance medication. Am J Psychiatry 139: 918–922

19. Ho BC, Andreasen NC, Flaum M, Nopoulos P, Miller D (2000) Untreated initial psychosis: its relation to quality of life and symptom remission in first-episode schizophrenia. Am J Psychiatry 157 (5): 808–815

20. Hoff AL, Sakuma M, Razi K, Heydebrand G, Csernansky JG, DeLisi LE (2000) Lack of association between duration of untreated illness and severity of cognitive and structural brain deficits at the first episode of schizophrenia. Am J Psychiatry 157 (11): 1824–1828

21. Huber G (1986) Psychiatrische Aspekte des Basisstörungskonzepts. In: Süllwold L, Huber G (eds). Schizophrene Basisstörungen. Springer, Berlin, Heidelberg, New York, pp 39–143

22. Huber G, Gross G, Schüttler R (1979) Schizophrenie. Verlaufs- und sozialpsychiatrische Langzeituntersuchungen an den 1945–1959 in Bonn hospitalisierten schizophrenen Kranken. Springer, Berlin, Heidelberg, New York

23. Humphreys MS, Johnstone EC, MacMillan JF, Taylor PJ (1992) Dangerous behaviour preceding first admissions for schizophrenia. Br J Psychiatry 161: 501–505

24. Jackson HJ, McGorry PD, McKenzie D (1994) The reliability of DSM-III prodromal symptoms in first episode psychotic patients. Acta Psychiatrica Scandinavica 90: 375–378

25. Jackson HJ, McGorry PD, Dudgeon P (1995) Prodromal symptoms of schizophrenia in first-episode psychosis. Prevalence and specificity. Compr Psychiatry 36: 241–250

26. Jackson HJ, McGorry PD, Dakis J et al. (1996) The inter-rater and test-retest reliabilities of prodromal symptoms in first-episode psychosis. Australian and New Zealand Journal of Psychiatry 30: 498–504

27. Johnstone EC, Crow TJ, Johnson AL, McMillan JF (1986) The Northwick Park study of first episodes of schizophrenia: I. Presentation of the illness and problems relating to admission. Br J Psychiatry 148: 115–120

28. Johnstone EC, Macmillan JF, Frith CD, Benn DK, Crow TJ (1990) Further investigation of the predictors of outcome following first schizophrenic episodes. Br J Psychiatry 157: 182–189

29. Koreen AR, Siris SG, Chakos M, Alvir J, Mayerhoff D, Lieberman J (1993) Depression in first-episode schizophrenia. Am J Psychiatry 150 (11): 1643–1648

30. Klosterkötter J, Ebel H, Schultze-Lutter F, Steinmeyer EM (1996) Diagnostic validity of basic symptoms. Eur Arch Psychiatry Clin Neurosci 246: 147–154

31. Klosterkötter J (1998) Von der Krankheitsbekämpfung zur Krankheitsverhütung – ist ein solcher Paradigmenwandel auch für schizophrene Störungen möglich? Fortschr Neurol Psychiatr 67: 316–328

32. Klosterkötter J, Hellmich M, Schultze-Lutter F (2000) Ist die Diagnose schizophrener Störungen schon in der initialen Prodromalphase vor der psychotischen Erstmanifestation möglich? Fortschr Neurol Psychiatr 68 (Sonderheft 1): S13–S21

33. Klosterkötter J, Hellmich M, Steinmeyer EM, Schultze-Lutter F (2001) Diagnosing schizophrenia in the initial prodromal phase. Arch Gen Psychiatry 58: 158–164

34. Larsen TK, McGlashan TH, Moe LC (1996) First-episode schizophrenia: I. Early course parameters. Schizophr Bull 22: 241–256

35. Larsen TK, Johannessen JO, Opjordsmoen S (1998) First-episode schizophrenia with long duration of untreated psychosis. Pathways to care. Br J Psychiatry 172 (Suppl 33): 45–52

36. Lieberman JA, Kinon BJ, Loebel AD (1990) Dopaminergic mechanisms in idiopathic and drug-induced psychoses. Schizophr Bull 16: 97–110
37. Loebel AD, Lieberman JA, Alvir JM, Mayerhoff DI, Geisler SH, Szymanski SR (1992) Duration of psychosis and outcome in first-episode schizophrenia. Am J Psychiatry 149 (9): 1183–1188
38. Loebel AD, Lieberman JA, Alvir JMJ, Mayerhoff DI, Geisler SH, Szymanski SR (1996) Duration of psychosis and outcome in first-episode schizophrenia. Am J Psychiatry 149: 1183–1188
39. Malla AK, Norman RMG (1999) Facing the challenges of intervening early in psychosis. Annals RCPSC 32: 394–397
40. Malla AK, Norman RMG, Voruganti LP (1999) Improving outcome in schizophrenia: the case for early intervention. Canadian Medical Association Journal 160: 843–846
41. Maurer K, Häfner H (1995) Methodological aspects of onset assessment in schizophrenia. Schizophr Res 15: 265–276
42. McGlashan TH, Johannessen JO (1996) Early detection and intervention in schizophrenia. Schizophrenia Bulletin 22: 201–222
43. McGorry PD, McFarlane C, Patton GC et al. (1995) The prevalence of prodromal features of schizophrenia in adolescence: a preliminary survey. Acta Psychiatrica Scandinavica 92: 241–249
44. McGorry PD, Edwards J, Mihalopoulos SM (1996) EPPIC: an evolving system of early detection and optimal management. Schizophr Bull 22: 305–326
45. McGorry PD, Edwards J (1997) Early Psychosis Training Pack. Victoria Mill, Gardiner-Caldwell Communications, Australia
46. McGorry PD, McKenzie D, Jackson HJ, Waddell F, Curry C (2000) Can we improve the diagnostic efficiency and predictive power of prodromal symptoms for schizophrenia? Schizophr Res 42 (2): 91–100
47. Miller TJ, McGlashan TH, Woods SW, Stein K, Driesen N, Corcoran CM, Hoffman R, Davidson L (1999) Symptom assessment in schizophrenic prodromal states. Psychiatr Q 70: 273–287
48. Stirling J et al. (1991) Expressed emotion and early onset schizophrenia: a one-year follow-up. Psychol Med 21: 675–685
49. Stirling J, Tantam D, Thomas P, Newby D, Montague L, Ring N, Rowe S (1993) Expressed emotion and schizophrenia: the ontogeny of EE during an 18-month follow-up. Psychol Med 23 (3): 771–778
50. Strakowski SM, Keck PE Jr, McElroy SL, Lonczak HS, West SA (1995) Chronology of comorbid and principal syndromes in first-episode psychosis. Compr Psychiatry 36 (2): 106–112
51. Wing JK, Cooper JE, Sartorius N (1974) Measurement and Classification of Psychiatric Symptoms. An Introduction Manual for the PSE and Catego-program. Cambridge Press, London
52. Wyatt RJ (1991) Neuroleptics and the natural course of schizophrenia. Schizophr Bull 17 (2): 325–351
53. Yung AR, Phillips LJ, McGorry PD, McFarlane CA, Francey S, Harrigan S, Patton GC, Jackson HJ (1998) Prediction of psychosis. Br J Psychiatry 172 (suppl 33): 14–20

The early course of schizophrenia*

H. Häfner[1], K. Maurer[1], W. Löffler[2], W. an der Heiden[1], R. Könnecke[1], M. Hambrecht[3]

[1]Schizophrenia Research Unit, Central Institute of Mental Health, Mannheim, Germany
[2]formerly CIMH Schizophrenia Research Unit, now Institute for Cardiac Infarct Research Foundation at the Ludwigshafen Clinical Center, Germany
[3]formerly CIMH Schizophrenia Research Unit, now Department of Psychiatry and Psychotherapy, Elisabethenstift Hospital, Darmstadt, Germany

■ Introduction

It is usually the dramatic symptoms of the first psychotic episode that trigger the first treatment contact and, thus, determine the chances for effective treatment. First contact, however, is frequently preceded by a long period of incipient illness. Among the first whose interest was attracted to this fact were Sullivan [44], Cameron [8] and still earlier Emil Kraepelin [32] and Eugen Bleuler [6]. Like the further course of the disorder, the initial phase of schizophrenia varies greatly in type and length of time from illness onset until the climax of the first episode. The delayed beginning of treatment seems to be a problem which is encountered, throughout the world, even in countries with well-developed mental health care systems. Table 1 lists nine selected studies, which, however, are not fully comparable because of their methodological differences in assessing illness onset and because of different definitions used. Despite their flaws the studies all show a timespan of several years between onset and first treatment contact and a duration of at least one year for untreated psychosis. Because of fewer difficulties involved, the latter assessment can be considered fairly reliable. These results have triggered a great number of studies into the consequences that duration of untreated illness (DUI) and psychosis (DUP) might have.

Most of these studies have shown, though not consistently, that DUP is associated with indicators of an unfavorable course of schizophrenia [10, 35, 36, 50]. For this reason numerous research groups are making great efforts to develop instruments that would permit us to recognize schizophrenia earlier and predict psychosis onset as a prerequisite of appropriate early intervention.

At the same time numerous early intervention programs have been launched (see Klosterkötter, this volume).

---

* This contribution, not presented at the symposium, has been included in this volume to fill the void left by W. an der Heiden's cancelled contribution and to provide an adequate representation of the topic. It is not dealt with in the discussion and the concluding remarks.

Table 1. Duration of the prephase of schizophrenia from onset – 1st sign, 1st psychotic symptom – until first contact or first admission by selected studies[1]

Author	N	Duration from 1st sign (in years)	Duration from 1st psychotic symptom (in years)
Gross 1969 (Germany) [13]	290	3.5	
Lindelius 1970 (Sweden) [34]	237		4.4[2]
Huber et al. 1979 (Germany) [28]	502	3.3	
Loebel et al. 1992 (USA) [35]	70	2.9	1.0
Beiser et al. 1993 (Canada) [3]	70	2.1	1.0
McGorry et al. 1996 (Australia) [36]	200	2.1	1.4
Lewine 1980 (USA) [33]	97		1.9
Häfner et al. 1995 (Germany) [21]	232	5.0[3]	1.1
Johannessen et al. 1999 (Norway) [29]	43		2.2

[1] slightly different diagnostic definitions and methodological standards
[2] age at first psychotic symptoms or marked personality changes indicative of mental illness
[3] Prodromal phase until appearance of first psychotic symptom only
Source: [22], modified

■ The ABC study sample

In 1987 we commenced our research into the onset, early and further course of schizophrenia with a controlled study design. The results of the ABC Schizophrenia Study, funded by the German Research Association over a period of 15 years, have been published successively. Currently, we are about to complete a 12-year follow-up of our first-episode sample and to enter data analysis.

The population-based ABC study sample was recruited from a semirural, semiurban geographical region in Central Germany. It comprised 232 first illness episodes of broadly defined schizophrenia (ICD-9: 295, 297, 298.3, 298.4) (= 84% of 276 first admissions) from a German population of about 1.5 million (for further details of the sample see [19, 20]).

Individual demographic and social development, onset and early course of the illness were assessed retrospectively using the IRAOS interview [17, 24]. A characteristic of this instrument is that it allows relevant events to be entered in a time matrix based on objectively verifiable or reliably remembered "anchor events" such as the birth of a child, a holiday spent abroad, etc. Using this instrument we collected parallel data from three different sources (the patient, a close relative, medical records). By comparing the information provided by these sources we were able to test what type of data on the milestones of the evolving disorder were of good to satisfactory reliability. Concerning single symptoms, observable behavior showed the highest degree of agreement between the three sources. For the purpose of a multidimensional assessment of the disorder and its further course the following instruments were used: PSE (Present State Examination

[49]), the SANS (Scale for the Assessment of Negative Symptoms [2]), the PIRS (Psychiatric Impairments Rating Schedule [5]), the DAS (Disability Assessment Scale [30, 47] and FU-HSD (Follow-up History and Sociodemographic Description Schedule [46]).

The prospective part of the study was based on a representative ABC subsample of 115 first-episode cases, who were assessed both retrospectively at first admission to trace their case histories back to illness onset and prospectively at 6 cross sections: at first admission and 6 months, 1, 2, 3 and 5 years after. These cases were compared with controls randomly drawn from the population register and matched by age, sex and place of residence.

■ Results

When the number of symptoms in the three clinical symptom categories nonspecific, negative and positive is depicted on a yearly basis and in the year preceding first admission on a monthly basis, the course of illness over time and its gradients become plain to see (Fig. 1).

Nonspecific and negative symptoms precede the first psychotic symptoms by several years. At illness onset, symptoms increase exponentially. In the psychotic episode, as Fig. 1 shows, negative and nonspecific symptoms also increase steeply. After the climax of the episode, symptoms diminish on all three dimensions. Psychotic symptoms, which respond to neuroleptic medication most clearly, usually subside more rapidly than negative symptoms, which frequently take more time to remit.

Eighteen percent of the sample had an acute type of early illness course, i.e., there was a timespan of four weeks at the most between first illness sign and first admission. Characteristic of these cases was a predominance of positive symptoms without a preceding prodromal stage. A subacute type of onset with a prodromal stage of four weeks to one year was observed in 15% of cases. A total of 68% of the sample had a chronic type of onset with more than a year elapsing between illness onset and first admission. The three types of early illness course, acute, subacute and chronic, are equally frequent in men and women. In developing countries acute cases are almost twice as frequent as in industrialized countries [45, 48].

A prodromal stage marked by negative and nonspecific symptoms is seen in 73% of cases. Only 7% experience illness onset with purely positive symptoms and 20% with both positive and negative symptoms occurring within the same month. Unlike Angloamerican studies and textbooks on the topic, most of which report a predominance of the chronic type of onset with mainly negative symptoms in men and a predominance of the acute type of onset with primarily positive symptoms in women, we did not observe such a sex difference in our systematically studied epidemiological sample. But throughout the milestones of incipient illness – first illness sign, first negative symptom, first positive symptom and climax of the first episode – there was a significant sex difference of about four years. The higher age of women at onset and their second peak of

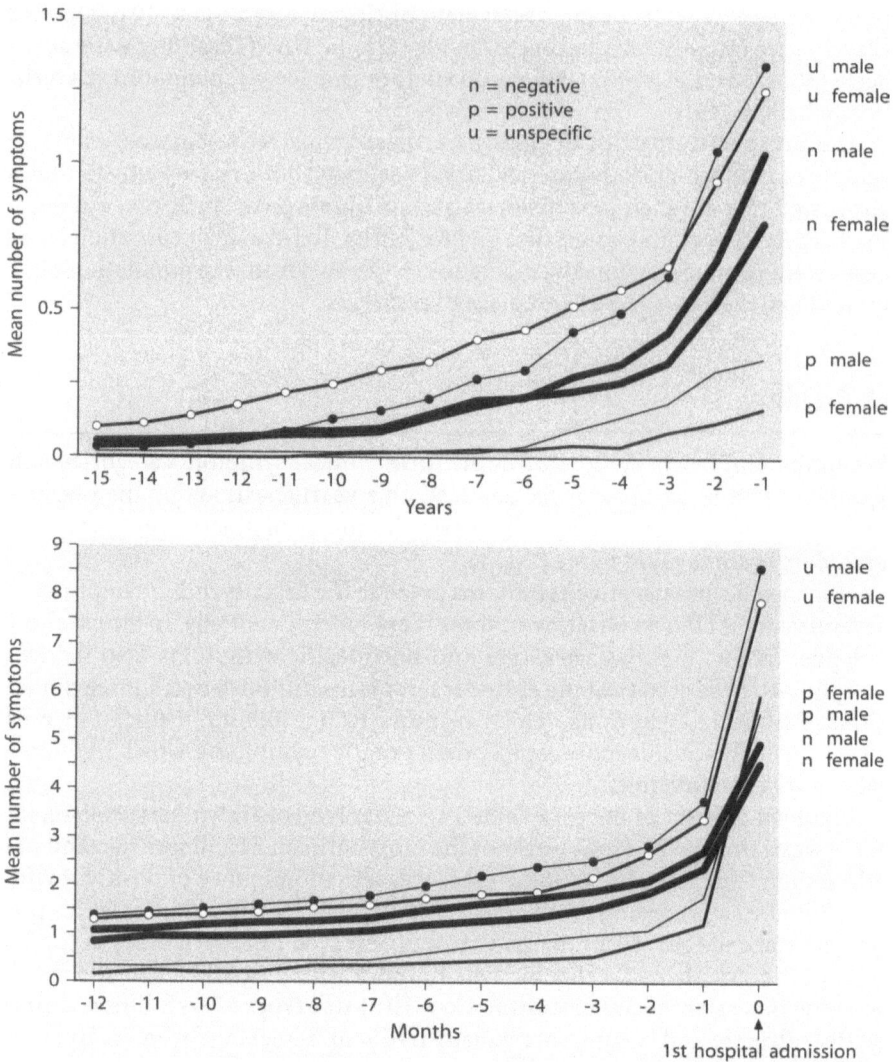

Fig. 1. Cumulative numbers of positive, negative and unspecific symptoms from onset until first hospital admission for schizophrenia (males = 108, females = 124); top: per year until one year before 1st admission; bottom: per month in the last year before 1st admission (Source: [21]).

onsets around menopause were accounted for by the sensitivity reducing effect of estrogen, a potent neuromodulator, on D2 receptors. We were able to demonstrate this in both animal experiments [18] and in a controlled clinical study [39, 40]. The sex difference in age of onset, it will be demonstrated, has consequences for course and outcome.

In Fig. 2 are depicted, on the basis of mean values from the ABC study data, age of onset and duration of the prodromal stage, psychotic prephase until the climax of the first episode as well as time to first admission.

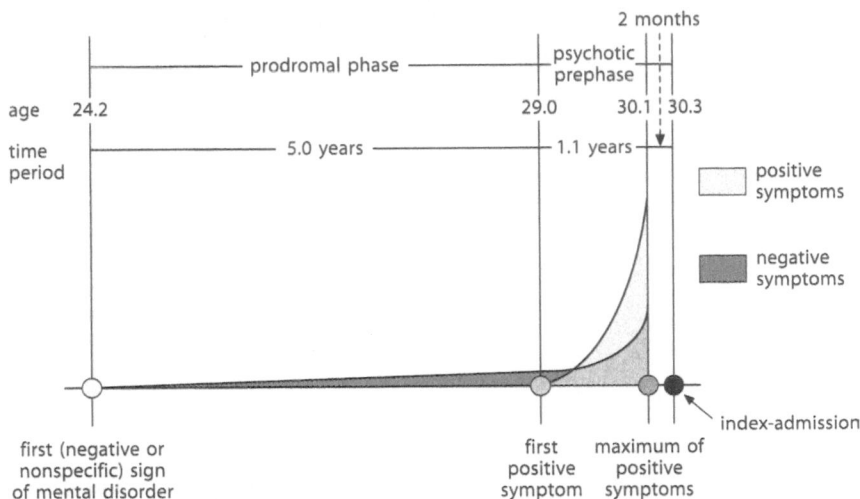

Fig. 2. The prephases of schizophrenia from first sign of mental disorder to first admission – N = 232 (108 males, 124 females) – for both sexes together (Source: [21]).

The durations of the prodromal phase and psychotic prephase, as mentioned above, show a highly skewed distribution with a predominance of short durations and medians of 2.33 years for the prodromal phase and of 0.8 years for the psychotic prephase.

▦ Development of symptoms, social disability and substance abuse

Initial symptoms

Among the 10 most frequent initial symptoms, equally frequent in men and women except worrying, there were no positive symptoms (Table 2). Two symptom dimensions clearly predominated: *affective* symptoms, such as depressive mood, feelings of guilt and anxiety, and *negative* symptoms, such as trouble with thinking and concentration, loss of energy, slowness, poor work performance and social withdrawal.

When first symptom occurrence was depicted purely descriptively on the basis of four categories in a simplified additive model – not taking symptom persistence in subsequent stages into account – the crude clusters depicted in Fig. 3 emerged.

First to appear, 4.5 to 4 years – showing a second peak 3 to 2.5 years – before first admission, were affective symptoms. Next to emerge, 4 to 1.5 years before first admission, were negative symptoms, which showed considerable overlap with affective symptoms. Dysthymic symptoms, including menstrual disturbances and disturbances of appetite and sleep, headache, etc., appeared about 3

Table 2. The ten most frequent earliest signs of schizophrenia (independent of the course) reported by the patients[1]

	Total (n = 232) %	Men (n = 108) %	Women (n = 124) %	p
Restlessness	19	15	22	
Depression	19	15	22	
Anxiety	18	17	19	
Trouble with thinking and concentration	16	19	14	
Worrying	15	9	20	*
Lack of self-confidence	13	10	15	
Lack of energy, slowness	12	8	15	
Poor work performance	11	12	10	
Social withdrawal, distrust	10	8	12	
Social withdrawal, communication	10	8	12	

[1] Based on closed questions, multiple counting possible. All items tested for sex differences; *: $p < 0.05$
Source: [21], modified

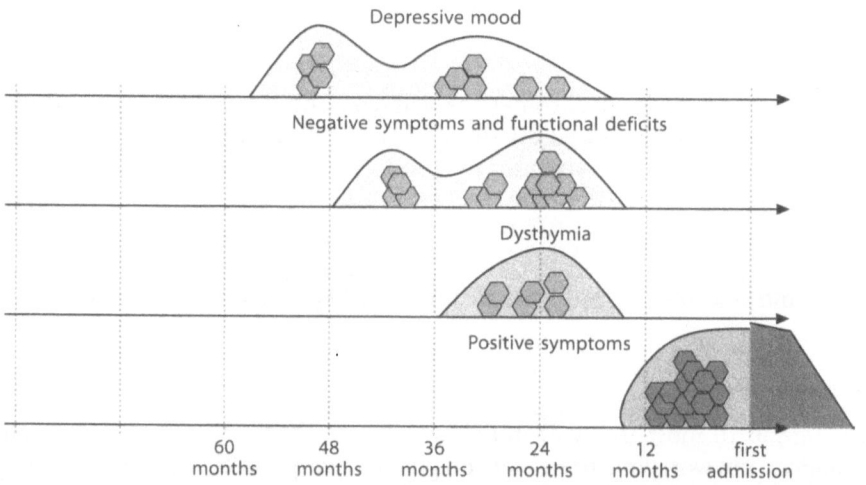

Fig. 3. First onset of pre-psychotic symptoms prior to first admission – IRAOS data of 170 first illness episodes with four clinical types of prodromal phases.

to 1.5 years before first admission. Finally, about one year before first admission, psychotic symptoms manifested themselves. Based on mean values, this pattern of course cannot be regarded as characteristic of schizophrenia, i.e., invariably encountered in all cases.

Early depression

We chose four depressive symptoms presumed to show only little overlap with negative symptoms: depressive mood, feelings of guilt, lack of self-confidence

Table 3. Comparison of 4 depressive IRAOS items in patients and controls – lifetime prevalence by age at first admission of schizophrenic patients – continuously present or recurrent symptoms only

IRAOS item	Schizophrenics (n = 57) %	Controls (n = 57) %	Chi² test	Relative risk
Depressive mood	70.2	19.3	***	3.6
Feelings of guilt	33.3	10.5	**	3.2
Lack of self-confidence	59.4	12.3	***	4.8
Suicide attempt	12.3	8.8	n.s.	1.4

n.s. not significant, **: $p < 0.01$, *** $p < 0.001$
Source: [25]

and attempted suicide. 83 % of the total first-episode sample (N = 232) and 81 % of the cases with a restrictive ICD 295 diagnosis of schizophrenia (N = 203), except for schizoaffective disorder, suffered from depressive mood for at least two weeks before first admission. 39 % showed a continuous presence of depressive symptoms, 34 % recurring depressive episodes and 8 % only one depressive episode. Only 19 % experienced no episode of depressive mood of at least 14 days' duration in the early course of schizophrenia.

A comparison of a representative subsample of 57 schizophrenic patients from the city of Mannheim with 57 healthy controls matched for age and sex and place of residence showed a 3 to almost 5 times higher cumulative prevalence of depressive symptoms for schizophrenics (Table 3). Attempted suicide with a 40 % excess, which did not reach significance presumably because of the small numbers, pointed to an early suicide risk before the first treatment contact.

A descriptive analysis of the illness course showed that after the remission of the first episode the frequency of depression, as based on the CATEGO [49] depressive syndrome, remained fairly stable (see Table 4), and the same held true, when other criteria for depression, e.g., the broad ICD-10 research criteria or the ICD-10 clinical criteria of depression, were used.

Table 4. Prevalence of depressive episodes over 5 years after first admission according to ICD-10 research criteria (N = 115)

	1st admission n	%	6 months n	%	1 year n	%	2 years n	%	3 years n	%	5 years n	%
a All criteria for F32:												
F32	26	22.6	12	13.5	7	7.9	7	9.0	1	1.3	6	7.0
b Severity of symptoms according to criterion C for F32:												
C ≥ 4	85	73.9	24	27.0	26	29.2	25	31.6	20	26.3	19	22.1

Source: [22]

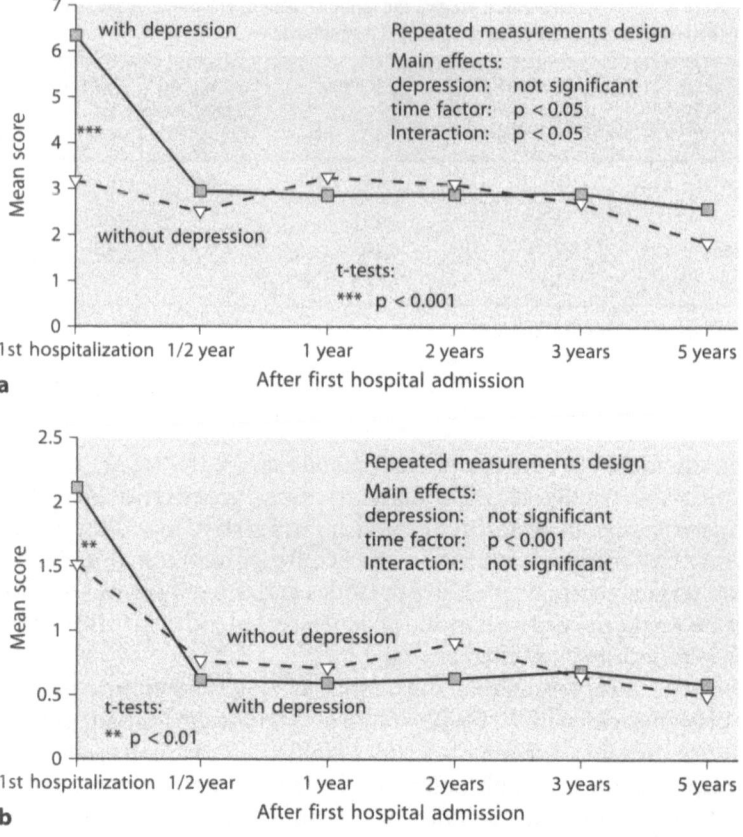

Fig. 4. a The course of depressive CATEGO syndrome over 5 years in patients with and without early-course depressive mood (n = 115). **b** The course of symptoms (CATEGO total score) over 5 years in patients with and without early-course depressive mood (n = 115) (Source: [25]).

To study the power of early depressive symptoms as predictors of the first illness episode and of the following 5-year course, we divided our sample of restrictively defined schizophrenia (n = 203) into 39 (= 19%) patients without and 164 (= 81%) with depressive mood in the early course of schizophrenia. The group experiencing depressive mood in the prephase had significantly elevated CATEGO depression, and CATEGO total scores in the first psychotic episode (Fig. 4) and elevated SANS global ratings in the psychotic episode (Fig. 5a). Hence, early-course depression seemed to be a predictor of the overall severity of the first psychotic episode, but not of the further course of psychotic symptoms.

Using a repeated measurements design we found that early depression predicted neither positive nor non-specific symptoms, but it did predict negative symptoms by exerting a significantly negative effect particularly on affective flattening up to the one-year and at the 5-year assessment (Fig. 5b).

The causal mechanism producing depressive symptoms long before antipsychotic treatment is initiated and before the illness produces its first consequences

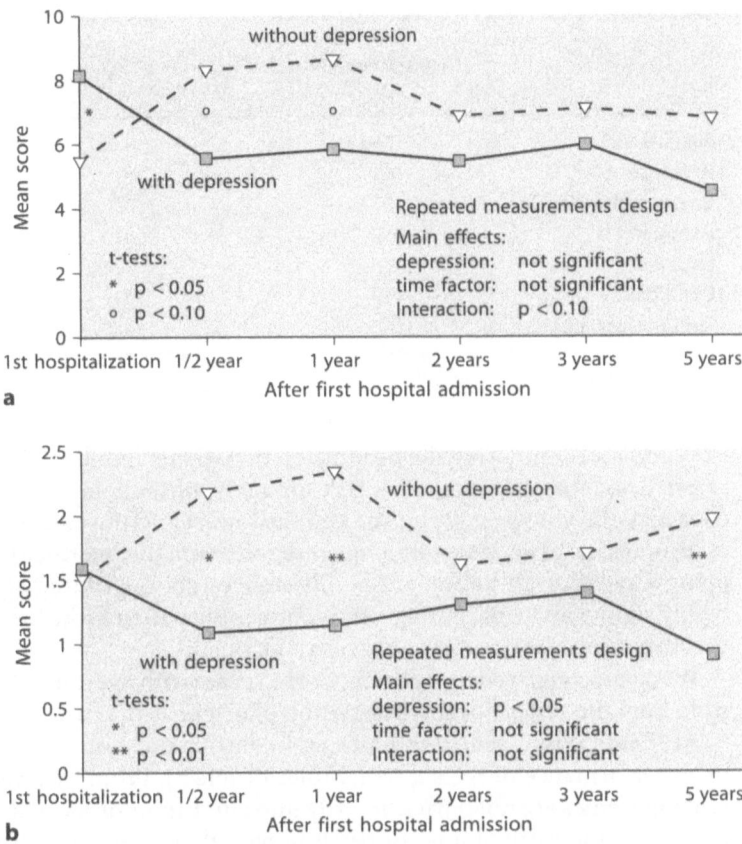

Fig. 5. a The course of negative symptoms (SANS total score) over 5 years in patients with and without early-course depressive mood (n = 115). **b** The course of affective flattening (SANS global rating) over 5 years in patients with and without early-course depressive mood (n = 115) (Source: [25]).

makes both pharmacogenic and reactive explanations seem unlikely. We rather presume that what we are dealing with here are premonitory signs of the pathophysiological process that subsequently brings forth depressive, negative and positive symptoms and leads to a psychotic episode.

Negative symptoms and social impairment in the early illness stages and their consequences for further illness

To be able to measure changes and to control for temporal effects emanating, for example, from unemployment rates in the population at large, studies into the social consequences of a disorder must take a baseline into account, e.g., the patients' social status at illness onset, but only few longitudinal studies into schizophrenia do so.

We assessed the level of social development at illness onset by dividing our first-episode sample (N = 232) into three age groups (12 to 20, 21 to 35 and 36 to

Table 5. Social-role performance at the emergence of the first sign of mental disorder (percentages)

	Schizophrenics (n = 57) %	Controls (n = 57) %	p[1]
Age (in years)	24.0	4.0	
School education	65	61	n.s.
Occupational training	37	44	n.s.
Employment	33	42	n.s.
Own income	37	42	n.s.
Own accommodation	46	51	n.s.
Marriage or stable partnership	47	58	n.s.

1: *n.s.* not significant
Source: [25]

59 years) and comparing the proportion of patients fulfilling six key roles characteristic of the main period of risk for schizophrenia in these age groups. As expected, the youngest group showed the lowest and the oldest group the highest proportion of patients fulfilling these roles with the intermediate group occupying a position in between. The differences between three age groups were highly significant. Our finding – the younger the patients, the lower their level of social development at onset – was a trivial one.

We again compared the subsample of 57 cases with age- and sex-matched controls from the same city and population of origin as the patients.

At illness onset, schizophrenics and controls did not differ significantly in their performance of the six social roles (Table 5). From this we conclude that schizophrenics are not born primarily into conditions of social disadvantage. At the end of the early illness course, however, there were significant differences (Table 6). This means that the social consequences of the disorder emerge between illness onset and first contact, i.e., in the early illness course. The gap was most pronounced in marriage and stable partnership: a look at the patients' development between illness onset and first admission showed nearly equal initial values for both schizophrenic and healthy men and women. The proportion

Table 6. Social-role performance at first admission (percentages)

	Schizophrenics (n = 57) %	Controls (n = 57) %	p[1]
Age (in years)	30.0	30.0	
School education	93	95	n.s.
Occupational training	63	65	n.s.
Employment	44	58	t
Own income	49	74	**
Own accommodation	63	75	n.s.
Marriage or stable partnership	25	68	***

1: *n.s.* not significant; t: $p < 0.1$; **: $p < 0.01$; ***: $p < 0.001$
Source: [25]

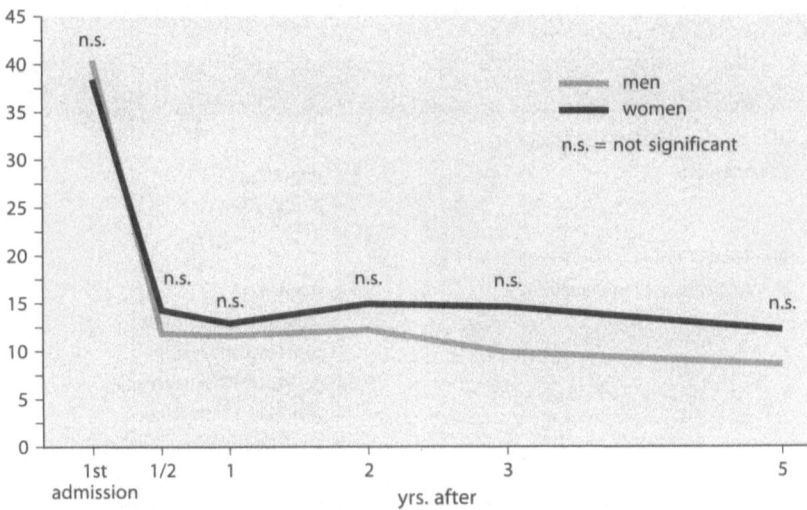

Fig. 6. Five-year course from first admission on (6 cross sections) for men and women by the CATEGO total score (n = 115), (Source: [14]).

of married patients of either sex declined steadily and significantly, whereas for healthy controls it kept increasing with the result of marked differences at first admission: at age defined by the appearance of the first sign of illness in patients, 36.7% of the male patients and 43.3% of the male controls, 59.3% of the female patients and 74.1% of the female controls were married or in a stable partnership. By age at first admission the corresponding figures were 16.7% for the male patients, 60.0% for male controls, 33.3% for female patients and 77.8% for female controls.

Their lower level of social development at illness onset due to the 3 to 4 years lower age at illness onset and men's 2.5 years earlier age of marrying in the population at large placed male schizophrenics at a considerable disadvantage compared with their female counterparts. We wondered whether this might be a factor contributing to the consistent finding of the epidemiological 5-year outcome studies [4, 41, 42] reporting a poorer social course for men despite an equal symptom-related course for both sexes (Fig. 6).

Gender differences in illness behaviour and their consequences

We compared symptomatology and behavior in the first episode between men and women. While no differences emerged with the positive and negative core symptoms, we found a significant excess of 8 socially adverse behavioral items for men: self-neglect, reduced interest in a job, deficits in personal hygiene etc. and a higher cumulative prevalence of alcohol and drug abuse (Table 7). In contrast, women showed a significant excess of only two items: restlessness and over-adaptiveness/conformity. The latter, a socially favorable behavior, probably indicates women's better compliance and more favorable social behavior in

Table 7. Behavioral items with significant sex differences (from a total of 303 PSE, PIRS, SANS, DAS and IRAOS items)* – ABC first-episode sample, N = 232

More frequent in women:	More frequent in men:
a) cumulative until first admission	
≋ restlessness	≋ drug abuse
	≋ alcohol abuse
b) cross-sectional: at first admission	
≋ overadaptiveness/conformity	≋ self-neglect
	≋ reduced interest in a job
	≋ social inattentiveness
	≋ deficits of free time activities
	≋ deficits of communication
	≋ social disability (overall estimate)
	≋ loss of interests
	≋ deficits of personal hygiene

* Validated by split-half method for Å-correction
Source: [14]

schizophrenia. In all population studies on the topic [9, 11] conduct disorders, aggressive behavior, antisocial personality, drug and alcohol abuse are consistently overrepresented in adolescent and young adult males. These findings suggest that we might here be dealing with sex- and age-specific illness behavior rather than symptoms of the disorder in a stricter sense. A look at the presence of the 8 socially adverse behavioural items over the 5-year course made plain that the poorer social course of schizophrenia in men than women is explained by the

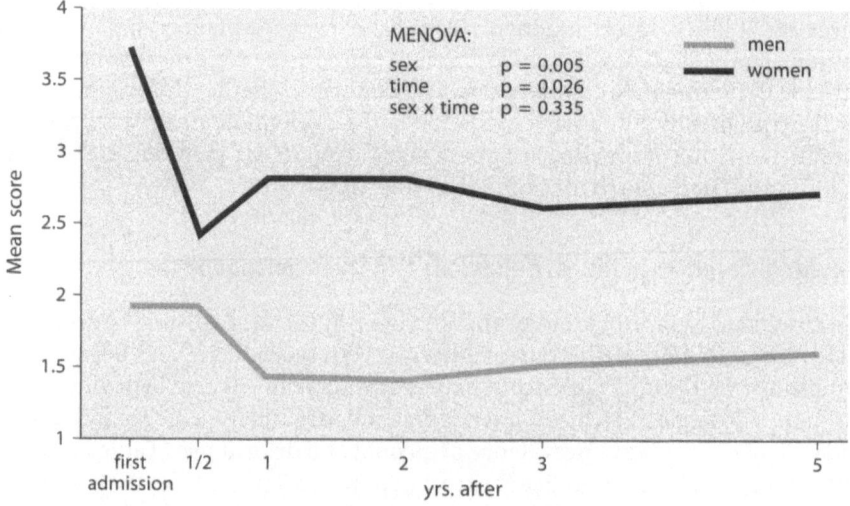

Fig. 7. Socially negative behavior over 5 years after first admission by sex (n = 115) (Source: [15]).

great difference in men and women's illness behavior (Fig. 7), because the symptom-related course, as already demonstrated, showed no significant sex differences.

Testing the heuristic explanation of a better five-year social outcome in women

As factors predicting social outcome, operationalized by the proportion of patients earning their living 5 years after first admission, two variables (number of social roles not fulfilled at illness onset out of the 6 roles mentioned and socially adverse behavior [by number of items] at psychosis onset) were tested in a predictor model of stepwise logistic regression. Other relevant variables taken into account were symptoms measured by the PSE at first admission, type of onset, age at first psychotic symptom and sex. As Fig. 8 shows on the right, the only factors predicting 5-year social outcome were level of social development, operationalized by the number of non-fulfilled social roles at psychosis onset, and socially adverse illness behavior. Symptomatology, type of onset, age and sex had no significant effect beyond that mediated by the first two variables. In a second step of testing our hypotheses, we used a path-analytical model to analyze how age at onset and gender influenced socially adverse behavior at first admission and the number of non-fulfilled social roles at psychosis onset and, via these effects, also social outcome. As the section on the left in Fig. 8 demonstrates, male gender showed significant associations, which attained medium to high partial correlation coefficients, with the two mediating variables and age at onset with the number of non-fulfilled social roles. Hence, our results confirmed the decisive indirect effect, mediated by the two variables mentioned, of age at onset and gender on social outcome.

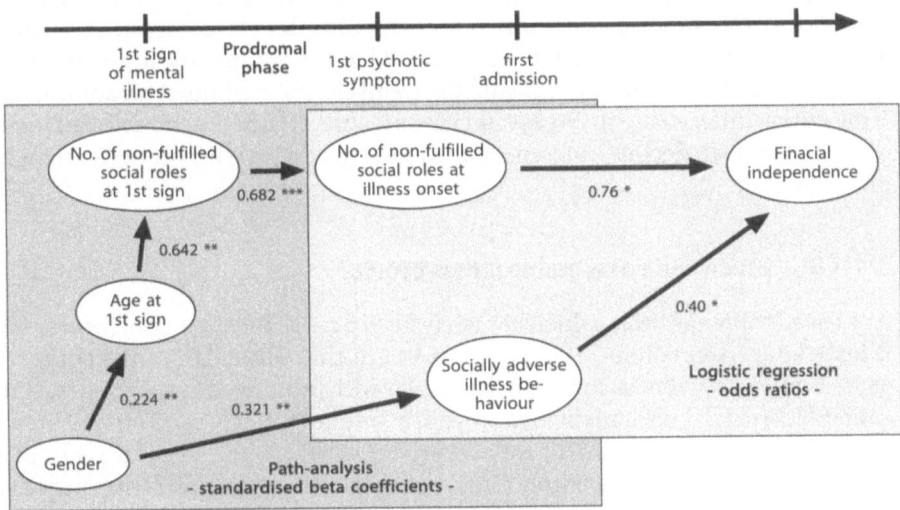

Fig. 8. Prediction of 5-year social outcome (financial independence) – First-episode sample n = 115 (Source: [16]).

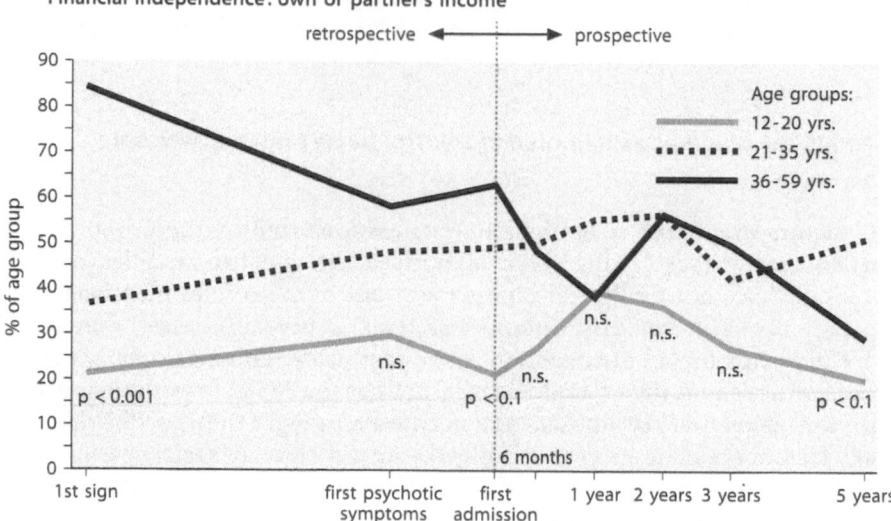

Fig. 9. Social course: financial independence (ABC follow-up sample n = 115) (Source: [23]).

Finally, we tested the alternative hypothesis of social stagnation versus social decline by comparing level of social development – as based on financial autonomy or capability to earn one's living – at illness onset in the three age groups (Fig. 9). Slight, non-significant upward movement occurred only in the youngest group. This slight ascent in the two years following first admission was accounted for by rehabilitative measures, but this was not a truly lasting effect. Eleven years after illness onset social outcome in this group reflected almost exactly the patients' social status at the outbreak of the disorder. In contrast, the oldest group as early as the prodromal phase started to suffer rapid decline from their high social status at illness onset, and the trend clearly continued for some time. The group differences in 5-year social outcome attained a statistical trend. Despite the steep decline outcome in the oldest group was slightly better than in the youngest.

Does DUP predict an unfavorable illness course?

We tested the hypothesis, which has lately been a cause for some controversy (cf. Klosterkötter, this volume; Häfner, this volume), that DUI or DUP might be associated with a poor illness course, in particular with prolonged first episodes, considerable social consequences and more frequent relapses. The result we obtained, depicted in Fig. 10, was surprising. DUI, in the mean 6 years and mainly characterized by a chronic course and gradually accumulating negative symptoms, turned out to be a significant predictor of nonspecific and negative symptoms at five-year follow-up. DUP, characterised by a predominance of

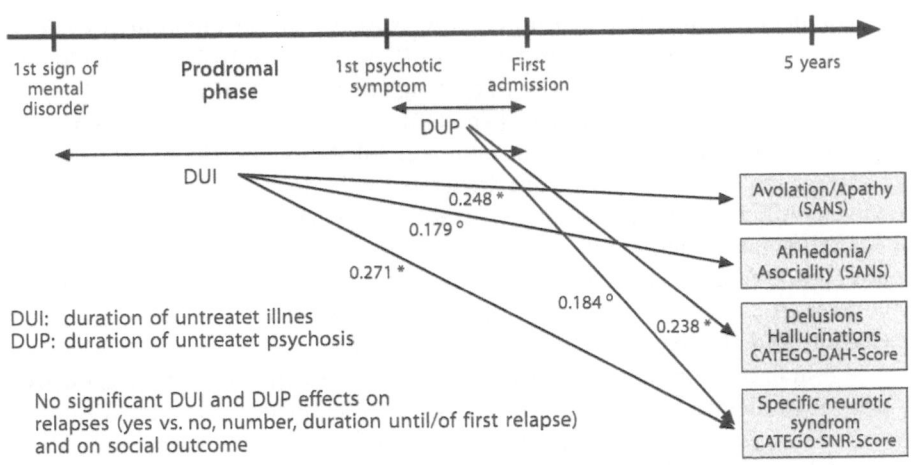

Fig. 10. Prediction of positive and negative symptoms five years after first admission by DUI and DUP – first-episode follow-up sample n = 115.

psychotic episodes of mostly short duration and acute type, was a significant predictor of nonspecific symptoms, frequent in both periods, as well as of positive symptoms.

In contrast, none of the factors discussed in the literature as predicting an unfavorable further course, such as number of relapses, time to or duration of first relapse, were significantly correlated either with DUI or DUP. The most fiercely debated question, whether shortening DUI and DUP would lead to a more favorable illness course, cannot be answered in a valid way on the methodological basis applied in the studies published so far on the topic (cf. Häfner, this volume).

Comorbidity with alcohol and drug abuse

A series of recent studies has shown that comorbidity with alcohol and drug abuse influences course and outcome in schizophrenia [1, 31, 37, 38, 43]. Our IRAOS data on the milestones of developing illness enabled us to analyze the sequence of onset of alcohol and drug abuse.

Table 8. Alcohol and drug abuse in first-episode patients of schizophrenia and general population controls. Lifetime prevalence until age at first admission

	Patients (n = 232)	Controls (n = 57)	RR
Alcohol abuse	23.7 % (n = 55)	12.3 % (n = 7)	2*
Drug abuse	14.2 % (n = 33)	7.0 % (n = 4)	2*

*χ^2 tests: alcohol abuse: $p < 0.06$, drug abuse: $p < 0.15$
Source: [26]

For alcohol abuse until age at first admission, we found a lifetime prevalence of about 24% for the patients and of about 12% for the controls matched for age, sex and population of origin [27]. For drug abuse the figures were 14% for the patients and 7% for the controls (Table 8). Consequently, the relative risk for comorbidity at first admission was about 2. Substance and alcohol abuse in the early course of schizophrenia are associated with dissocial behavior, interpersonal conflicts, expansive mood and emotional instability.

Of the male patients 39%, but only 22% of the females, had a history of alcohol and/or drug abuse at first admission. Of the patients with drug abuse 88% consumed cannabis – without any greater sex difference – and 58% alcohol. Cocaine and amphetamines played a minor role.

Age at first admission at 24.6 years was at its lowest for patients suffering from drug abuse before first admission, at 29.5 years second lowest for alcohol abusers and at 31.1 years significantly higher for those free of any type of abuse. At 27.6 years the figure for patients with both alcohol and drug abuse lay in between. When age at onset was defined by the first sign of the disorder the same relation emerged with cannabis abusers and abstinent patients showing a difference of 8 years.

This temporal pattern suggests that substance abuse might speed up schizophrenia onset [12]. To test this hypothesis we analyzed at which point substance abuse started in relation to illness onset, which in 3/4 of the cases was marked by a prodromal phase. Thirty-three percent of the patients started with alcohol abuse (Fig. 11) and 28% with drug abuse (Fig. 12) mostly long before illness onset. Remarkably, in a large proportion of the cases, both illness onset and

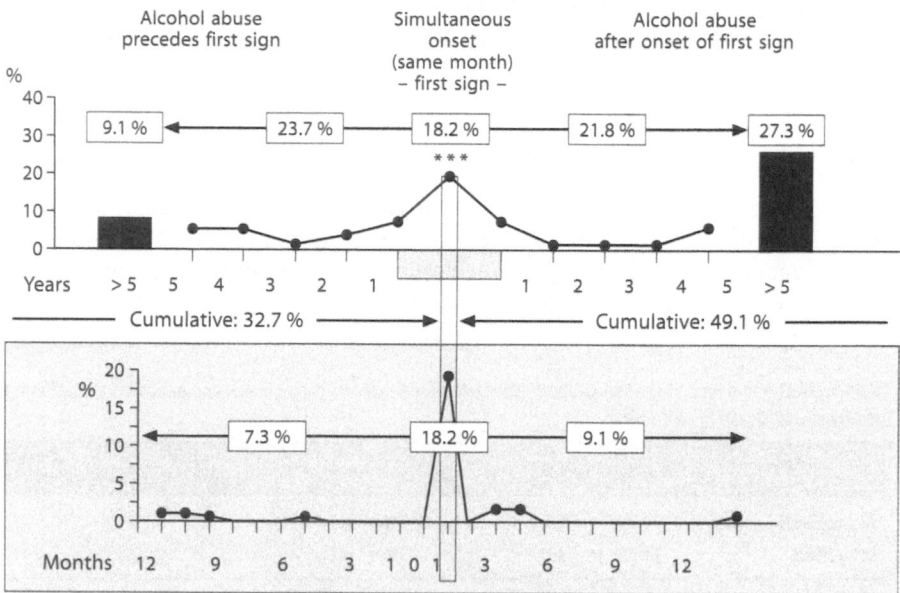

Fig. 11. Sequence of onset of alcohol abuse and first sign of mental disorder (Source: [7]).

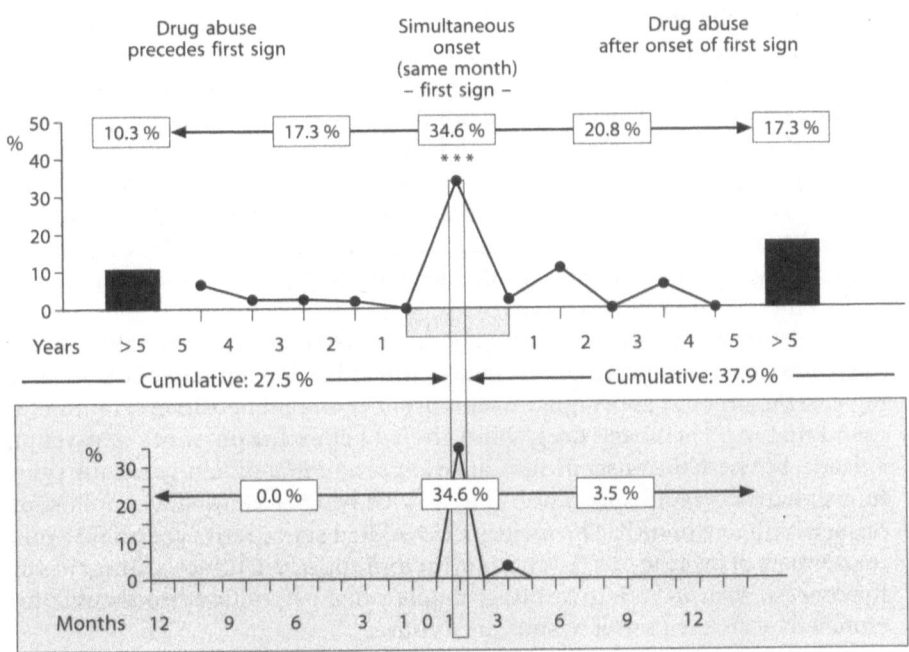

Fig. 12. Sequence of onset of drug abuse and first sign of mental disorder (Source: [7]).

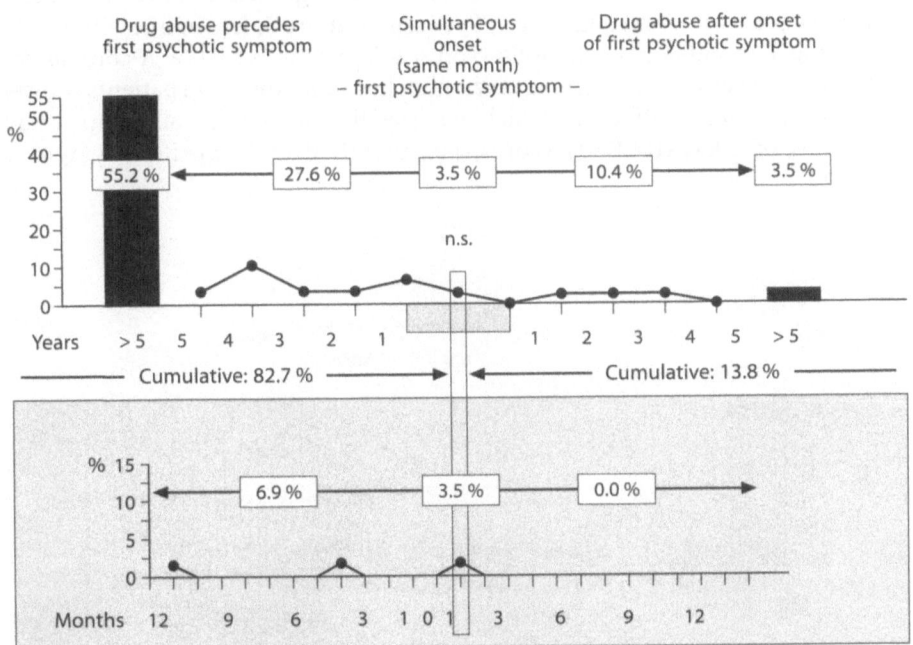

Fig. 13. Sequence of onset of drug abuse and first psychotic symptom (Source: [7]).

beginning of the abuse took place in the same month: for alcohol in 18 % and drugs in no fewer than 35%. The scale at the top depicts years, except for the month of simultaneous onset, the scale at the bottom the months of the year preceding and of that following illness onset. The graphs at the bottom make the simultaneous increase in both abuse and illness onsets particularly plain. In these cases a precipitation of illness onset – predominantly that of prodromal symptoms – is conceivable, as for example Gardner and Lowinson [12] and Addington and Addington [1], looking at their own results, suggest. In 38 % of the alcohol-abusing and in about 50% of the drug-abusing patients, however, comorbidity emerged after illness onset.

We also analyzed whether drug abuse – in 88% of cases cannabis abuse – might have triggered psychotic episodes via possible dopaminergic effects. Looking into the order of appearance of comorbidity and first positive symptom, we found that in 83% indeed drug abuse started before the onset of the psychotic episode, but here the onset of substance abuse and that of first psychotic symptom showed no rapid succession (Fig. 13). Only 3.5% showed a simultaneous onset within one month. The majority (55%) had started with drug abuse more than 5 years before the first psychotic symptom appeared. Hence, contrary to our hypothesis, it turned out to be rather unlikely that psychotic episodes were precipitated by a recent onset of substance abuse.

Consequences of alcohol and drug abuse

We also studied the consequences of alcohol and drug abuse in the further course over five years after first admission. The result is more or less in line with results from the few epidemiological follow-up studies so far available. A comparison of comorbid patients with age- and sex-matched non-comorbid patients showed a highly significant difference, which persisted throughout the follow-up period, in terms of CATEGO DAH scores, i.e., they had more positive symptoms (Fig. 14).

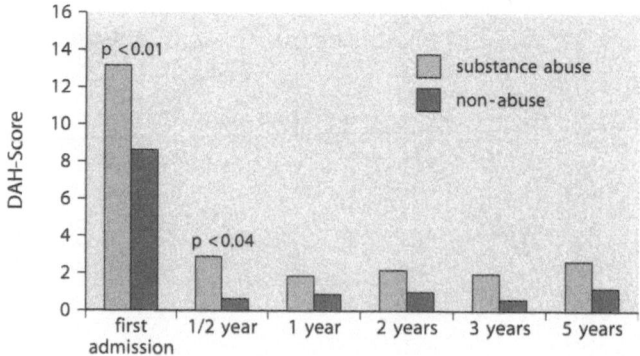

Fig. 14. Five-year course of positive symptoms (CATEGO DAH score) in patients by substance abuse in the early course – first episode follow-up sample n = 115 (Source: [7]).

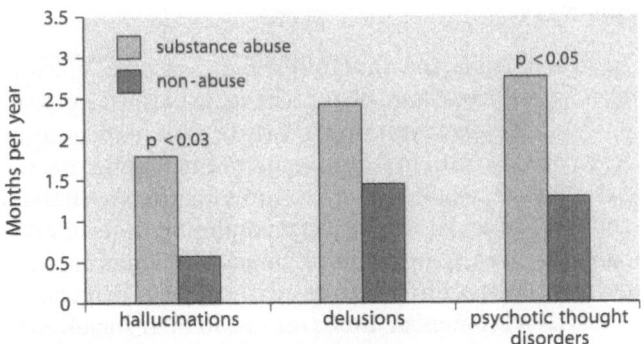

Fig. 15. Prediction of psychotic symptoms 5 years after first admission (symptoms present in month per year) by substance abuse in the early course – first-episode follow-up sample n = 115 (Source: [7]).

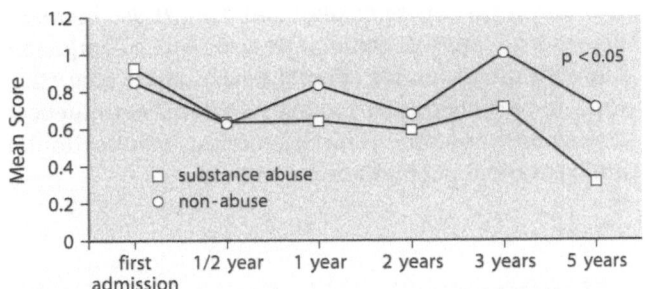

Fig. 16. Five-year course of affective flattening by substance abuse in the early course – first-episode follow-up sample n = 115 (Source: [7]).

Looking at this effect in detail, we found that early substance abuse predicted elevated levels of all the three categories of positive symptoms, hallucinations, delusions and thought disorder, in the 5 years after first admission (Fig. 15).

At the same time, drug abuse (mainly cannabis abuse) significantly predicted lower scores for affective flattening (Fig. 16).

The association between substance abuse, on the one hand, and increased positive symptoms, on the other hand, sounds plausible. It may be mediated by a poor compliance and by dopaminergic effects. Some evidence emerged for the hypothesis that drug abuse might decrease certain negative symptoms. This also reflects the need for some schizophrenics to alleviate by cannabis abuse in particular the unpleasant negative symptoms such as indifference and poor ability to accept new experiences, especially since an increase in positive symptoms is usually not experienced as particularly distressing [1].

We also found that comorbid patients showed significantly reduced compliance with neuroleptic medications and rehabilitative measures in comparison with non-comorbid patients.

Summary

In 73 % of cases, the onset of the first psychotic episode is preceded on average by a 5-year prodromal phase. The main earliest signs of the disorder are depressive and negative symptoms. Early depressive symptoms at a cumulative prevalence of 81 % until first admission predict higher overall symptom scores in the first illness episode and lower scores for affective flattening in the medium-term course. The social course of schizophrenia is decided before the first treatment contact – in early-onset illness by social stagnation, in late-onset illness by social decline. The sex difference in social course is determined by men's lower level of social development at illness onset and their socially adverse illness behavior. In most cases comorbidity with alcohol and drug abuse, with a relative risk of 2 for both men and women, begins after illness onset, but before first admission. In a small proportion of cases, the onset of substance abuse and, more rarely, the onset of alcohol abuse might trigger the onset of schizophrenia prematurely, but astonishingly, they do not seem to precipitate the onset of psychosis. In the medium-term course alcohol and drug abuse increase positive symptoms and decrease affective flattening, but also reduce compliance and utilization of rehabilitative measures. Except in the early illness phase the disorder, positive symptoms in particular, seem to have no decisive influence on the gradient of social course and outcome. This has serious implications for treatment, currently aimed at reducing psychotic symptoms.

■ References

1. Addington J, Addington D (1998) Effect of substance abuse in early psychosis. Br J Psychiatry 172 (Suppl 33): 134–136
2. Andreasen NC (1983) The Scale for the Assessment of Negative Symptoms (SANS). Iowa City: University of Iowa
3. Beiser M, Erickson D, Flemming JAE, Iacono WG (1993) Establishing the onset of psychotic illness. Am J Psychiatry 150: 1349–1354
4. Biehl H, Maurer K, Schubart C, Krumm B, Jung E (1986) Prediction of outcome and utilization of medical services in a prospective study of first onset schizophrenics – results of a prospective 5-year follow-up study. Eur Arch Psychiatry Neurol Sci 236: 139–147
5. Biehl H, Maurer K, Jablensky A, Cooper JE, Tomov T (1989) The WHO Psychological Impairments Rating Schedule (WHO/PIRS). I. Introducing a new instrument for rating observed behaviour and the rationale of the psychological impairment concept. Br J Psychiatry 155 (Suppl 7): 68–70
6. Bleuler E (1911) Dementia praecox oder Gruppe der Schizophrenien. In: Aschaffenburg, G (ed) Handbuch der Psychiatrie. Deuticke: Leipzig, pp 1–420
7. Bühler B, Hambrecht M, Löffler W, an der Heiden W, Häfner H (2002) Precipitation and determination of the onset and course of schizophrenia by substance abuse – a retrospective and prospective study of 232 population-based first illness episodes. Schizophrenia Res 54: 243–251
8. Cameron DE (1938) Early schizophrenia. Am J Psychiatry 95: 567–578
9. Choquet M, Ledoux S (1994) Epidémiologie et adolescence. In: Confrontations psychiatriques, vol 27 (no 35). Paris: Rhone-Poulenc rorer specia, pp 287–309
10. Crow TJ, MacMillan JF, Johnson AL, Johnstone EC (1986) A randomised controlled trial of prophylactic neuroleptic treatment. Br J Psychiatry 148: 120–127

11. Döpfner M, Pluck J, Berner W, Fegert JM, Huss M, Lenz K, Schmeck K, Lehmkuhl U, Poustka F, Lehmkuhl G (1997) Mental disturbances in children and adolescents in Germany. Results of a representative study: age, gender and rater effects. Zeitschrift für Kinder- und Jugendpsychiatrie Psychotherapie 25: 218–233

12. Gardner EL, Lowinson JH (1991) Marijuana's interaction with brain reward systems: update 1991. Pharmacol Biochem Behav 40: 571–580

13. Gross G (1969) Prodrome und Vorpostensyndrome schizophrener Erkrankungen. In: Huber G (ed) Schizophrenie und Zyklothymie. Ergebnisse und Probleme. Stuttgart: Thieme, pp 177–187

14. Häfner H (1998) Ist es einzig die Krankheit? In: Möller HJ, Müller N (eds) Schizophrenie – Moderne Konzepte zu Diagnostik, Pathogenese und Therapie. Wien: Springer, pp 37–59

15. Häfner H (1998) Neues zum Verlauf der Schizophrenie. In: Fleischhacker WW, Hinterhuber H, Meise U (eds) Schizophrene Störungen. State of the Art II. Innsbruck: Verlag Integrative Psychiatrie, pp 20–55

16. Häfner H (2000) Ist es alles nur die Krankheit? (Schriften der Mathematisch-naturwissenschaftlichen Klasse der Heidelberger Akademie der Wissenschaften Nr. 7). Berlin Heidelberg New York: Springer-Verlag

17. Häfner H, Riecher-Rössler A, Hambrecht M, Maurer K, Meissner S, Schmidtke A, Fätkenheuer B, Löffler W, an der Heiden W (1992) IRAOS: an instrument for the retrospective assessment of the onset of schizophrenia. Schizophr Res 6: 209–223

18. Häfner H, Behrens S, Vry J de, Gattaz WF (1992) An animal model for the effects of estradiol on dopamine-mediated behavior: implications for sex differences in schizophrenia. Psychiatry Res 38: 125–134

19. Häfner H, Maurer K, Löffler W, Riecher-Rössler A (1993) The influence of age and sex on the onset and early course of schizophrenia. Br J Psychiatry 162: 80–86

20. Häfner H, Nowotny B, Löffler W, an der Heiden W, Maurer K (1995) When and how does schizophrenia lead to social deficits? Eur Arch Psychiatry Clin Neurosci 246: 17–28

21. Häfner H, Maurer K, Löffler W, Bustamante S, an der Heiden W, Riecher-Rössler A, Nowotny B (1995) Onset and early course of schizophrenia. In: Häfner H, Gattaz H (eds) Search for the Causes of Schizophrenia, vol III. Berlin: Springer-Verlag, pp 43–66

22. Häfner H, an der Heiden W, Löffler W, Maurer K, Hambrecht M (1998) Beginn und Frühverlauf schizophrener Erkrankungen. In: Klosterkötter J (ed) Frühdiagnostik und Frühbehandlung psychischer Störungen. Bayer-ZNS Symposium XIII. Berlin: Springer-Verlag, pp 1–28

23. Häfner H, Hambrecht M, Löffler W, Munk-Jørgensen P, Riecher-Rössler A (1998) Is schizophrenia a disorder of all ages? A comparison of first episodes and early course across the life-cycle. Psychol Med 28: 351–365

24. Häfner H, Löffler W, Maurer K, Riecher-Rössler A, Stein A (1999) Instrument für die retrospektive Erfassung des Erkrankungsbeginns und -verlaufs bei Schizophrenie und anderen Psychosen. Instrument for the retrospective assessment of the onset of schizophrenia and other psychosis. Bern: Huber

25. Häfner H, Maurer K, Löffler W, an der Heiden W, Könnecke R, Hambrecht M (1999) Onset and prodromal phase as determinants of the course. In: Gattaz WF, Häfner H (eds) Search for the causes of schizophrenia, vol. IV: Balance of the century. Darmstadt: Steinkopff-Verlag, Berlin: Springer, pp 1–24

26. Häfner H, Maurer K, Löffler W, an der Heiden W, Könnecke R, Hambrecht M (2001) Onset and early course of schizophrenia – a challenge for early intervention. Psychiatria Fennica 32 (Suppl 2): 81–108

27. Hambrecht M, Häfner H (1996) Substance abuse and the onset of schizophrenia. Biol Psychiatry 40: 1155–1163

28. Huber G, Gross G, Schüttler R (1979) Schizophrenie. Eine Verlaufs- und sozialpsychiatrische Langzeitstudie. Berlin: Springer

29. Johannessen JO, Larsen TK, McGlashan T (1999) Duration of untreated psychosis: an important target for intervention in schizophrenia? Nord J Psychiatry 53: 275–283

30. Jung E, Krumm B, Biehl H, Maurer K, Bauer-Schubart C (1989) Mannheimer Skala zur Einschätzung von sozialer Behinderung (DAS-M). Weinheim: Beltz

31. Kovasznay B, Fleischer J, Tanenberg-Karant M, Jandorf L, Miller AD, Bromet E (1997) Substance use disorder and the early course of illness in schizophrenia and affective psychosis. Schizophr Bull 23: 195–201
32. Kraepelin E (1909–1915) Psychiatrie. (Vol. 1-4). Leipzig: Barth
33. Lewine RJ (1980) Sex differences in age of symptom onset and first hospitalization in schizophrenia. Am J Orthopsychiatry 50: 316–322
34. Lindelius R (1970) A study of schizophrenia. Acta Psychiatr Scand Suppl 216
35. Loebel AD, Lieberman JA, Alvir JMJ, Mayerhoff DI, Geisler SH, Szymanski SR (1992) Duration of psychosis and outcome in first-episode schizophrenia. Am J Psychiatry 149: 1183–1188
36. McGorry PD, Edwards J, Mihalopoulos C, Harrigan SM, Jackson JH (1996) EPPIC: An evolving system of early detection and optimal management. Schizophr Res 22: 305–326
37. Mueser KT, Bellack AS, Blanchand JJ (1992) Comorbidity of schizophrenia and substance abuse: implications for treatment. J Consult Clin Psychol 60 (6): 845–856
38. Perkins KA, Simpson JC, Tsuang MT (1986) Ten-year follow-up of drug abusers with acute or chronic psychosis. Hosp Comm Psychiatry 37: 481–484
39. Riecher-Rössler A, Häfner H, Stumbaum M, Maurer K, Schmidt R (1994) Can estradiol modulate schizophrenic symptomatology? Schizophr Bull 20: 203–214
40. Riecher-Rössler A, Häfner H, Dütsch-Strobel A, Oster M, Stumbaum M, van Gülick-Bailer M, Löffler W (1994) Further evidence for a specific role of estradiol in schizophrenia? Biol Psychiatry 36: 492–495
41. Salokangas RKR, Stengard E, Räkköläinen V, Kaljonen IHA (1987) New schizophrenic patients and their families (English summary). In: Reports of Psychiatria Fennica, No. 78: Skitsofrenian tutkimuksen, hoidon ja kuntoutuksen valtakunnallinen kehittämisohjelma. Foundation for psychiatric research in Finland, pp 119–216
42. Shepherd M, Watt D, Falloon I, Smeeton N (1989) The natural history of schizophrenia: a five-year follow-up study of outcome and prediction in a representative sample of schizophrenics. Psychol Med Monograph (Suppl 15). Cambridge: Cambridge University Press
43. Smith J, Hucker S (1994) Schizophrenia and substance abuse. Br J Psychiatry 165: 13–21
44. Sullivan SH (1927) The onset of schizophrenia. Am J Psychiatry 6: 105–134
45. Varma VK, Malhotra S, Yao ES (1996) Course and outcome of acute non-organic psychotic states. Indian Psychiatric Quarterly 67: 195–207
46. WHO (1980) World Health Organization, WHO. Follow-up history and sociodemographic description schedule (FU-HSD). 2nd unpublished draft
47. WHO (1988) World Health Organization. Psychiatric Disability Assessment Schedule (WHO/DAS). Geneva: WHO
48. Wig NN, Parhee R (1989) International Classification in Psychiatry. In: Mezzich JE, Cranach M (eds). Cambridge: Cambridge University Press, pp 115–121
49. Wing JK, Cooper JE, Sartorius N (1974) Measurement and classification of psychiatric symptoms. An instruction manual for the PSE and CATEGO Program. London: Cambridge University Press
50. Wyatt RJ, Henter ID (1998) The effects of early and sustained intervention on the long-term morbidity of schizophrenia. J Psychiatr Res 32: 169–177

Testing models of the early course of schizophrenia

F. Schultze-Lutter, W. Löffler, H. Häfner
Department of Psychiatry and Psychotherapy, University of Köln, Germany

■ Introduction

The main rationale for an early detection and intervention in schizophrenia are findings of a positive correlation between the duration of untreated psychosis and various indicators of a negative outcome [18, 19]. Furthermore, it was shown that social deficits already occur prior to the first psychotic symptom during the initial prodrome [see Häfner et al., this volume] and that the deterioration of functioning is not linear but tends to worsen for the first few years, often plateauing in the later course [19]. Consequently, by an earlier detection of the illness and an earlier intervention, it is hoped to reduce the psychological, social and possibly biological disruption leading to poor outcome. Therefore, not only a detailed characterization of the symptoms and disturbances of the initial prodrome but also a study of the evolution of prodromal to psychotic symptoms are necessary [23].

Psychopathological models of the development of schizophrenia and descriptions of the prodromal phenomena date back to the very beginning of schizophrenia research – until recently – mainly employing a retrospective approach with patients already having developed manifest schizophrenia. Of these models, the one of Conrad [4] originating in the clinical data and self-reports of 107 German soldiers with a psychotic diagnosis as well as the one of Docherty and colleagues [5] based on three case reports and a review of literature on the development of schizophrenia between 1938 and 1975 including Conrad's work were probably the most influential. Both assumed that the sequence of illness stages is unidirectional and compelling with nonspecific changes being followed by more specific prepsychotic and finally psychotic symptoms, independent of the subtype of schizophrenia.

However, a retrospective approach bears the risks of problems of recall and effort after meaning, which are probably aggravated by the variable time interval between the prodrome and the interview. In an attempt to control these problems, the Instrument for the Retrospective Assessment of the Onset of Schizophrenia, IRAOS [10, 11], was developed for the systematic collection of data on individual social development, onset features, symptom accumulation and early course of psychosis (see Häfner et al., this volume).

Based on data of this study, the question of whether and how the social and clinical early course of schizophrenia can be modeled will be addressed. Therefore, the models of Conrad [4] and Docherty et al. [5] will be empirically tested using data of the Mannheim Age-Beginning-Course (ABC) schizophrenia study, and a causal model of the social course from first sign of illness until five years after first admission based on findings of the same study will be estimated.

■ Methods

Sample

Data is part of the Mannheim ABC schizophrenia study with a population-based sample of 232 first illness episodes of broadly defined schizophrenia according to ICD 9 diagnoses 295, 297, 298.3/.4 [for details see 7, Häfner et al., this volume]. To model the early clinical course, a subsample of 170 patients (73 %) of the ABC study with an initial prodromal state characterized by unspecific and/or negative symptoms was used; to model the social course, a subsample of 115 first-episode patients re-examined after 5 years [for details see 9,12] was used.

Instruments and procedure

Onset, social and clinical course until first admission were assessed retrospectively using a semi-structured instrument, the Instrument for the Retrospective Assessment of the Onset of Schizophrenia, IRAOS [10, 11]. Furthermore, psychopathology and social adjustment was cross-sectionally assessed with the Present State Examination, PSE [21], the Scale for the Assessment of Negative Symptoms, SANS [1], Psychological Impairment Rating Schedule, PIRS [3], and the Disability Assessment Schedule, DAS [16].

Besides detailed sociodemographic data and treatment history, the IRAOS assesses 65 unspecific, negative and positive symptoms for their presence, time of first occurrence and continuity (present once, recurrently present, continuously present from first occurrence to first admission for schizophrenia). Thereby, it was aimed at an avoidance/minimization of confounding memory effects by using a time matrix with anchor events for each patient [20].

The course of illness after first admission was assessed prospectively in a subsample of 115 first-episode cases at five follow-ups over five years using the same cross sectional instruments and, additionally, the FU-HSD [22]. An overview of the instruments, procedures and results of the ABC study is given in Häfner and an der Heiden [9], Häfner et al. [12] and Häfner et al. (this volume).

Data analyses

To test existing or hypothesized complex models of the early clinical and social course of schizophrenia at a higher level of abstraction, a structural equation modeling (SEM) technique was applied using the computer program LISREL8 (Linear Structural Relationships; [15]). Unlike ANOVA and multiple regression that are concerned with means and intercorrelations among observed variables, respectively, but do not offer a differentiation between observed and latent variables, SEM tests a priori specifications about the effects between variables and their directionalities (system of hypotheses) simultaneously allowing to define common domains of certain observed variables, i.e., latent variables [17]. Being theoretical constructs, latent variables can represent a wide range of phenomena, e.g., different stages of the clinical course as proposed by Conrad [4] or Docherty et al. [5], and thus differ from factors derived from factor analyses, e.g., symptom dimensions as described by Andreasen et al. [2], which account for pairwise but not for higher order correlations between observed variables [6].

Although SEM is a priori, requiring the specification of an unequivocal model, it is not exclusively confirmatory and can assist in model generation when the initial model does not fit the data, is repeatedly modified (sensibly relocating, deleting or adding variables) and re-tested. Thereby it is aimed to 'detect' a model that makes theoretical sense as well as has a reasonable statistical correspondence to the data [17].

To test the clinical models of Conrad [4] and Docherty et al. [5], the time between first occurrence of a symptom and first admission regardless of its persistence or recurrence was considered. Because of the great interindividual variance in the duration of (pre-)psychotic symptoms before hospitalization and for reasons of interindividual comparison, these data were z-transformed separately for each patient with exclusion of symptoms never present in the individual course. These systematically missing data were handled with pairwise deletion in the SEM calculation process.

Model specifications

Model of the social course of schizophrenia. The onset of the first sign of the disorder and, hence, of schizophrenia, and, in fact, all the subsequent milestones of the early illness course display a meanwhile well-known sex difference of 3 to 4 years in favor of women [7]. Furthermore, comparing the social adjustment between the Mannheim subsample of 57 patients of the ABC study and 57 age- and gender-matched healthy controls, it showed that social adjustment did not differ by the time of the first sign of illness. Social adjustment was operationalized by six key social roles, usually fulfilled during the period of maximum risk for schizophrenia: finished school education, finished occupational training, employment, own accommodation, own income and marriage or stable partnership. However, differences in social adjustment, especially with regard employment, own income and marriage or stable partnership, occurred in the prodromal phase prior to the onset of the first psychotic symptom [13]. As regards gender differences in patients, women performed better than men in terms of employment, own accommodation, and marriage or stable partnership already by the time of first sign of illness [7]. However, this effect is probably related to the higher age at illness onset in women [13, Häfner et al., this volume].

Significant gender differences were also demonstrated for social aspects of illness behavior, restlessness and overadaptiveness – more frequent in women – and for substance abuse, reduced interest in acquiring a job, loss of interest, lack

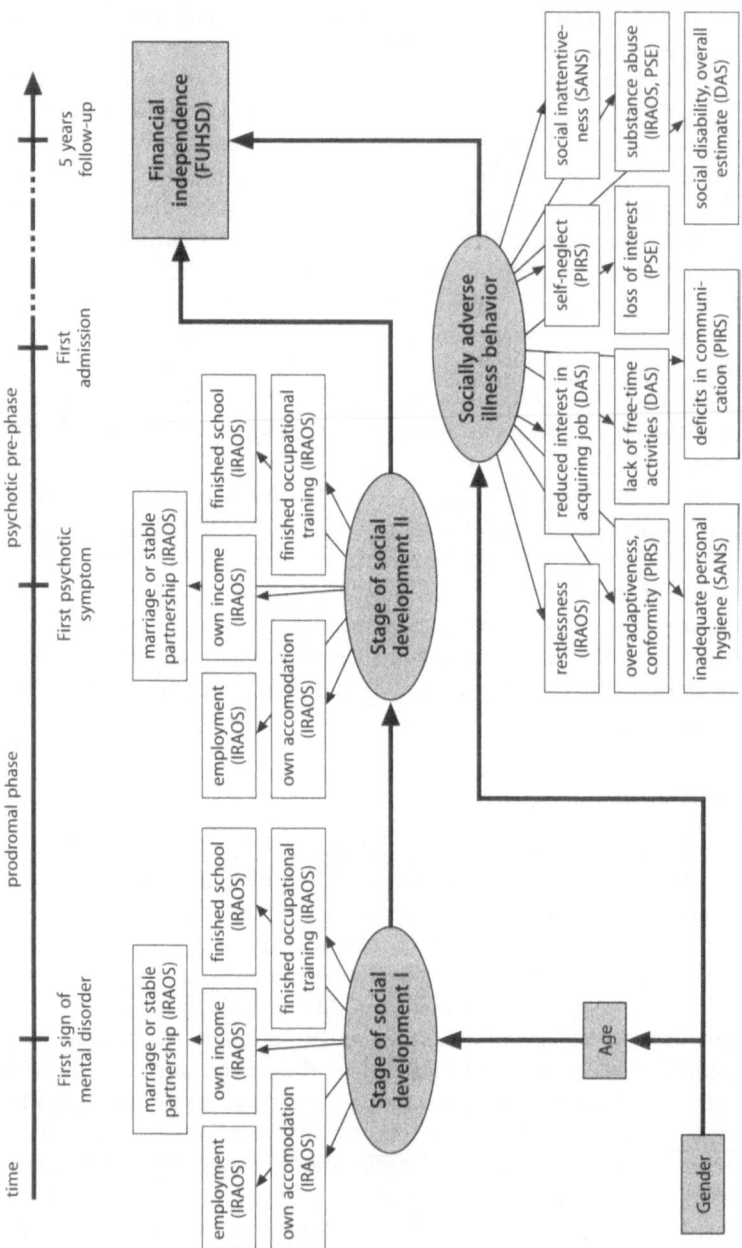

Fig. 1. Prediction of 5-year social outcome: model specification – First-episode sample, n = 115.

of free-time activities, social inattentiveness, deficits of communication, self-neglect, inadequate personal hygiene and an overall estimation of social disability – more pronounced in men [7, 13]. On the basis of these results we developed a model, which we tested in two steps: stepwise logistic regression was applied to test the prediction of 5-year social outcome by four traditional prognostic indicators together with the two social variables "social development at psychosis onset" and "social behavior in the first psychotic episode". A path analytic approach was adopted to test the effects of age at onset and gender on the two significant predictors. To briefly summarize the results, the number of social roles not fulfilled by the time of the first psychotic symptom and socially adverse illness behavior were significant predictors of the social development at 5 year-follow up defined in terms of financial independence, whereas gender, age at first sign of mental illness, type of onset and symptomatology at first admission were not. The effects of age at onset and gender on social outcome were mediated by the two social variables [13; for a detailed discussion of the results see Häfner et al., this volume.]. In fact, symptomatology – either prodromal or psychotic – did not show any gender-related peculiarities – neither at the time of first sign of illness, of first psychotic sign nor admission or of the 5 year-follow up [7]. To establish the validity of these results obtained in a two-step analysis, we entered them in a comprehensive "causal" model, which we tested using the SEM approach. This model of the determinants of the social course of schizophrenia is illustrated and specified in Fig. 1.

Conrad's stage model. Based on clinical data of 107 German soldiers with a diagnosis of a psychotic episode of schizophrenia, Conrad [4] postulated four stages of beginning and two of remitting schizophrenia, these latter two were not included in our analysis. He called the first, prodromal stage *trema* and reported that it could last for years. It is characterized by uncertainty, depression, suspiciousness, anxiety and social withdrawal. The second stage, *apopheny*, is marked by the appearance of psychotic symptoms and derealization. Insight and reality control are lost. The next stage is called *anastrophae*. In it formal thought disorders and the attribution of unexplainable experiences to external causes in secondary delusions occur. The fourth and *apocalyptic* stage is identical with a full-blown, severe psychosis associated with disorganization, severe anxiety, restlessness and catatonic symptoms. Table 1 shows the IRAOS items attributed to the symptoms described for each of Conrad's four stages and, thus, serves as the initial specification of his phase model to be tested.

In an earlier analysis, we [14] had tested on IRAOS data the sequence of the symptoms described by Conrad [4] as characterizing the four stages of schizophrenia. In that study, 16% of the sample comprising 267 first-admission cases were in their second or further episodes and only 73% had experienced a prodromal stage. The results confirmed Conrad's model only with respect to *trema* as the first stage of illness (in 76% of the sample), failing to provide any evidence for the sequence of the other stages. For this reason, it seemed reasonable to take another shot at testing the two stage models in a more comprehensive way on the basis of a sample comprising only cases with prodromal stages.

Table 1. IRAOS items attributed to each stage of Conrad's model [4]

Conrad	ABC study (IRAOS symptoms)
Trema (as latent variable)	
absurd behavior	antisocial behavior, self injury, other behavioral abnormalities
depression, melancholy with disgust with life	depressed mood, suicide attempt
anxiety	anxiety
torturing feelings of guilt	feelings of guilt and self-blame
suspiciousness, gap between self and surrounding world (social withdrawal)	communication, distrust/social withdrawal
delusional mood	delusional mood
feeling high-spirited and expectant	expansive mood
apathy, loss of drive	insufficient energy
Apophany (as latent variable)	
abnormal experiences of reference	delusions of reference
delusions of various contents	delusions of persecution, of influence
hallucinations	visual hallucinations, other hallucinations
thought disturbances	thinking and concentration, weakness of focused thinking
experiences of jamais and déjà vu	derealization, depersonalization
feelings of grandiosity (delusion)	expansive delusions
Anastrophae (as latent variable)	
feelings of alien influence, thought insertion	thought insertion, delusions of influence, of control
thought broadcasting, becoming audible	thought broadcast
verbal hallucinations	auditory hallucinations, verbal hallucinations not based on depression or elation
other delusions and illusions	delusions of persecution, delusions concerning appearance, further delusions
thought disorders	psychotic thought disturbances, thought block or withdrawal, echo or commentary
abnormal somatic complaints	Further perceptual disturbances (not hallucinations)
Apocalypse (as latent variable)	
catatonic symptoms	motor block/hyperkinesia and dyskinesia
unusual speech (neologisms, incoherence)	unusual speech
other disintegrative symptoms	other changes in affect
severe restlessness	tension, irritability

Table 2. IRAOS items attributed to each stage of Docherty and colleagues' model [5]

Docherty et al.	ABC study (IRAOS symptoms)
Overextension (as latent variable)	
sense of being overwhelmed, increased mental effort required even for every-day demands	leisure activities, speed of coping with normal daily activities, household roles/participation in family life, behavior in emergencies
overstimulation	increased distractibility/disturbance of attention
persisting anxiety	anxiety
parapraxes	other behavioral abnormalities
distractibility	increased distractibility/disturbance of attention
decreasing performance, efficiency	speed of coping with normal daily activities, work relationships
irritability	irritability, lack of consideration and friction in dealings with other people
Restricted consciousness (as latent variable)	
limitation of the range of thought	thinking and concentration, weakness of focused thinking, preoccupation with secret things/unusual thoughts
apathy, listlessness	insufficient energy
deterioration of personal appearance and upkeep	self-care
boredom, hopelessness	depressed mood
social withdrawal	social withdrawal, oversensitivity
obsessional symptoms	obsessions
phobic symptoms	anxiety
somatization	aches and pains, further perceptual disturbances
Disinhibition (as latent variable)	
hypomania, elevation of mood	expansive mood
ideas of reference (may appear)	delusional mood
Psychotic disorganization (as latent variable)	
perceptual disorganization	further perceptual disturbances
cognitive disorganization	psychotic thought disturbance, thought insertion, broadcast, echo, commentary, block or withdrawal
hallucinatory phenomena	auditory, visual, other hallucinations and verbal hallucinations not based on depression or elation
difficulties finding the right word	unusual speech
ideas of reference	delusions of reference
loss of sense of self-identity, self and control	delusions of control, of influence, concerning appearance
catatonia	motor block/hyperkinesia and dyskinesia
Psychotic resolution (as latent variable)	
decreased anxiety	anxiety
increased psychotic organisation, delusional system	delusions of persecution, expansive and further delusions

Stage model of Docherty and colleagues. Docherty et al. [5] had formulated their five-stage model on the basis of three case descriptions and a survey of available literature, including Conrad's work [4]. According to their model, the illness begins with a stage of *overextension*, characterized by experiencing a sense of being overwhelmed and first signs of cognitive impairment. It is followed by *restricted consciousness* involving apathy, social withdrawal, hopelessness and somatization. The third stage is *disinhibition*, marked by hypomania, dissociation and reduced impulse control. It is followed by the onset of full-blown psychosis, "psychotic disorganization" characterized by positive and catatonic symptoms and disorganization. The final stage, *psychotic resolution*, is defined by a psychotic organization involving the development of an organizing delusional system or the massive denial of all unpleasant affect and responsibility. Table 2 shows the IRAOS items attributed to the symptoms described for each of the five stages and, thus, serves as the initial specification of Docherty's stage model to be tested.

▓ Results

As regards the model of the social course (Fig. 1), the initially specified model converged after 64 iterations and was validated by the data (testing H_0: $\Delta = 0$; $\chi^2 = 370.88$, df = 348, p = 0.19). It explained about two thirds of the variance in the data (goodness of fit index (GFI) = 0.80; adjusted GFI = 0.76; root mean square residual (RMR) = 0.23). However, following changes as suggested by the modification indices, a slightly different model was generated that converged after 147 iterations (Fig. 2), was more clearly supported by the data ($\chi^2 = 280.31$, df = 293, p = 0.69), but added only an additional 3% to the explained variance of the initial model (GFI = 0.82; adjusted GFI = 0.79; RMR = 0.16). These results confirmed what had been shown by our two-step analysis of the interaction of social and biological factors as determinants of the medium-term social outcome of schizophrenia (cf. Häfner et al., this volume).

As regards the stage models, neither Conrad's nor Docherty et al.'s model was empirically supported or even converged (Conrad's model: $\chi^2 = 498.32$, df = 205, p = 0.0; Docherty's model: $\chi^2 = 909.67$, df = 373, p = 0.0). Modified and simplified models – although still far from reaching significance – were able to explain a considerable proportion of the variance of the z-standardized ABC data: Conrad's model explained 74% (GFI = 0.79; adjusted GFI = 0.74; RMR = 0.053; Fig. 3), Docherty et al.'s model 71% (GFI = 0.75; adjusted GFI = 0.71; RMR = 0.054; Fig. 4). Yet, both models still failed to attain the conventional level of a good fit of $\geq 90\%$ [16] required in case of a nonsignificant goodness-of-fit χ^2 statistic.

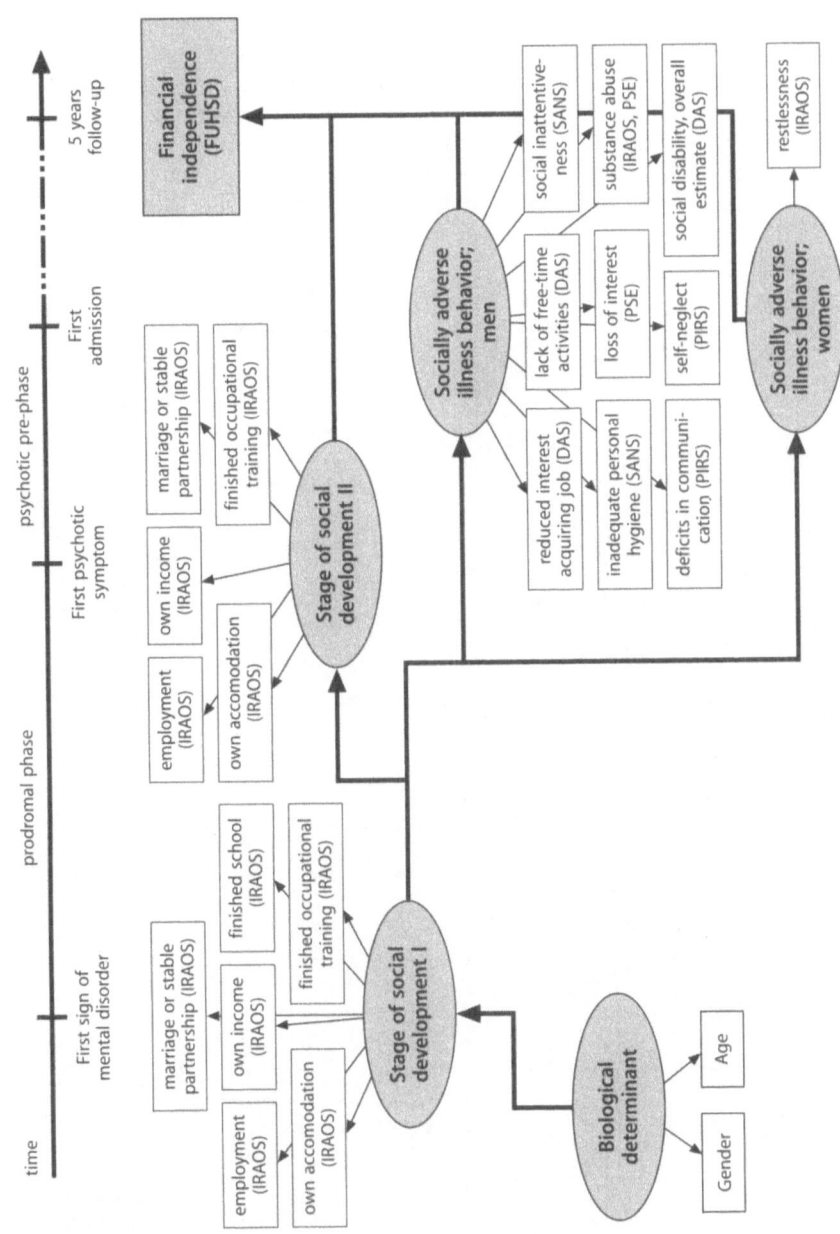

Fig. 2. Prediction of 5-year social outcome: empirical model – First-episode sample, n = 115.

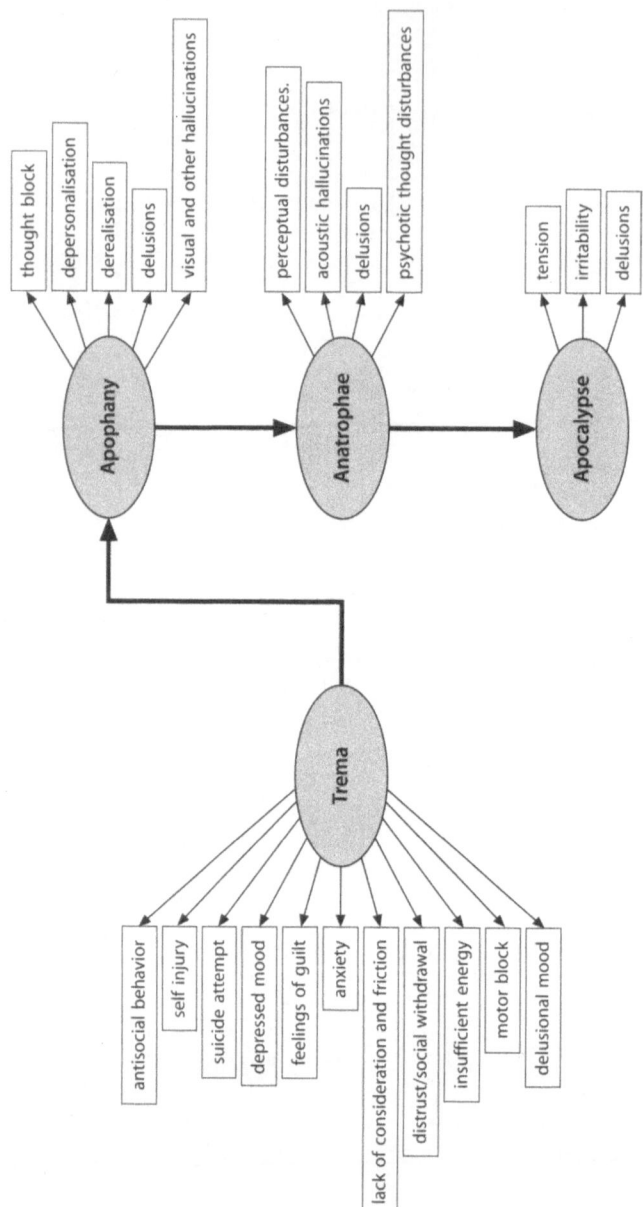

Fig. 3. Conrad's stage model: empirical model.

▒ Discussion

Our analyses failed to confirm the models of the early stages of schizophrenia as proposed by Conrad [4] and Docherty and colleagues [5], respectively. There are several reasons for this result: Conrad's model is based on a highly selected clin-

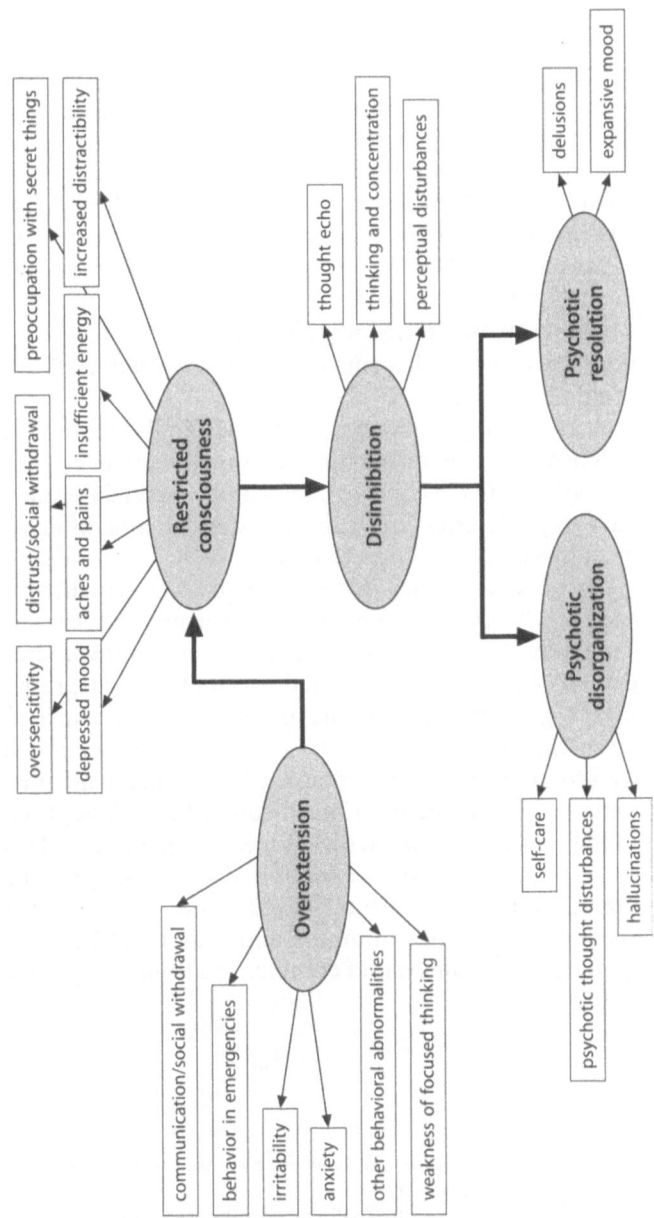

Fig. 4. Docherty et al.'s model: empirical model.

ical group – young soldiers with acute psychosis – and that of Docherty et al. has a very small data base. Neither Conrad nor Docherty and colleagues give a clear description of the symptoms and their selection. For this reason, the operationalization of the two models with IRAOS symptoms is somewhat arbitrary. Furthermore, some symptoms considered in the models have no equivalent in the IRAOS, e.g., dissociative phenomena, and changes in severity, e.g., in the level of anxiety as proposed by Docherty, could not be modeled.

Another problem arises from the systematically missing data resulting from individual clinical pictures for that no statistical 'fix' exists [17]. Choosing pairwise deletion as the best of all insufficient options to handle this problem – listwise deletion would have resulted in no data, imputation of mean scores in a great distortion of the symptom patterns, produced nonpositive definite covariance matrices with mathematically out-of-bound values that caused estimations to fail and led to the dismissal of the respective variables from the model. And the high interindividual variance even in the z-transformed data with standard deviations between 1.5 for 'pains and aches' and 0.3 for non-acoustic hallucinations will lead to rather small bivariate covariances, thus impeding mathematical proof of the model.

A theoretical problem is presented by the model assumption of a subtype-independent, general and unidirectional sequence of illness stages. Considering the variance in the clinical picture and course, different transition models might have to be described for subgroups of patients differing, e.g., in psychopathology, time course and/or etiology.

Irrespective of this unanswered question, cognitive and social dysfunctions and, parallel to them, functional impairment increase in the early course illness depending on age at onset of first sign of illness and gender. This could be demonstrated by the evaluated social model integrating different earlier findings. It gives further support to the main aims, especially of early intervention research, the avoidance or at least delay and reduction of social disruptions that lead to poor outcome. Perhaps it is also this general aspect of the progressive nature of an incipient serious disorder like schizophrenia that should be additionally focused in the striving for early detection and prognosis of illness onset. Yet, a prerequisite for a validation of any developmental model or models is an exact, detailed and prospective assessment of the occurrence, severity and persistence of clinical symptoms and functional impairments and an adequate method for the analysis of complex relations and patterns.

◼ References

1. Andreasen NC (1983) The Scale for the Assessment of Negative Symptoms (SANS). University of Iowa, Iowa City
2. Andreasen NC, Arndt S, Allinger R, Miller D, Flaum M (1995) Symptoms of schizophrenia. Archives of General Psychiatry 52: 341–351
3. Biehl H, Maurer K, Jablensky A, Cooper JE, Tomov T (1989) The WHO Psychological Impairments Rating Schedule (WHO/PIRS). I. Introducing a new instrument for rating observed behaviour and the rationale of the psychological impairment concept. British Journal of Psychiatry 155: 68–70
4. Conrad K (1958) Die beginnende Schizophrenie. Thieme, Stuttgart New York
5. Docherty JP, van Kammen DP, Siris SG, Marder SR (1978) Stages of the onset of schizophrenic psychosis. American Journal of Psychiatry 135: 420–426
6. Formann AK (1984) Die Latent-Class-Analyse. Beltz, Weinheim Basel

7. Häfner H (2000a) Gender differences in first-episode schizophrenia. In: Frank E (ed) Gender and Its Effects on Psychopathology. American Psychiatric Press, Inc., Washington DC London, pp 187–228
8. Häfner H (2000b) Ist es alles nur die Krankheit? Neue Ergebnisse aus der Schizophrenieforschung. Springer, Berlin Heidelberg New York
9. Häfner H, an der Heiden W (1999) The course of schizophrenia in the light of modern follow-up studies: the ABC and WHO studies. European Archives of Psychiatry and Clinical Neuroscience 249 (Suppl 4): IV/14–IV/26
10. Häfner H, Riecher-Rössler A, Hambrecht M, Maurer K, Schmidtke A, Fätkenheuer B, Löffler W, an der Heiden W (1992) IRAOS: an instrument for the assessment of onset and early course of schizophrenia. Schizophrenia Research 6: 209–223
11. Häfner H, Löffler W, Maurer K, Riecher-Rössler A, Stein A (1999) Interview für die retrospektive Erfassung des Erkrankungsbeginns und -verlaufs bei Schizophrenie und anderen Psychosen. Huber, Bern
12. Häfner H, Maurer K, Löffler W, an der Heiden W, Munk-Jørgensen P, Hambrecht M, Riecher-Rössler A (1998) The ABC schizophrenia study: a preliminary overview of the results. Social Psychiatry and Psychiatric Epidemiology 33: 380–386
13. Häfner H, Löffler W, Maurer K, Hambrecht M, an der Heiden W (1999) Depression, negative symptoms, social stagnation and social decline in the early course of schizophrenia. Acta Psychiatrica Scandinavia 100: 105–118
14. Hambrecht M, Häfner H (1993) "Trema, Apophänie, Apokalypse" – Ist Conrads Phasenmodell empirisch begründbar? Fortschr Neurol Psychiat 61: 418–823
15. Jöreskog KG, Sörbom D (1993) LISREL 8: Structural Equation Modeling with the SIMPLIS Command Language. Scientific Software International, Chicago
16. Jung E, Krumm B, Biehl H, Maurer K, Bauer-Schubart C (1989) DAS – Mannheimer Skala zur Einschätzung sozialer Behinderung. Beltz, Weinheim
17. Kline RB (1998) Principals and Practice of Structural Equation Modeling. Guilford Press, New York London
18. Lieberman JA, Fenton WS (2001) Delayed detection of psychosis: causes, consequences, and effect on public health. American Journal of Psychiatry 157: 1727–1730
19. Malla AK, Norman RMG, Voruganti LP (1999) Improving outcome in schizophrenia: the case for early intervention. Canadian Medical Association Journal 160: 843–846
20. Maurer K, Häfner H (1995) Methodological aspects of the onset assessment in schizophrenia. Schizophrenia Research 15: 265–276
21. Wing JK, Cooper JE, Sartorius N (1974) Measurement and Classification of Psychiatric Symptoms. Cambridge University Press, London
22. World Health Organization, WHO (1980) Follow-up history and sociodemographic description schedule (FU-HSD). 2nd unpublished draft: January 1980
23. Yung AR, McGGorry PD (1996) The prodromal phase of first-episode psychosis: past and current conceptualizations. Schizophrenia Bulletin 22: 353–370

Discussion:* psychopathological predictors of onset and course of schizophrenia

H. Häfner
Schizophrenia Research Unit, Central Institute of Mental Health, Mannheim,
Germany

The two lectures discussed deal with predictors of the onset and early course of schizophrenia. Prof. Klosterkötter's contribution is based on a prospective, our own on a retrospecte design. Common to both are efforts to find ways to recognize and predict illness or psychosis onset earlier than at present. These goals can be subjected to the following questions: What is it that the authors want to predict, when, how and why?

The last question is the easiest to answer: both contributions pursue the goal of improving early recognition and prediction of schizophrenia onset as a basis for preventive intervention. But unlike our group, represented by Frauke Schultze-Lutter, Joachim Klosterkötter believes to have almost succeeded in attaining this goal.

The second goal is theoretical in nature: what information do the analyses of the early course provide on the disorder and the underlying neurobiological and psychological processes? There is no simple answer to this question yet.

▓ Early recognition of schizophrenia

If the aim is to obtain indication for a specific early intervention, such as early treatment with antipsychotic medications, it must be ensured in predicting the onset of schizophrenia that 1) the risk of schizophrenia is *recognized* and distinguished from that of other disorders (early diagnosing) and 2) the timepoint of this risk is reliably *predicted*. For the goal of distinguishing psychosis risk from risks for other illnesses the temporal dimension is of secondary importance. Early recognition of this type can be based on risk factors fairly remote in time such as familial load, as demonstrated by Wolfgang Maier (Maier et al., this volume), or pre-, peri- and postnatal complications (Verdoux & Sutter, this volume)

* As Wolfram an der Heiden was unable to present his talk on "DUI and DUP as predictors of schizophrenic course" because of illness, Joachim Klosterkötter kindly included the topic in his talk. As Patrick McGorry, too, the invited discussant of this session, had to cancel his participation at a short notice, I had no choice but to fill the gap myself. As a co-author of the second contribution to this session, I will mainly concentrate on discussing Joachim Klosterkötter's talk.

and developmental anomalies in childhood and youth, as shown in the birth cohort studies conducted by Done and Jones in Great Britain [7, 8, 17, 18], Isohanni et al. [15, 16] in Finland or Cannon et al. [3] and Poulton et al. [29] in New Zealand.

The prognostic and discriminating power of such tools for predicting schizophrenia risk can be improved by looking for additional risk factors closer to the illness onset, such as indicators of cognitive and social impairment in adolescence. This was done in the conscript studies conducted in Israel, on which Mark Weiser reported, and in Sweden [24]. For this reason early intervention centers, such as the EPPIC center in Melbourne [27] and the early-recognition and intervention center (FETZ) in Cologne (see Klosterkötter, this volume), make use of such discriminative predictors in selecting patients for their intervention programs [30].

To evaluate the effort described in Joachim Klosterkötter's paper to prospectively validate predictors of the timepoint of psychosis onset and to test the predictive power of certain features or clusters of early signs and symptoms, the first thing to look at is the individual period of risk covered in the study. In Klosterkötter's study this period had a mean length of 9.3 years. But we do not know yet how long the period of latency until psychosis onset is in individual cases.

Apart from the question of finding an appropriate design for testing the validity of predictors, it might well be possible to predict psychosis onset if it were possible to recognize signs or symptoms indicative of an incipient or progressing disease process. Such reliable signs or symptoms would be comparable, for example, to vomiting as a prodromal symptom of food poisoning. But, considering the fact that in most cases schizophrenia onset occurs with unspecific symptoms, as shown in the ABC Schizophrenia Study [12], it seems rather unlikely that such reliable indicators occur in schizophrenia. For this reason we have no choice but to concentrate on later stages of the incipient, progressing illness process.

An early indicator might be a characteristic sequence of single features or of symptom patterns. As shown in our contribution (cf. Schultze-Lutter et al., this volume), modeling the early illness course using the traditional models of symptom sequence [4, 6], which differ in their underlying concepts, has not been successful. This, however, does not mean that such patterns of sequence do not exist. But there is a third dimension of risk factors, functionally associated with the underlying disease process, that might contribute to predicting psychosis onset or a climax of psychotic symptoms: an accumulation of prodromal signs and symptoms in both number and severity, an increase in the distress experienced by the person affected as well as in cognitive and social impairment. One indicator of that type (a loss of 30 points or more in the Global Assessment of Functioning (GAF) scale for at least one month) was included in the set of composite criteria that Yung et al. [30] successfully tested in their prospective study of 40 cases presenting indicators of a high risk for psychosis.

The gradients of these processes are bound to show considerable variation, as illustrated by the survival analysis of the duration of illness from onset to first admission for schizophrenia [11, 25]. The distribution is highly skewed with short durations predominating (Fig. 1).

In view of the fact that it is before the first treatment contact that impairments lead to most of the social consequences associated with schizophrenia [13, Schultze-Lutter et al., this volume] early recognition is an objective of clear public-health relevance irrespective of the difficulties involved.

But how successful was Joachim Klosterkötter in his attempt to recognize schizophrenia early and to predict psychosis onset? In the 9.3-year period of risk, he succeeded in correctly recognizing a risk for schizophrenia in an extremely high proportion of 78% and in predicting psychosis onset in more than 50% of cases (positive predictive power). How was this possible? One reason is that risk for psychosis was highly enriched in that sample of patients who had been referred by their doctors to psychiatric university departments for diagnostic clarification because of "suspected schizophrenia". Another reason stems from the first: among the ten "basic symptoms" of the highest "prognostic accuracy" presented in Table 5 of Klosterkötter's contribution there are thought disorders, ideas of reference, visual and auditory disturbances, which are clearly indicative of mild or attenuated psychotic symptoms. When entered in the study, the patients, on average, probably were at an illness stage near to a full-blown psychosis irrespective of their clinical diagnosis. Consequently, the cluster of basic symptoms used represents a screening set that proved to be of a high predictive power for psychosis onset in this particular high-risk population. The result is not valid for at-risk persons in the general population. It is only valid for patients who have been ascertained as being at a high-risk for schizophrenia and who fulfill the clinical inclusion criteria of the population studied by Klosterkötter. To make these criteria easier to use at other centers, they should be described in greater detail.

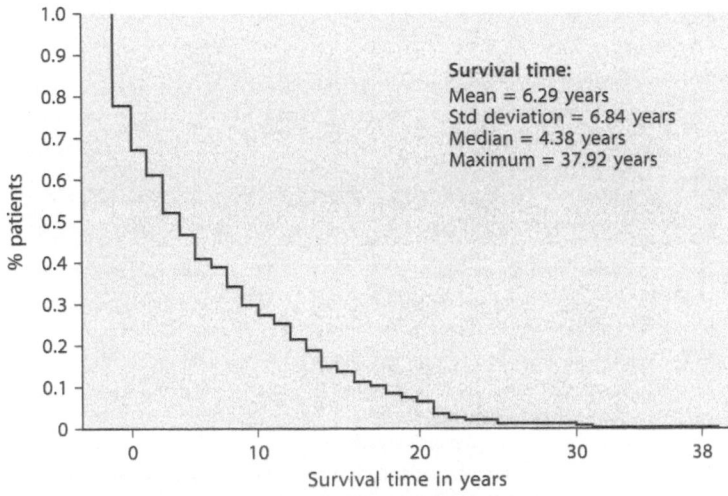

Fig. 1. Survival function for the duration of the early course (ABC first-episode sample N = 232) [11]

As the patients in the study were also administered PSE interviews, as mentioned by Joachim Klosterkötter, it would be interesting to analyze these data using the CATEGO algorithm independently of the set of basic symptoms. Such analyses would yield definitions of the patients' diagnosis and psychopathology that are in accordance with the ICD criteria, symptoms and syndromes.

Despite their weaknesses of external validity in predicting onset, Joachim Klosterkötter's results have important practical implications for early intervention. They show that persons who display the described cluster of early symptoms are not only at a high risk for schizophrenia, which may manifest itself at some point over a period of several years, but also clearly in need of treatment because of the overall severity of their psychopathology. The fact that the probands had been referred by their doctors to psychiatric university departments can be seen as an indication of their need for treatment. Even if the screening procedure were of a lower diagnostic accuracy, it would not have any negative consequences for the indication for therapy, as long as the intervention remains targeted to current symptomatology. An important point in treating patients who present prodromal symptoms of a low discriminative power, especially before any psychotic symptoms have occurred, is that the early intervention centers should provide treatment programs for other diagnostic outcomes as well, such as major depressive disorder or obsessive-compulsive disorder.

■ Self-observed symptoms and additional predictive criteria

From a theoretical point of view, it is remarkable that only one cross section of subjectively experienced symptoms, assessed at various, not precisely known stages before full-blown psychosis, showed such a high prognostic value independently of any behavioral, psychological or neurobiological indicators. Such

Table 1. Empirical subgroups at the beginning of schizophrenia – ABC first-episode sample N = 232

Prodromal phase (plus one month of psychotic phase		Psychotic phase (minus one month)	
Subgroups (cluster analysis)		Subgroups (cluster analysis)	
28 %	Low values on all dimensions	23 %	Low values on all dimensions
15 %	Delusional symptoms and depersonalization/ non-specific, negative depressive symptoms	14 %	Delusional symptoms
30 %	Non-specific, negative, depressive symptoms	26 %	Non-specific, negative, depressive symptoms
16 %	Delusional symptoms, psychotic thought disorders and hallucinations / non-specific, negative, depressive symptoms	14 %	Substance abuse and hallucinations
11 %	Psychotic thought disorders and hallucinations/ non-specific, negative, depressive symptoms	15 %	Psychotic thought disorders
		10 %	Disorganization

a result is conceivable if the signs or symptoms in question are sufficiently stable over the early illness course. To a limited extent this seems to be the case. In the first-episode sample of the ABC Study we studied symptom clusters at the prodromal stage, including one month of positive symptomatology to prevent positive symptoms from being excluded as prodromal signs, and in the subsequent psychotic prephase until first admission. As expected, non-specific, negative and depressive symptoms, which showed by far the highest frequencies at the prodromal stage, were associated with three clusters (Table 1). They continued to persist at the psychotic stage as a discrete cluster. Three other clusters, too, clearly persisted. What was new at the psychotic stage were mainly disorganizational symptoms, indicative of a full-blown psychosis, and comorbidity with substance abuse – the latter is of no relevance in this context. Consequently, the symptom clusters, including that of psychotic symptoms, can be presumed to be fairly stable at the stage that results in the first psychotic episode.

The 5-year course following first admission, prospectively assessed at 5 cross sections, presented a highly varied picture, as reflected in Liddle's three-factor model [19–21]. Figure 2 shows that all three factors were positively correlated with the factors of the subsequent cross sections. The negative factor, showing medium to high coefficients, was significantly correlated with that same – negative – symptom factor at each subsequent cross section, hence showing a high degree of stability. At the second assessment, which took place six months after first admission and in most cases after remission of psychosis, the negative factor also predicted social outcome and the amount of social impairment at the 5-year follow-up. In contrast, the psychotic and the disorganizational factors displayed a very low degree of stability over the five years following first admission, presumably because of their primarily episodic courses. The reason why the positive-symptom cluster also proved fairly stable in the first psychotic episode is

Fig. 2. Five-year course of the "psychomotor poverty syndrome", "disorganization syndrome" and "reality distortion syndrome" – ABC follow-up sample n = 115 [23]

presumably that this illness stage was artificially homogeneous due to the inclusion criterion "first psychotic episode". Hence, as in many previous longitudinal studies, after remission of the first psychotic episode only the negative symptom dimension turned out to be a good predictor of that same symptom dimension and of the social course of schizophrenia.

To facilitate an early recognition of the disorder not only the self-experienced symptoms tested in Klosterkötter's study can be used, but also additional indicators of incipient illness may be obtained from observed behavior, neuropsychological testing of perception, attention and memory [1, 5] as well as from neurobiological factors such as changes in morphological or functional brain anomalies and possibly also from changes in transmitter activity and neurophysiological variables (eye tracking, EVP, etc.). They might prove helpful in predicting psychosis onset. At present we are still far from having identified any good biological indicators of schizophrenia onset, but this might change soon.

Independently of expensive and time-consuming special examinations, we need an early recognition instrument that is easy to use in daily practice and enables us to reliably recognize the disorder and to predict the approximate timepoint of psychosis onset. Supplementing the interventions provided for high-risk groups there should be screening methods and instruments for identifying at-risk individuals in the general population at an earlier stage, so that they can be referred to specialist services for examination with instruments of a better diagnostic and predictive power and finally for the treatment they require. This means that the tools for early recognition and prediction must be designed as comprising at least two stages: 1) a screening stage to identify individuals at a slightly enhanced risk and 2) a specialist stage for a thorough and possibly also multi-level examination to recognize and predict the disorder and to identify indication for therapy.

▦ DUI and DUP

This leads us to the prognostic significance of DUI and DUP. Joachim Klosterkötter presented a list of studies that have demonstrated a lengthy DUP to predict an unfavorable course, but also three or so studies that have found no such correlation. Our own analysis based on the ABC subsample of 115 first illness episodes, retrospectively assessed back to the onset of the first sign of mental illness and prospectively followed up at 6 cross sections over five years from first admission on, yielded no clear-cut correlations. As Fig. 10 in Häfner et al. (this volume) shows, DUP was significantly correlated with positive and non-specific symptom scores at 5-year follow-up. In contrast, DUI – here cases with long prodromal stages characterized by negative and non-specific symptoms predominated – was significantly correlated only with negative and nonspecific symptom scores at five-year follow-up. Neither DUP nor DUI had any significant effects on relapses (their number, time to or duration of first relapse) and on social outcome. This result sounds absolutely plausible in view of the assumption that there is a certain degree of stability in the early illness course, in extended prodromal stages in particular, which tend to turn chronic early and to be associated with a predominance of an acute type of course of the first psychotic episode.

The main problem in comparing results from studies on the topic is that the criteria used for defining DUI and DUP and the exactness of assessing the onset and end of these periods differ greatly. For this reason comparisons across studies are difficult and inconsistencies of results quite understandable. However, since the majority of studies appear to show (cf. Klosterkötter, this volume, and Häfner et al., this volume) that the longer the duration of untreated psychosis, the more signs there seems to be of a poor further course of the disorder, it is conceivable that such an association exists, despite the methodological weaknesses involved.

Even if we take these results for granted, misgivings are justified about the evidence purportedly showing a causal association, e.g. concerning the highly speculative hypothesis of a neurotoxic effect of psychosis on the further illness course [22]. Norman & Malla [28] recently gave a detailed review of the methodological implications of the topic. Their core argument runs that early disease-inherent phenomena are responsible for different trends in the further course of the disorder. An acute onset with a short DUP and no lengthy period of negative symptoms and impairments is presumed to be associated with a good outcome. In contrast, a lengthy insidious prodromal stage characterized by a chronic early course of negative symptoms and persisting impairments is seen as indicative of a disease process turning chronic at an early stage.

The reason why the unfavorable consequences of DUI and DUP are being debated in such an intensive and controversial manner is that they are used as arguments for the need for early intervention. But the only thing that can be regarded as established according to Norman and Malla [28] is that „DUP may be related to easing or reducing psychotic symptoms, once treatment begins for first-episode patients". And there is no evidence available yet showing that the further course of schizophrenia can really be improved by early intervention, that is, by shortening DUI and DUP. Such evidence can only be obtained by testing the efficacy of early-intervention measures, i.e., in double blind studies with a random allocation of probands [26].

■ Modeling the early social course of schizophrenia

Our presentation (cf. Häfner et al., this volume) summarized the previously published results according to which most of the social consequences in schizophrenia occur before the climax of the first episode and, hence, before the current beginning of treatment. This was most clearly shown by the analysis of trends in the social role "marriage and stable partnership", particularly vulnerable in schizophrenia. At illness onset, 37% of the men and 59% of the women affected, compared with 43% and 74% of their healthy male and female counterparts respectively, are married. At the end of the early illness stage, i.e. at first admission, only 17% of male and 33% of female patients, compared with 60% and 78% of healthy controls respectively, are married.

The factors explaining the social course of schizophrenia in general and the poorer course in men than women seem not to be direct consequences of the disorder. They are mediated by the level of social development at psychosis onset and the socially adverse illness behavior of young men. In an earlier study we had analyzed this association in two steps: at first by stepwise logistic regression and using the ability to earn one's living as a variable of 5-year outcome [cf. 14]. The only variables with a significant effect on 5-year social outcome were "non-fulfilled social roles at psychosis onset" and "socially adverse illness behavior in the psychosis". The traditional predictors: age, gender, symptomatology and type of early illness course (acute versus chronic) had no direct effect of any significance on the outcome variable. In a second step we tested how the mediating variables – social status at illness onset and illness behavior – were associated with the traditional clinical predictors. In this analysis we used a path-analytical model. Fig. 8 in Häfner et al. (this volume) illustrates the expected highly significant partial correlations between gender, age at onset and socially adverse illness behavior on the one hand, and age and level of social development at illness onset, on the other hand [10].

The SEM model (Structural Equation Model and the computer program LIS-REL-8), entered as a new element in the analysis by Frauke Schultze-Lutter, allowed us to test the associations in an all-inclusive model. Irrespective of the question whether this model is appropriate to test the type of data in question, which I am unable to judge, the fact that the result coincided with the result of the previous two-step analysis can be seen as indicating the validity of the result from this earlier analysis.

The consequences for the social course of schizophrenia, depending as it does on age and level of social development at illness onset, which, too, is determined by age, were demonstrated in Fig. 9 of Häfner et al.'s contribution (this volume).

As a result, the course of schizophrenia as reflected in patients' social biographies is largely determined by factors not directly produced by the disorder or even specific to it. These factors are also important determinants of the social course of other chronic diseases, such as multiple sclerosis.

A factor more or less specific to schizophrenia, which is responsible for the later age of illness onset in women, is the protective effect of estrogen. But this protective effect disappears in women in the menopausal period. As a result, men, because of their lack of a protective effect and because of their sex-specific socially adverse behavior, develop the most severe types of schizophrenia at a young age and, at a later age, considerably milder types than postmenopausal women. In any case, looking at the course of schizophrenia, which we used to regard as determined by illness-related factors alone, we are now faced with a complex process of interacting biological, psychological and social factors. It is the interplay of these factors with the direct effects of the disorder that produces what we perceive as the illness course and the patients' social biographies.

■ Testing the stage models

As Frauke Schultze-Lutter showed, we failed in our attempt to apply Conrad's [4] and Docherty et al.'s [6] models of illness stages to the sequence of symptom occurrence in the early course of schizophrenia in the way described by the authors of these models in their publications. Nor did the models turn out to be applicable to the IRAOS data, collected in the ABC Study, on the period from illness onset until first admission in the first psychotic episode. With respect to the reasons mentioned by Schultze-Lutter et al. (this volume) for this negative result we can add that the information provided by Conrad and Docherty et al. allowed us to construct only an additive model. Consequently, as we also had to apply it to the IRAOS data, we could merely focus on the sequence of first symptom occurrence. It was not possible for us to test a cumulative model which would have allowed us to also consider at each new illness stage the persistence of symptoms from previous stages.

Finally, there is the fundamental question of the correctness of Conrad's and Docherty et al.'s core premise that the proposed sequence of illness stages is compelling and valid for all cases irrespective of the high variability of the speed of progress of incipient illness. It has not yet been tested whether individual illness courses may differ not only in the speed of their progress, but also in the type and sequence of their symptoms. The question of an appropriate stage model of incipient illness has not yet been resolved.

■ Lifetime trajectory of the course of schizophrenia

The model of a developmental trajectory of schizophrenia from birth to illness onset shows no clear-cut tendency to either a favorable or an unfavorable outcome compared with that of the healthy population over the same period of age. After remission of the first episode, mean symptom scores and neuropsychological test results more or less resettle on a plateau [9]. This trajectory of the illness course does not coincide with the deteriorating course of dementia praecox described by Kraepelin. But there are extremes that differ greatly from this picture based on mean values: a group with gradually progressing illness of a deteriorating course – the patients finally develop severe cognitive impairment and social disability, perhaps even dementia – and a group displaying a full and permanent recovery without any perceivable consequences after the first episode. The mean values show neither stepwise decline with each relapse after the first episode nor a later period of improvement, as suggested by Breier et al. [2], although their own data did not support this view. Between these two periods fairly stable in the mean, i.e., from birth to onset and from remission of the first episode until many years later, the onset of the disorder and the first episode occur. This illness stage is by far the most active period, as the increase in symptoms of any category (cf. Fig. 1 in Häfner et al., this volume) and in cognitive and social impairment with the devastating social consequences show. It is not yet known exactly what kind of degenerative or dysfunctional processes are at work in this phase. If we are ever going to succeed in intervening at this stage of the disorder earlier and better than by the current practice of an in fact belated treatment of the psychotic episode, we will presumably have to be able to prevent, halt or ameliorate the disease process. For this reason we will continue our efforts of finding ways of recognizing and predicting the disorder earlier and better. We are looking forward not only to early intervention programs embracing traditional therapeutic tools, but also to the prospects offered by methods of neuroprotection (Cf. Behl, this volume; Ehrenreich & Sirén, this volume).

■ References

1. Bilder RM, Reiter G, Bates JA, Willson DF, Lieberman JA (1995) Neuropsychological profiles of first-episode schizophrenia. Schizophrenia Res 15: 109
2. Breier A, Schreiber JL, Dyer J, Pickar D (1991) National Institute of Mental Health longitudinal study of chronic schizophrenia: prognosis and predictors of outcome. Arch Gen Psychiatry 48: 239–246
3. Cannon M, Caspi A, Moffitt T, Harrington H-L, Taylor A, Murray RM, Poulton R (2002) Evidence for early, pan-developmental impairment specific to schizophreniform disorder. Results from a longitudinal birth cohort. Arch Gen Psychiatry 59: 449–456
4. Conrad K (1958) Die beginnende Schizophrenie. Versuch einer Gestaltanalyse des Wahns. Thieme-Verlag: Stuttgart New York
5. Cornblatt BA, Keilp JG (1994) Impaired attention, genetics, and the pathophysiology of schizophrenia. Schizophrenia Bull 20: 31–46
6. Docherty JP, Van Kammen DP, Siris SG, Marder St. R (1978) Stages of onset of schizophrenic psychosis. Am J Psychiatry 135: 420–426
7. Done D, Crow TJ, Johnstone EC, Sacker A (1994) Childhood antecedents of schizophrenia and affective illness: social adjustment at ages 7 and 11. Br Med J 309: 699–703
8. Done DJ, Sacker A, Crow TJ (1994) Childhood antecedents of schizophrenia and affective illness: intellectual performance at ages 7 and 11. Schizophrenia Res 11: 96–97
9. Goldberg TE, Hyde TM, Kleinman JE, Weinberger DR (1993) Course of schizophrenia: neuropsychological evidence for a static encephalopathy. Schizophr Bull 19: 797–804
10. Häfner H (2000) Ist es alles nur die Krankheit? Schriften der Mathematisch-naturwissenschaftlichen Klasse der Heidelberger Akademie der Wissenschaften Nr. 7. Springer-Verlag, Berlin Heidelberg New York
11. Häfner H, Maurer K (2001) The prodromal phase of psychosis. In: Miller T, Mednick SA, McGlashan T, Libiger J, Johannsessen JO (eds) Early Intervention in Psychotic Disorders. Kluwer Acad Publ, Dordrecht, pp 71–100
12. Häfner H, Maurer K, Löffler W, Bustamante S, an der Heiden W, Riecher-Rössler A, Nowotny B (1995) Onset and early course of schizophrenia. In: Häfner H, Gattaz WF (eds) Search for the Causes of Schizophrenia III. Springer: Berlin Heidelberg, pp 43–66
13. Häfner H, Nowotny B, Löffler W, an der Heiden W, Maurer K (1995) When and how does schizophrenia lead to social deficits? Eur Arch Psychiatry Clin Neurosci 246: 17–28
14. Häfner H, Maurer K, Löffler W, an der Heiden W, Könnecke R, Hambrecht M (1999) Onset and prodromal phase as determinants of the course. In: Gattaz WF, Häfner H (eds) Search for the Causes of Schizophrenia, vol. IV: Balance of the Century. Steinkopff-Verlag, Darmstadt, Springer, Berlin, pp 1–24
15. Isohanni M, Jones PB, Kemppainen L, Croudace, T, Isohanni I, Veijola J, Räsänen S, Wahlberg KE, Tienari P, Rantakallio P (2000) Childhood and adolescent predictors of schizophrenia in the Northern Finland 1966 birth cohort – a descriptive life-span model. Eur Arch Psychiatry Clin Neurosci 250: 311–319
16. Isohanni M, Jones PB, Räsänen S, Järvelin M-R, Oja H, Koiranen M, Jokelainen J, Rantakallio P (2001) Early developmental milestones in adult schizophrenia. A 28-year follow-up of the North Finland birth cohort. Schizophrenia Res 52: 1–19

17. Jones PB, Done DJ (1997) From birth to onset: a developmental perspective of schizophrenia in two national birth cohorts. In: Keshavan MS, Murray RM (eds) Neurodevelopmental and Adult Psychopathology. Cambridge University Press, Cambridge, pp 119–136
18. Jones PB, Murray RM, Rodgers B (1995) Childhood risk factors for schizophrenia in a general population birth cohort at age 43 years. In: Mednick SA, Hollister J (eds) Neural Development in Schizophrenia: Theory and Practice. Plenum Press, New York, pp 151–176
19. Liddle PF (1987) Schizophrenic syndromes, cognitive performance and neurological dysfunction. Psychol Med 17: 49–57
20. Liddle PF (1987) The symptoms of chronic schizophrenia. A re-examination of the positive-negative dichotomy. Br J Psychiatry 151: 145–151
21. Liddle PF, Barnes TRE (1990) Syndromes of chronic schizophrenia. Br J Psychiatry 157: 558–561
22. Loebel AD, Lieberman JA, Alvir JMJ, Mayerhoff DI, Geisler SH, Szymanski SR (1992) Duration of psychosis and outcome in first-episode schizophrenia. Am J Psychiatry 149: 1183–1188
23. Löffler W, Häfner H (1999) Dimensionen der schizophrenen Symptomatik. Nervenarzt 70: 416–429
24. Malmberg A, Lewis G, David A, Allebeck P (1998) Premorbid adjustment and personality in people with schizophrenia. Br J Psychiatry 172: 308–313
25. Maurer K (2001) Prodromal symptoms as indicators of psychosis transitions. Results from the Mannheim ABC study (Abstract). The World Journal of Biological Psychiatry 2 (Suppl 1): 99
26. McGorry PD, Jackson HJ (eds) (1999) The Recognition and Management of Early Psychosis. Cambridge University Press, Cambridge
27. McGorry PD, Edwards J, Mihalopoulos C, Harrigan SM, Jackson JH (1996) EPPIC: an evolving system of early detection and optimal management. Schizophrenia Bull 22: 305–326
28. Norman RM, Malla AK (2001) Duration of untreated psychosis: a critical examination of the concept and its importance. Psychol Med 31: 381–400
29. Poulton R, Caspi A, Moffitt TE, Cannon M, Murray R, Harrington H (2000) Children's self-reported psychotic symptoms and adult schizophreniform disorder: a 15-year longitudinal study (In Process Citation). Arch Gen Psychaitry 57: 1053–1058
30. Yung AR, Phillips LJ, McGorry PD, McFarlane CA, Francey S, Harrigan S, Patton GC, Jackson HJ (1998) Prediction of psychosis. A step towards indicated prevention of schizophrenia. Br J Psychiatry 172 (Suppl 33): 14–20

Perspectives of Neuroprotective Interventions

Neuroprotection in schizophrenia – What does it mean? – What means do we have?

H. Ehrenreich, A.-L. Sirén

Departments of Psychiatry and Neurology, Georg-August University, and Max-Planck Institute for Experimental Medicine, Göttingen, Germany

Putative cellular mechanisms in the etiology/pathogenesis of schizophrenia

The molecular and cellular mechanisms responsible for schizophrenic psychosis are far from being understood. Imbalance of neurotransmitters, particularly of the dopaminergic system, accounting for the often dramatic clinical features, has been uncovered and is successfully repressed by dopamine antagonists [5, 26]. Other neurotransmitter systems are affected as well [5, 26]. Imbalance is caused by profound neuronal dysfunction due to neurodevelopmental/neurodegenerative dysregulation and is also detectable in less spectacular and therefore initially often ignored symptoms [36, 38]. In fact, a remarkable worsening of cognitive/mental performance can be observed during early episodes of the psychosis [20, 36], supporting the concept of a major neuronal damage occurring at that time.

Post-mortem and neuroimaging studies of schizophrenia have revealed changes in brain structure and volume that seem to reflect a reduction of dendritic and synaptic connections rather than purely neuronal or glial cell loss [1, 16, 21, 30]. These findings are in agreement with a pathophysiological model of reduced synaptic connectivity arising from disturbances of brain development active during perinatal and adolescent periods [21]. Various cytoarchitectural abnormalities in the brains of schizophrenic patients hint to abnormal neural cell proliferation/migration, abnormal glial and neuronal maturation and formation of axonal/dendritic connections, abnormal axonal myelination, and aberrant apoptosis/neuronal pruning during development [1, 15]. A reduction in interneuronal neurophil in the prefrontal cortex has been shown to be a prominent feature of cortical pathology in schizophrenia suggesting that subtle changes in cellular architecture and brain circuitry may have a devastating impact on cortical function [27].

Progressive deterioration of cognitive functions together with progressive ventricular enlargement as shown in imaging studies [6, 23, 32] support a neurodegenerative component in the pathophysiology of schizophrenia. A recent study using high-resolution MRI demonstrated dynamic patterns of accelerated gray matter loss in the brains of childhood-onset schizophrenia with earliest defects in the parietal association cortex. Here, gray matter loss is known to be strongly associated with environmental risk factors [4, 32]. Interestingly, the deficits spread and intensified over 5 years of disease progression frontally to prefrontal cortex and to temporal brain regions [32] indicative of continuous degenerative processes. Accordingly, an increased postnatal (adult) rate of neuronal apoptosis/pruning, metabolic alterations in neurons and reduced synaptic sprouting/altered neuroplasticity have been proposed [1, 15, 16, 36].

Etiology of schizophrenia: risk factors of manifestation of disease

Epidemiologists and clinicians have repeatedly reported on a dramatic worsening of the cognitive/mental performance as early as during the first episode of the psychosis. During further episodes a slowly progressing or long-term stable course of the disease is usually observed. Despite general agreement on the significance of a genetic predisposition [10, 11, 16, 33, 38], the etiology/etiologies of schizophrenic psychosis remain(s) obscure. There is, however, strong evidence [8, 9, 12, 19, 24, 25, 33, 35] for a number of co-factors (e.g., neurotrauma, drug abuse) that influence manifestation and course of schizophrenia (Fig. 1). Again, this observation underlines the dual origin of the disease-determining processes: neurodevelopmental and neurodegenerative, and urges the early application of neuroprotective strategies as "add-on therapy" to the predominantly symptomatic neuroleptic treatment of schizophrenic psychosis.

What is neuroprotection?

Neuroprotection may be defined as an attempt to maintain the highest possible integrity of cellular interactions in the brain resulting in an undisturbed neural function. Loss of brain function can be detrimental, whereas loss of brain cells may not even be measurable. In fact, mere prevention of cell death can be undesired: elimination of dysfunctional or transformed cells may contribute to the preservation of the best possible function, perhaps at the price of increased cell death. Neuroprotection may be prophylactic or therapeutic. In the first case, it means prevention of functional loss before it occurs. Identification of risk factors (genetic or environmental) is essential for prevention. Therapeutic neuroprotection means maintenance or amelioration of remaining function as much as possible. Here, erythropoietin and estrogens, among others, may be interesting candidates for therapeutic strategies since these agents can influence a spectrum of pathways presumably involved in the neurodegenerative aspects of schizophrenic psychosis, i.e., apoptosis, metabolic status of neurons, synaptic connections and axonal sprouting/pruning.

Means of neuroprotection

Imitation of brain endogenous protective mechanisms may be the key to future successful approaches to neuroprotection. Thus, a major aim of research in this

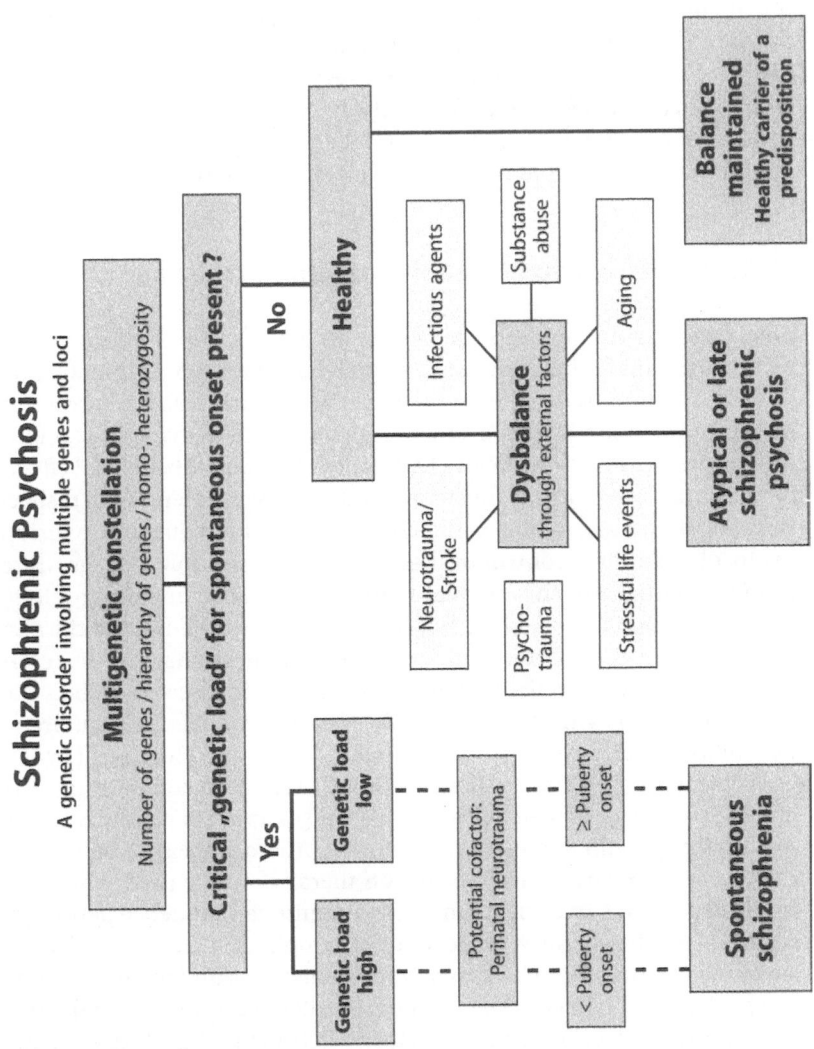

Fig. 1. A schema summarizing the complexity of etiology/pathogenesis of schizophrenic psychosis. Identification of risk factors, both genetic and environmental, may help in designing future neuroprotective add-on therapies to the symptomatic neuroleptic treatment.

respect has to be to gain a more precise understanding of endogenous mechanisms of protection, defense against and response to damage, adaptation to and coping with new situations. We presume that activation/mimicry of endogenous mechanisms will be efficient and well tolerated. An example of endogenous neuroprotection is the development of relative ischemic tolerance in response to repeated transient ischemic events [2, 13]. Preconditioning obviously (re)activates silent genetic programs of cellular defense/survival strategies thereby leading to a modulation of neuronal tissue vulnerability [2, 14, 17]. Another example of endogenous neuroprotection may be adult neurogenesis upon physical exercise [34]. In fact, this phenomenon may also explain how alterations in behavior or even psychotherapy can exert actions at a cellular level associated with a gain of brain function. Inactivity, in contrast, has long been known to lead to a loss of function ("use it or lose it"). Lack of input to the sensory cortex upon amputation of a finger in monkeys results in restructuring of the cortex [18, 22].

◼ Application of neuroprotective concepts in the clinic

For schizophrenia, neuroprotection is an entirely novel approach. Neuroprotection has thus far been an issue in hypoxic/ischemic or traumatic brain injury. In these conditions, despite promising experimental studies, hardly any concept of neuroprotection has been convincingly efficient in man [7]. It is important to understand why these strategies have failed. The lack of beneficial effects in many clinical trials can be attributed to methodological problems with respect to selection of patients and a non-sufficient adherence to inclusion/exclusion criteria. Protocol violations, control of therapeutic time window, dosage, duration and safety/potential toxicity of treatments have created major problems [7, 37]. Moreover, animal models are limited in their power to imitate the clinical situation with respect to heterogeneity of population, risk factors and complicating diseases. This is in particular true with psychiatric diseases such as schizophrenia with no satisfying animal models. Existing models, at best, are capable of exemplifying certain aspects of the disease. Thus, introduction of promising new concepts, based on the application of well-tolerated compounds, directly into clinical treatment of schizophrenic psychoses appears justified. In schizophrenia, erythropoietin and estrogens, among others, appear to be interesting candidates for a "neuroprotective add-on therapy" to the predominantly symptomatic neuroleptic treatment since these agents can influence pathways involved in the neurodegenerative aspects of schizophrenic psychoses, i.e., apoptosis, metabolic status of neurons, synaptic connections and axonal sprouting/pruning [3, 28, 29, 31]. In Göttingen, a neuroprotective approach to the treatment of schizophrenic psychosis using erythropoietin (EPO) as "experimental add-on therapy" to a standardized neuroleptic regimen is presently in preparation. Prophylactic application of EPO in persons at risk to develop a psychosis (e.g., high genetic load, neurotrauma, psychotrauma, etc.) or in a presumable prodromal phase will also have to be considered for future studies.

◼ References

1. Arnold SE, Trojanowski JQ (1996) Recent advances in defining the neuropathology of schizophrenia. Acta Neuropathol (Berl) 92: 217–231
2. Barone FC, White RF, Spera PA, Ellison J, Currie RW, Wang X, Feuerstein GZ (1998) Ischemic preconditioning and brain tolerance: temporal histological and functional outcomes, protein synthesis requirement, and interleukin-1 receptor antagonist and early gene expression. Stroke 29: 1937–1950; discussion 1950–1951

3. Campana WM, Misasi R, O'Brien JS (1998) Identification of a neurotrophic sequence in erythropoietin. Int J Mol Med 1: 235–241

4. Cannon TD, Thompson PM, van Erp TGM, Toga AW, Huttunen M, Lönnqvist J, Standertsköld-Nordenstam C-GA (2001) A probabalistic Atlas of Cortical Gray Matter Changes in Monozygotic Twins Discordant for Schizophrenia. International Congress on Schizophrenia Research; Whistler, Canada

5. Carlsson A (1988) The current status of the dopamine hypothesis of schizophrenia. Neuropsychopharmacology 1: 179–186

6. Davis KL, Buchsbaum MS, Shihabuddin L, Spiegel-Cohen J, Metzger M, Frecska E, Keefe RS, Powchik P (1998) Ventricular enlargement in poor-outcome schizophrenia. Biol Psychiatry 43: 783–793

7. De Keyser J, Sulter G, Luiten PG (1999) Clinical trials with neuroprotective drugs in acute ischaemic stroke: are we doing the right thing? Trends Neurosci 22: 535–540

8. Freed EX (1975) Alcoholism and schizophrenia: the search for perspectives. A review. J Stud Alcohol 36: 853–881

9. Fujii DE, Ahmed I (2001) Risk factors in psychosis secondary to traumatic brain injury. J Neuropsychiatry Clin Neurosci 13: 61–69

10. Hafner H (2000) Epidemiology of schizophrenia. A thriving discipline at the turn of the century. Eur Arch Psychiatry Clin Neurosci 250: 271–273

11. Isohanni M, Jones P, Kemppainen L, Croudace T, Isohanni I, Veijola J, Rasanen S, Wahlberg KE, Tienari P, Rantakallio P (2000) Childhood and adolescent predictors of schizophrenia in the Northern Finland 1966 birth cohort – a descriptive life-span model. Eur Arch Psychiatry Clin Neurosci 250: 311–319

12. Karlsson H, Bachmann S, Schroder J, McArthur J, Torrey EF, Yolken RH (2001) Retroviral RNA identified in the cerebrospinal fluids and brains of individuals with schizophrenia. Proc Natl Acad Sci U S A 98: 4634–4639

13. Kitagawa K, Matsumoto M, Tagaya M, Hata R, Ueda H, Niinobe M, Handa N, Fukunaga R, Kimura K, Mikoshiba K et al. (1990) 'Ischemic tolerance' phenomenon found in the brain. Brain Res 528: 21–24

14. Kuhn GH, Palmer TD, Fuchs E (2001) Adult neurogenesis: a compensatory mechanism for neuronal damage. European Archives of Psychiatry and Clinical Neuroscience 251: 152–158

15. Lieberman J, Chakos M, Wu H, Alvir J, Hoffman E, Robinson D, Bilder R (2001) Longitudinal study of brain morphology in first episode schizophrenia. Biol Psychiatry 49: 487–499

16. Lieberman JA (1999) Is schizophrenia a neurodegenerative disorder? A clinical and neurobiological perspective. Biol Psychiatry 46: 729–739

17. Liu J, Ginis I, Spatz M, Hallenbeck JM (2000) Hypoxic preconditioning protects cultured neurons against hypoxic stress via TNF-alpha and ceramide. Am J Physiol Cell Physiol 278: C144–153

18. Manger PR, Woods TM, Jones EG (1996) Plasticity of the somatosensory cortical map in macaque monkeys after chronic partial amputation of a digit. Proc R Soc Lond B Biol Sci 263: 933–939

19. McAllister TW (1992) Neuropsychiatric sequelae of head injuries. Psychiatr Clin North Am 15: 395–413

20. McCarley RW, Niznikiewicz MA, Salisbury DF, Nestor PG, O'Donnell BF, Hirayasu Y, Grunze H, Greene RW, Shenton ME (1999) Cognitive dysfunction in schizophrenia: unifying basic research and clinical aspects. Eur Arch Psychiatry Clin Neurosci 249: 69–82

21. McGlashan TH, Hoffman RE (2000) Schizophrenia as a disorder of developmentally reduced synaptic connectivity. Arch Gen Psychiatry 57: 637–648

22. Merzenich MM, Nelson RJ, Stryker MP, Cynader MS, Schoppmann A, Zook JM (1984) Somatosensory cortical map changes following digit amputation in adult monkeys. J Comp Neurol 224: 591–605

23. Rapoport JL, Giedd J, Kumra S, Jacobsen L, Smith A, Lee P, Nelson J, Hamburger S (1997) Childhood-onset schizophrenia. Progressive ventricular change during adolescence. Arch Gen Psychiatry 54: 897–903

24. Sachdev P, Smith JS, Cathcart S (2001) Schizophrenia-like psychosis following traumatic brain injury: a chart- based descriptive and case-control study. Psychol Med 31: 231–239

25. Schneier FR, Siris SG (1987) A review of psychoactive substance use and abuse in schizo-phrenia. Patterns of drug choice. J Nerv Ment Dis 175: 641–652
26. Schwartz JC, Diaz J, Pilon C, Sokoloff P (2000) Possible implications of the dopamine D(3) receptor in schizophrenia and in antipsychotic drug actions. Brain Res Brain Res Rev 31: 277–287
27. Selemon LD, Goldman-Rakic PS (1999) The reduced neuropil hypothesis: a circuit based model of schizophrenia. Biol Psychiatry 45: 17–25
28. Sirén A-L, Ehrenreich H (2001) Erythropoietin – a novel concept of neuroprotection. Euro-pean Archives of Psychiatry and Clinical Neuroscience 251: 179–184
29. Sirén AL, Fratelli M, Brines M, Goemans C, Casagrande S, Lewczuk P, Keenan S, Gleiter C, Pasquali C, Capobianco A, Mennini T, Heumann R, Cerami A, Ehrenreich H, Ghezzi P (2001) Erythropoietin prevents neuronal apoptosis after cerebral ischemia and metabolic stress. Proc Natl Acad Sci U S A 98: 4044–4049
30. Sowell ER, Toga AW, Asarnow R (2000) Brain abnormalities observed in childhood-onset schizophrenia: a review of the structural magnetic resonance imaging literature. Ment Retard Dev Disabil Res Rev 6: 180–185
31. Tabira T, Konishi Y, Gallyas F, Jr. (1995) Neurotrophic effect of hematopoietic cytokines on cholinergic and other neurons in vitro. Int J Dev Neurosci 13: 241-252
32. Thompson PM, Vidal C, Giedd JN, Gochman P, Blumenthal J, Nicolson R, Toga AW, Rapoport JL (2001) From the cover: Mapping adolescent brain change reveals dynamic wave of accelerated gray matter loss in very early-onset schizophrenia. Proc Natl Acad Sci U S A 98: 11650–11655
33. Thurm I, Haefner H (1987) Perceived vulnerability, relapse risk and coping in schizophre-nia. An explorative study. Eur Arch Psychiatry Neurol Sci 237: 46–53
34. van Praag H, Kempermann G Gage FH (1999) Running increases cell proliferation and neu-rogenesis in the adult mouse dentate gyrus. Nat Neurosci 2: 266–270
35. van Reekum R, Cohen T, Wong J (2000) Can traumatic brain injury cause psychiatric dis-orders? J Neuropsychiatry Clin Neurosci 12: 316–327
36. Velakoulis D, Wood SJ, McGorry PD, Pantelis C (2000) Evidence for progression of brain structural abnormalities in schizophrenia: beyond the neurodevelopmental model. Aust N Z J Psychiatry 34 (Suppl): S113–126
37. Windisch M, Gschanes A, Hutter-Paier B (1998) Neurotrophic activities and therapeutic experience with a brain derived peptide preparation. J Neural Transm Suppl 53: 289–298
38. Woods BT (1998) Is schizophrenia a progressive neurodevelopmental disorder? Toward a unitary pathogenetic mechanism. Am J Psychiatry 155: 1661–1670

Neuroprotective effects of estrogens in the central nervous system: mechanisms of action

C. Behl

Max-Planck-Institute of Psychiatry, Munich, Germany

▩ Introduction

The pathogenesis of various multi-factorial diseases including Parkinson's disease, stroke and Alzheimer's disease (AD) is characterized by genetic disposition and additional external and sometimes environmental factors. Despite the obvious differences in the basic processes that lead to neurodegeneration (AD as a chronic, neurodegenerative disorder as compared to stroke as an acute neurodegenerative insult), final common pathogenetic pathways may be defined. Such pathways are frequently characterized by the activation of certain genes that mediate programmed cell death (or: apoptosis). One frequently occurring common feature in neurodegenerative conditions and disorders is the occurrence of *oxidative stress*. In the search for novel pharmaceutical agents that can interfere with oxidative stress-associated neurodegenerative disorders molecular mechanisms of neuroprotection have been described. Such mechanisms include extracellular as well as intracellular pathways. Extracellular neuroprotection may be defined as the addition of certain compounds to neuronal tissue (e.g., antioxidants, neurotrophic factors) and endogenous neuroprotection can be mediated by the induction of novel neuroprotective gene transcription. A powerful physiological mediator that drives both possible pathways of neuroprotection (extracellular and endogenous) is the female sex hormone estrogen.

AD is the most frequent type of dementia in the human elderly population. It is characterized histopathologically through the occurrence of extracellular protein aggregates, which are built up by the amyloid β protein and by the intracellular hyperphosphorylation of the cellular tau-protein [for review: 21]. A minority of AD cases are characterized by mutations in certain genes (APP, PS1, PS2), but the majority of AD cases are strictly age-associated, so that age and the aging process itself can be addressed as the real risk factor of this deadly neurodegenerative disorder. During aging, various intrinsic physiological neuroprotective and neurotrophic systems are decreasing in their activity, including neurotrophic factor expression itself, certain neuropeptides (e.g., CRH, AVP), neurotransmitters (mainly acetylcholine) and hormones. Among the hormones, the female sex hormone estrogen is the most prominent, which almost drops to zero female menopause with the start. Based on the fact that neurotrophic input decreases with age, AD may also be defined as a disease of decreasing and lost neuroprotection [for review: (1)]. One major end point of nerve cell death occurring in AD tissue is oxidative stress.

Oxidative stress is defined by the misbalance of the generation of the reactive oxygen species versus the physiological detoxification and removal of these oxygen radicals. *Reactive oxygen species (ROS)* are a normal and regular by-product of our daily living under molecular oxygen. In fact, ROS including the superoxide radical, the hydroxyl radical, and hydrogen peroxide, perform even physiological roles including signal transduction. Most prominently, nitric oxide has been found to be an important signaling molecule in nervous tissue. The accidental overflow of ROS production, which mostly occurs in the mitochondria during electron transport, is regularly controlled by cellular intrinsic antioxidant systems including superoxide dismutase (SOD), catalase, and glutathione peroxidase. This physiological balance can be disturbed by either the overproduction of ROS or the impairment of the antioxidant systems as occurring during aging. Exogenous sources including UV light, ionizing radiation, and certain environmental toxins generate an increased oxidative environment which then leads to damage of vital molecules in the cells. This oxidative damage may effect proteins, DNA and lipids. While oxidized proteins may form aggregates and precipitates in cells or may create dysfunctional enzymes, the oxidations of DNA may lead to mutations (and finally tumor formation) and the oxidation of lipids directly leads to the disintegration of membrane structures. Indeed, it is the peroxidation reaction mediated by the hydroxyl radical leading to the oxidation of non-saturated carbohydrate site chains in membrane lipids that induces dysfunction of the membrane and cell lysis [5, 8].

The amyloid β-protein (A β), which is found aggregated in nerve tissue of AD patients, is believed to be the sensual mediator of neurodegeneration in AD [21]. A β is derived from a larger transmembranal precursor protein (APP = amyloid β precursor protein), and the biochemical processing of APP which is performed by α-, β-, and gamma-secretases is in the major focus of pharmaceutical neurobiological research. A β aggregates in vitro as well as in vivo may induce an over all oxidative environment. A β can directly interact with the neuronal membranes leading to the accumulation of ROS or may indirectly attract and activate inflammatory cells (e.g., microglial cells) which then leads to a ROS accumulation. The experimental evidence for a potent role in the pathogenesis and progression of AD is overwhelming [3, 13, 15, 18, 20]. It has been clearly shown that A β protein induces intracellular oxidase systems that lead to the generation of superoxides and subsequently to the accumulation of intracellular peroxides which then may be the substrate for the formation of the highly reactive hydroxyl radical. A β induces the oxidation of membrane lipids which is believed to be the cause of nerve cell death in certain in vitro models [3]. In addition, whether intracellular A β causes some damage via oxidative pathways is being discussed. In addition to A β the excitatory amino acid glutamate as well as other potential neurotoxins are believed to induce similar oxidative events in nerve cell death. Ultimately, this may lead to direct oxidative damage and dysfunction of these cells. Moreover, a slow and chronic build-up of oxidative stress may induce secondary envents such as oxidative apoptosis [1]. In the search for novel approaches that prevent oxidative nerve cell death associated with neurodegenerative disorders, such as AD, one goal is to find novel more powerful and pharmacologically better antioxidants and on the other hand novel genetic neuro-protective modulators. The female sex hormone estrogen is believed to be a mul-titalent with respect to this.

■ The female sex hormone estrogen as a neuroprotectant

The rationale for looking into estrogen as a neuroprotective compound has been recently fuelled by clinical reports demonstrating that replacement of estrogen in post-menopausal women decreases the incidence of certain neurodegenerative conditions including mild cognitive impairment, Parkinson's disease, and AD. It is known that sex hormones like estrogen effect brain structure and function. Var-ious gender differences in cognitive functions exist, like women having better ver-bal abilities, perceptual speed, and accuracy. High estrogen levels support verbal skills in females, and with post-menopausal, estrogen replacement therapy explicit memory is improved: thus, it may be concluded that estrogen specifically maintains verbal memory in women and may prevent of forestall a deterioration in short- and long-term memory that occurs with normal aging and perhaps with AD [22]. Summaries of case controls and cohort studies show that estrogen replacement therapy indeed decreases the relative risk of AD and it is concluded that estrogen has an in vivo protective effect with respect to AD [9].

Estrogen is by far much more than just a sex hormone. In addition to its clas-sical effects during sex differentiation and maturation, estrogen has been shown to act also in nervous tissue and the brain. Indeed, estrogen has been described as a neuroactive steroid which acts in both a genomic and non-genomic manner. Activities of estrogen in nervous tissue include effects on the basal forebrain cholinergic activity and integrity, the dendritic plasticity, the NMDA receptor density, neurotrophic signaling, APP processing, synaptic connectivity, and finally estrogen may act as direct and neuroprotective antioxidant [2].

Estrogen is a steroid (17β-estradiol) and is able to bind to cognate intracellu-lar steroid receptors. These receptors are nuclear transcription factors that, upon binding their ligand, they translocate into the nucleus inducing or repressing the transcription of certain estrogen receptor target genes. In addition to the genomic mode of action, which is called the genomic estrogen activity, estrogen may also act in a non-classical way which does not directly involve estrogen receptors.

Estrogen as a structural antioxidant:
receptor-independent protection (non-genomic, rapid)

In 1995 we were able to show that 17β-estradiol protects cultured neuronal cells against direct oxidative insults induced by hydrogen peroxide, A β, and gluta-mate.

A follow-up study has clearly shown that it is the phenolic structural nature of 17β-estradiol that mediates the direct antioxidant effect of 17β-estradiol. On the one hand, 17α-, 17β-, and ethinyl estradiol directly prevent oxidative damage in clonal hippocampal HT22-cells, while on the other hand, mestranol, the methyl ether of ethinyl estradiol, lacks this antioxidant activity [4]. Indeed, 17β-estradiol has a chemical structure which is quite similar to that of the most prominent lipophilic cellular antioxidant a-tocopherol (vitamin E). Both molecules consist of a phenolic free radical scavenging group and a lipophilic tail that mediates the incorporation into membranes. 17β-estradiol protects just like vitamin E against oxidative damage in cultured neuronal cells as well as in organotypic hippocampal preparations [4]. The antioxidant effect of phenolic groups in general is due to the donation of a proton by the antioxidant which leads to the direct detoxification of the free radical-bearing molecule (e.g., hydroxyl radicals). In a second step recycling of the antioxidant radical is possible, for instance, through vitamin C [8]. This antioxidant neuroprotection performed by 17β-estradiol is independent of estrogen-receptor activity. This has been demonstrated by comparing various different estrogen-derivative molecules with respect to their estrogen receptor binding and activating potency compared to their in vitro antioxidant activity. Molecules such as 4-dodecylphenol, 4,4-biphenol, and 2,4,6-trimethylphenol (TMP) were directly compared with this respect to 17β-estradiol. We found for instance, that, TMP has no affinity to the estrogen receptor and also does not activate estrogen receptor-dependent gene transcription, but does protect neurons against oxidative cell death. Moreover, TMP is also acting as an antioxidant in cell-free paradigms (e.g., LDL-oxidation assays) just like 17β-estradiol [14]. TMP may represent a phenolic antioxidant molecule which has almost ideal pharmacological features. With respect to the blood-brain barrier, penetration of TMP appears to be very good due to its very low molecular mass, its high lipophilicity, and other characteristics. Therefore, TMP is currently used in a variety of acute and chronic neurodegenerative model systems in vivo. Initial results with respect to the protective potential of TMP are very encouraging.

Since the occurrence of an intact phenolic group and some lipophilic features are the basic requirements of antioxidant neuroprotective molecules and since for estradiol's direct antioxidant activities no estrogen receptors are necessary, other phenolic physiological and non-physiological compounds can be defined and investigated with respect to their neuroprotective antioxidant potential. Considering this, we recently identified that delta9-tetrahydrocannabinol, a neuroactive cannabinoid and other related cannabinoid phenolic compounds are also acting as antioxidants in paradigms of neuronal cell death. Again no receptor systems, such as the cannabinoid receptor CB1, is necessary for the direct antioxidant neuroprotective activity [14].

Recently we suggested that nature itself also follows the principle of using phenolic groups as protective structures. It is obvious that membranes from different tissues in the body contain different amounts of transmembrane and integral proteins. Mitochondrial membranes, for instance, are highly enriched in transmembrane proteins, while neuronal membranes, in general, are less enriched in proteins. Indeed, the transmembrane domains of integral membrane proteins show an astounding accumulation of tyrosine and tryptophan residues, especially in the region of the highest lipid density. We found that these residues perform vital antioxidant functions inside these lipid bilayers and protect cells from oxidative destruction. Tyrosin- and tryptophan-containing peptides representing stretches from the transmembrane domains of different integral membrane proteins have been selected and used in in vitro antioxidant assays. The antioxidant functions of tyrosine, a phenolic amino acid, and tryptophan may provide a specific explanation for their unique transmembrane distribution pattern as well as for the increased vulnerability of low protein neuronal membranes to oxidative stress [17]. Again, phenolic groups inside peptide structures are able to prevent oxidative damage. In a further development of this idea tyrosine- and tryptophan-headed lipids were designed and used in paradigms of oxidative apoptosis. It became clear that comparing the EC50-values of such lipids to other standard antioxidants, such as N-acetyl-cysteine and β-carotin, they are much better and are acting in the lower micromolar range [17].

■ Receptor-dependent protection by estrogen (genomic, delayed)

While the above-mentioned neuroprotective activities of estrogen are completely independent of estrogen receptor and are exclusively dependent on the chemical structure of 17β-estradiol, various other neuroactivities of estrogen are strictly dependent on the activation of estrogen receptors expressed in nervous tissue. Up to now, two different estrogen receptor types have been identified and cloned, human estrogen receptor α and estrogen β [7, 10]. While there is an up to 69 % identity in the DNA binding sites of these receptors, there is a up to 85 % identity in the hormone binding site. Nevertheless, there are also structural differences in various co-activator and co-repressor binding sites. There is also a minimal sequence requirement at the DNA (estrogen response elements) which is shared by both types of receptors. The activation of estrogen receptors and the translocation of these receptors into the nucleus where they act as transcription factors is called the classical pathway which leads to the induction or repression of gene transcription. In addition, there is also a non-classical, but nevertheless, also genomic pathway where activated estrogen receptors directly interact with other intracellular signaling processes including the cAMP/CREB-mitogen-activated protein kinase – as well as other pathways. Consequently, estrogen receptors may therefore influence gene transcription of non-estrogen receptor-dependent genes. In addition to that membrane, estrogen receptors that are structurally related or distinct from the already known receptors are being studied by various researchers thus, allowing estrogen to act at the membrane site inducing a genomic intracellular response. Moreover, various interactions of estrogen receptors with cellular structures, such as caveolae or orphan receptors, can be proposed. In summary, the interaction possibilities of estrogen via receptors with different intracellular signaling systems manifold and are occur at different levels.

Estrogen receptor α and β are co-expressed in the central nervous system and, with respect to target tissues of neurodegenerative events, are co-expressed in the neocortex and the hippocampus as well as in various other brain regions [23]. The hippocampus is the brain region which is believed to be the site of the co-ordination of higher cognitive functions including learning and memory, but it is interesting to note that besides the traditional sites of estrogen action, such as the hypothalamus, various extra-hypothalamic sites in the brain and also in the spinal cord show estrogen receptor expression.

In order to identify genes that are dependent on estrogen receptor activity and that may mediate neuroprotective effects, we choose a molecular approach. Human clonal neuroblastoma cells were selected and transfected with estrogen receptor α and β, respectively. With these cell lines differential displays at the mRNA level were performed in order to find genes that are specifically induced in their transcription by estrogen receptor activity. Similar approaches have been successfully used in the past and apoptosis-related genes have been identified [11]. With the advent of novel molecular high through-put tools including DNA array chip analysis, we have extended our studies and used a commercially available Incyte human gene chip with approximately 9,000 expression DNA elements for hybridization experiments. Cells that over-express estrogen receptor a and that were treated with estrogen have been isolated, the mRNA purified and used for hybridizations of the gene chip. A wide range of differentially expressed genes have been found. Such genes include neuronal extracellular matrix proteins, signaling factors such as certain transcription factors as well as apoptosis-related genes (caspases). Experiments that verify a potential neuroprotective activity of these certain target genes are on-going and the over-expression of such cloned genes is currently being performed. Obviously, members of the mitogen-activated protein kinase (MAPK) signalling pathway also are target genes of estrogen receptor α activity. Therefore, we further investigated the effect of estrogen on the activity of this MAPK. Neuronal cells that over-express estrogen receptor α show increased ERK1/ERK2 phosphorylation compared to untreated control cells. Surprisingly this effect is not directly dependent on estrogen receptor α activity, since it also occurs in cells that do not show a classical genomic ER α response [12]. Other strictly estrogen receptor α-dependent genes, which are not effected in cells that do not express estrogen receptors, are currently being investigated in further detail.

Nevertheless, the estrogen-MAPK connection revealed a highly interesting link to basic processes of AD. The processing of APP can be effected by estrogen which has been shown in previous investigations by other researches. Here we found that the so-called non-amyloidogenic APP processing (α-secretase activity) is promoted by estrogen and the secretion of non-amyloidogenic forms of APP are increased in the supernatant of the estrogen-treated cells. Surprisingly these effects occur after applying a single dose of physiological concentrations of estrogen (10^{-8} M) and are completely blocked when inhibiting MAPK ERK 1/ERK 1 by specific inhibitors. Therefore, we could establish a direct link between estrogen, APP α processing and the activation of MAPK in these neuronal cells [12]. Whether theses events contribute to the potential neuroprotective effects of estrogen during estrogen replacement therapy with respect to the onset and incidence of AD is highly speculative. But it is intriguing to believe that long-term treatment of neuronal tissues with estrogen will also inhibit AD-associated biochemical pathways such as the detrimental APP processing. With our experiments we could not define the estrogen receptor as the ultimate prerequisite of this estrogen activity, since it also occurs in the absence of estrogen receptors. In addition, we were able to show that similar effects are performed by the male sex hormone testosterone in physiological doses (10^{-8} M) [6]. Interestingly enough, testosterone may only fulfill its APP α processing promoting effect when it is converted to estradiol which is mediated by the aromatase reaction.

■ Summary and outlook

Estrogen is a highly interesting structure and is far more than just a female sex hormone, but rather is a highly neuroactive molecule [2]. The modes of action range from the structural effects of estradiol's phenolic group to act as a neuroprotective antioxidant in models of oxidative apoptosis and oxidative cell damage to strictly estrogen receptor-dependent activities and may include additional interactions with various intracellular signaling pathways. Thus, the network of interactions of estrogen and estrogen receptors inside the cells is highly complex. In the search for novel neuroprotective compounds which may ultimately be used as neuroprotective compounds in the human, one approach is to use estradiol as the blue print structure of antioxidant neuroprotection and to define structures that are similar to estradiol, but lacking the estrogen hormone side effect. Such a structure may be TMP which has been introduced here and is currently under intensive investigation in various in vivo models of neurodegeneration. Novel antioxidant structures that are based on aromatic imines and aromatic amines have been recently introduced and it has been shown that they are even more potent than estradiol and estradiol derivatives such as TMP in various paradigms of oxidative apoptosis [19]. A completely separate approach is the genetic search for estrogen-regulated neuroprotective target genes that are effected during the physiological effects of estrogen in the nervous tissue as well as during estrogen replacement therapy in post-menopausal women. One approach to search for such estrogen-dependent genes is the use of DNA arrays which is currently ongoing and highly promising. In summary, we are far from understanding the whole range of neuroactivities of estrogen and it is a matter of intensive discussion about the Pro's and Con's of estrogen use in post-menopausal women. But nevertheless, estrogen is a model molecule that is well described as being neuroprotective and is a physiological modulator rather than being a pharmaceutical drug. Estradiol could lead us to novel pharmaceutical structures that act as neuroprotective antioxidants and on the other hand may pave the way for the identification of powerful new neuroprotective genes.

Acknowledgments I would like to thank all the members of the Behl Laboratory for their hard work in elucidating the neuroprotective potential of the female sex hormone estrogen. The present script of the talk held at the International Wissenschaftsforum of the University of Heidelberg, October 25-27, 2001, will be also published in Progress in Brain Research, Elsevier, Amsterdam 2002.

▨ References

1. Behl C (2000) Apoptosis and Alzheimer's disease. J Neur Transm 107: 1325–1344
2. Behl C (2001) Estrogen – Mystery Drug for the Brain? The Neuroprotective Activities of the Female Sex Hormone. Springer, Wien-NewYork
3. Behl C, Davies JB, Lesley R et al. (1994) Hydrogen peroxide mediates amyloid β protein toxicity. Cell 77: 817–827
4. Behl C, Skutella T, Lezoualch F, Post A, Widmann M, Newton C, Holsboer F (1997) Neuro-protection against oxidative stress by estrogens: structure-activity relationship. Mol Pharm 51: 535–541
5. Finkel T, Holbrook NJ (2000) Oxidants, oxidative stress and the biology of ageing. Nature 408 (6809): 239–247
6. Goodenough S, Engert S, Behl, C (2000) Testosterone stimulates rapid secretory amyloid pre-cursor protein release from rat hypothalamic cells via the activation of the mitogen-activated protein kinase pathway. Neurosci Lett 296 (1): 49–52
7. Green S, Walter P, Kumar V, Krust A, Bornert JM, Argos P, Chambon P (1986) Human oestrogen receptor cDNA: sequence, expression and homology to v-erb-A. Nature 320: 134–139
8. Halliwell B, Gutteridge JMC (1999) Free Radicals in Biology and Medicine. 3rd ed Oxford University Press
9. Henderson VW (2000) Oestrogens and dementia. In: Novartis Found Symp 230: 254–265
10. Kuiper GG, Enmark E, Pelto-Huikko M, Nilsson S, Gustafsson JA (1996) Cloning of a novel receptor expressed in rat prostate and ovary. Proc Natl Acad Sci USA 93: 5925–5930
11. Maggi A, Vegeto E, Brusadelli A, Belcredito S, Pollio G, Ciana P (2000) Identification of estro-gen target genes in human neural cells. J Steroid Biochem Mol Biol 74 (5): 319–325
12. Manthey D, Heck S, Engert S et al. (2001) Estrogen induces a rapid secretion of amyloid β precursor protein via the mitogen-activated protein kinase pathway. Eur J Biochem 268: 1–8
13. Markesbery WR (1999) The role of oxidative stress in Alzheimer disease. Arch Neurol 56: 1449–1452
14. Marsicano G, Moosmann B, Hermann H, Lutz B, Behl C (2002) Cannabinoids act as neuro-protectants independent of the cannabinoid receptor type I. (submitted)
15. McGeer PL, McGeer EG, Yasojima K (2000) Alzheimer disease and neuroinflammation. J Neural Transm Suppl 59: 53–57
16. Moosmann B, Behl C (1999) The antioxidant neuroprotective effects of estrogens and phe-nolic compounds are independent from their estrogenic properties. Proc Natl Acad Sci USA 96: 8867–8872
17. Moosmann B, Behl C (2000) Cytoprotective antioxidant function of tyrosine and tryptophan residues in transmembrane proteins. Eur J Biochem 267: 5687–5692
18. Moosmann B, Behl C (2002) Antioxidants as treatment for neurodegenerative disorders. Exp Opin Invest Drugs (in press)
19. Moosmann B, Skutella T, Beyer K, Behl C (2002) Protective activity of aromatic amines and imines against oxidative nerve cell death. Biol Chem (in press)
20. Rogers J, Cooper NR, Webster S, Schultz J, McGeer PL, Styren SD, Civin WH, Brachova L, Bradt B, Ward P, Lieberburg I (1992) Complement activation by β-amyloid in Alzheimer disease. Proc Natl Acad Sci USA 89: 10016–10020
21. Selkoe DJ (2001) Alzheimer's disease: genes, proteins, and therapy. Physiol Rev 81 (2): 741–766
22. Sherwin BB (2000) Oestrogen and cognitive function throughout the female lifespan. In: Novartis Found Symp 230: 188–201
23. Shughrue PJ, Lane MV, Merchenthaler I (1997) Comparative distribution of estrogen recep-tor α and β mRNA in the rat central nervous system. J Compar Neurol 388: 507–525

Results of two controlled studies on estrogen: avenue to neuroprotection in schizophrenia

J. Kulkarni, A. de Castella, M. Downey, S. White, J. Taffe, P. Fitzgerald, H. Burger
Alfred Psychiatry Research Centre, Monash University, Melbourne, Australia

Clinical estrogen trials in schizophrenia

Introduction

Estrogen is hypothesized to be protective for women against the early onset of severe symptoms of schizophrenia [13, 25]. This 'estrogen hypothesis' was derived from epidemiological, clinical and animal studies. Epidemiological studies [14] have shown that women with schizophrenia present with first-episode psychosis, on average, about 5 years later than men with schizophrenia. Clinical studies reveal greater differences in the symptoms suffered, with men having more negative symptoms of schizophrenia and women experiencing more affective and paranoid symptoms [10, 11]. Life-cycle studies have also shown that women are more vulnerable for either a first episode of psychosis or relapse of an existing illness at two major periods of hormonal change; first during the postpartum period and second during menopause [24, 26]. There have also been case reports of women whose schizophrenia symptoms were exacerbated at low estrogen phases of the menstrual cycle [8]. Riecher-Rossler et al. [23] conducted a study in which they demonstrated that psychotic symptoms in a group of 32 women with schizophrenia improved during the high estrogen phase of their menstrual cycle. These clinical findings fit well with animal studies in which estrogen has been shown to reduce the dopamine concentration in the striatum and modulate sensitivity as well as the number of dopamine receptors [2, 6, 12, 17]. Estrogen has also been reported to have dose-dependent effects on the modulation of dopaminergic systems [5]. Sumner and Fink [27] have also shown that estrogen can modulate serotonin systems by increasing the expression of genes for the 5-HT_{2A} receptor and the serotonin transporter in the dorsal raphe nucleus and forebrain of rats.

Following these epidemiological, clinical and animal study results, we conducted an open label pilot study [19] in which 11 women of child-bearing age with schizophrenia were given 0.02 mg oral ethinyl estradiol as an adjunct to antipsychotic drug treatment for 8 weeks, and compared their progress with a similar group who received antipsychotic drugs only. The group receiving estrogen made a significantly more rapid recovery from acute psychotic symptoms and also reported improvement in their general health status.

Subsequent to this, we conducted a dose-finding study for the optimal use of estradiol in women with schizophrenia [21]. This was a 3 arm double blind placebo controlled 28 day study in which 12 women received 50 mcg transdermal estradiol plus standardized antipsychotic drug, 12 women received 100 mcg transdermal estradiol plus standardized antipsychotic drug and 12 women received placebo plus standardized antipsychotic drug. All of the women had a diagnosis of DSM IV schizophrenia.

The main finding from this study was that the addition of 100 mcg transdermal estradiol provided the best outcome for women with schizophrenia compared with a group who received 50 mcg transdermal estradiol and a group who received antipsychotic drugs alone. The clinical improvement was significantly greater in the adjunctive 100-mcg-estrogen group with respect to key psychotic symptoms.

Currently, we are conducting a follow-up trial of 100-mcg transdermal estradiol in women with schizophrenia. An interim report is given below.

Method

Thirty-six women of childbearing age with acute schizophrenia have been recruited from the Dandenong Area Mental Health Service over the past 9 months. The targeted number of subjects for this study is 90 women over 3 years, commencing December 2000.

All patients in this study had a diagnosis of DSM IV schizophrenia. Women were excluded from the trials if they had any known endocrine abnormalities, were pregnant or lactating, were currently taking synthetic steroids, including the oral contraceptive pill, or were using illicit drugs. The Southern Health Care Network, Dandenong Hospital Ethics Committee approved the study. All patients gave written informed consent.

Each subject was enrolled in the trial for 28 days (one menstrual cycle) and received a baseline psychopathology and hormone assessment followed by assessments at days 4, 7, 14, 21 and 28. At each assessment, psychopathology was measured using the Positive and Negative Syndrome Scale (PANSS [15]). The PANSS is comprised of three subscales: the positive symptom subscale, the negative symptom subscale and the general symptom subscale. Hormone assays for serum estrogen (E2), progesterone (Prog), prolactin (PRL), luteinizing hormone (LH), follicle stimulating hormone (FSH) and testosterone (Test) were performed. Separate radio-immuno-assay tests were performed on each individual sample. A menstrual cycle interview (MCI [20]) was used to stage the patients' menstrual cycle phase.

Cognitive testing for each patient included the following:
- California Verbal Learning Test – Immediate
- Visual Reproduction (WMS-III) – Immediate
- Controlled Oral Word Association Test
- Stroop
- Trails A and B
- Digit Span
- California Verbal Learning Test – Delayed
- Visual Reproduction (WMS-III) – Delayed

This battery of cognitive tests was chosen as representative of measures of higher brain function most likely to be affected by estrogen. The areas of visuospatial skills and verbal memory skills were targeted along with more general cognitive testing.

All patients were randomized into the active 100 mcg estradiol skin patch treatment groups or an identical placebo patch group. The transdermal delivery systems utilized were adhesive skin patches containing 8 mg estradiol patches with a release rate of 100-mcg estradiol per 24 h. Both estrogen and placebo patches were changed every 4 days. Placebo patches were also adhesive, but had no active substance. All patients received antipsychotic drug treatment, which was administered according to a protocol that indicated doses of between 3 and 7 mg per day of risperidone. The dose of risperidone was dependent on the patient's clinical state.

For each patient, her change from baseline in total, positive, negative and general PANSS scores at each visit was calculated. These change scores formed a time sequence, beginning with zero at baseline.

Results

Demographic data. There were no statistically significant differences between the 18 women receiving 100-mcg adjunctive transdermal estradiol and 18 women receiving adjunctive transdermal placebo in terms of age, menstrual cycle phase, race, illness duration, diagnosis or antipsychotic drug dose (Figs. 1–3).

Mean Baseline PANSS for the two groups were 86.3 ± 27.7 for the 100-mcg estradiol group, and 73.3 ± 12.3 for the placebo group. This difference is statistically significant ($p < 0.05$). To allow for correction of this difference in the baseline scores, the change across time was calculated.

Change from baseline in the total PANSS, positive, negative and general subscales across time are shown (Figs. 4–7). The group receiving estrogen (100 mcg) had a more significant decrease in psychotic symptoms as measured by the

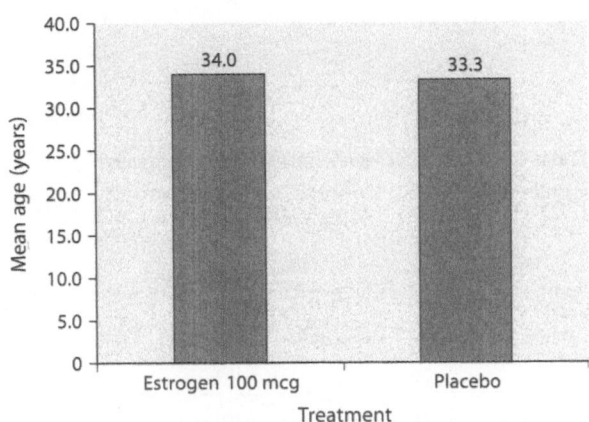

Fig. 1. Mean age of subjects in estrogen and placebo groups.

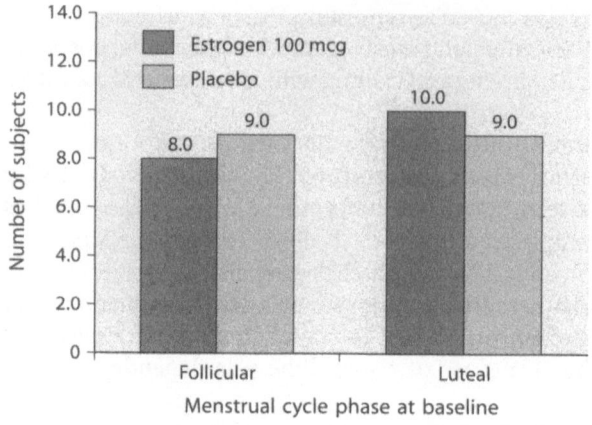

Fig. 2. Menstrual cycle phase of subjects at baseline.

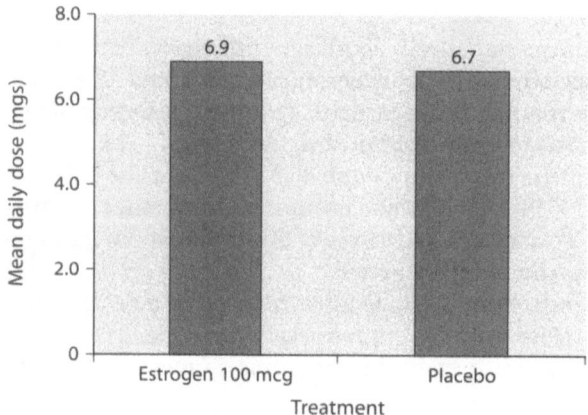

Fig. 3. Mean daily dose of anti-psychotic medication in risperidone equivalents.

Table 1. The mean hormone levels at baseline for both groups

	100 mcg Estradiol N = 18	Placebo N = 18
E2 Pmol/L	609.7 ± 564.4	498.9 ± 725.2
LH IV/L	11.1 ± 12.5	10.4 ± 14.2
PRL MIV/L	448.6 ± 672.1	203.3 ± 367.8

E2 serum estrogen; *LH* luteinizing hormone; *PRL* prolactin

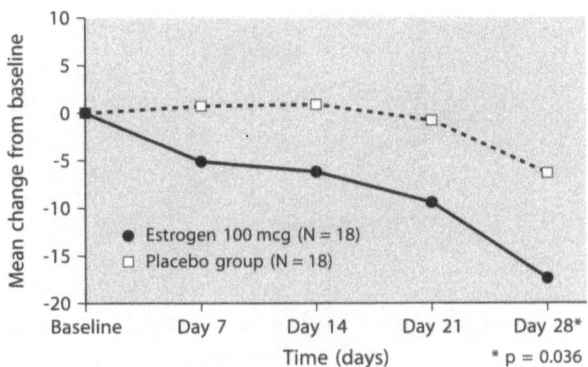

Fig. 4. Mean change from baseline in total PANSS scores for both groups.

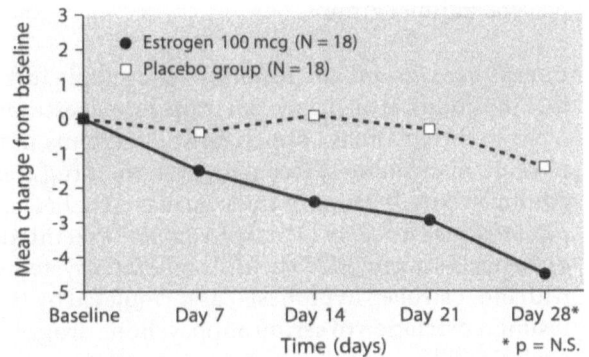

Fig. 5. Mean change from baseline in PANSS positive subscale scores for both groups.

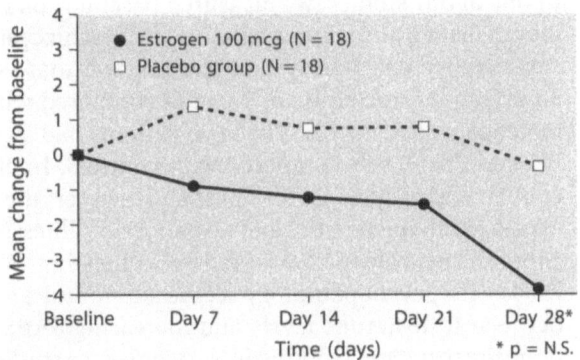

Fig. 6. Mean change from baseline in PANSS negative subscale scores for both groups.

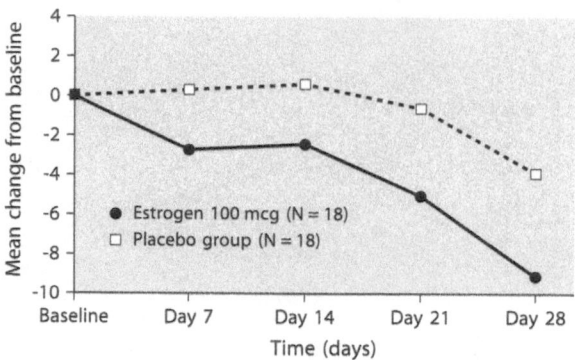

Fig. 7. Mean change from baseline in PANSS general subscale scores for both groups.

PANSS rating scale. The changes in hormone data across 28 days for the 2 groups (Table 1) revealed that the estrogen group had significantly higher mean estrogen levels, and lower LH levels. There were no significant differences in progesterone, FSH, prolactin or testosterone levels between the estrogen adjunct and placebo adjunct groups.

Interim conclusion. The results to date supply further evidence to again suggest that the addition of 100 mcg of transdermal estradiol provides greater improvement in the treatment of psychotic symptoms in women with DSM IV schizophrenia than standardized antipsychotic drug treatment alone. The impact of administering 100 mcg of transdermal estradiol, as indicated by its effect on the pituitary measured by LH assay, suggests that this dose and type of unconjugated estrogen is affecting CNS neurotransmitter systems positively. This is consistent with the "estrogen hypothesis" as formulated by Hafner [13] Results of cognitive testing, correlation of serum antipsychotic drug levels and further hormone data analysis will be described after more patients are recruited into this continuing study.

■ Clinical adjunctive estrogen trial in men with schizophrenia

In one of our studies, we measured baseline gonadotropin and sex steroid hormones in men and women suffering from schizophrenia compared with age- and sex-matched controls. A major finding was that 19 men with schizophrenia had an average testosterone of 26.6 mg compared with 17.7 mg in 18 healthy age-matched male controls. The male patients had significantly higher testosterone LH and FSH levels compared with controls. In effect, the male patients had a "puberty-like" gonadal axis profile. However, the patients had normal secondary sexual characteristics and no endocrine illnesses. The patients were all at least 3 months neuroleptic free at the time of testing. We also correlated testosterone levels with psychopathology scores and found a significant positive correlation between testosterone levels and increasing SAPS and SANS scores. The exact opposite results were found in the women we studied. Female patients had lower estrogen levels and higher LH levels compared to age and cycle-phase matched female controls. In effect, the female patients had a "menopause-like" gonadal axis profile – even though the average age for the patient group was 26.4 years and they were not menopausal. Estrogen levels correlated inversely with psychopathology scores.

From this data, clinical and pre-clinical studies, estrogen appears to have a potentially positive effect on psychotic symptoms most likely due to its dopamine modulating effect. In view of the positive response found in our adjunctive estrogen trials in women, we believe that adding short-term low dose estradiol to standardized antipsychotic drug treatment in men with schizophrenia could improve their response to neuroleptics.

Precedents for using estradiol as a treatment in men can be found in treatments for Alzheimer's disease and other types of dementia. Kyomen et al. [22] described a study in which 1.25 mg/day conjugated estrogen was given for 2 weeks with a marked improvement in agitation and physical aggression. Arnold [1] described similar use of 1.25 mg/day estradiol in young male patients with agitation and aggression post-traumatic brain injury. Diethylstibestrol (DES), which is an estrogen derivative, is commonly used in men to treat prostate cancer and as described by Kyomen [22] also was effective in treating aggressive behavior in an elderly man. Serum testosterone levels have been correlated with aggressive or violent behavior in men [7, 20] and the chronic administration of high doses of estrogen has been used to treat severe aggression and sexually offending behaviors in a small group of men [3]. A more positive study of the use of estradiol in men by Del Rio et al. [4] and Kirschbaum et al. [16] revealed that administering 0.1 mg estradiol to young male university students improved anxiety symptoms, suggesting that short-term treatment with estradiol leads to enhanced hypothalamic-pituitary-adrenal (HPA) and sympathetic responsiveness to psychological stress. Side effects of estrogen therapy in men such as gynecomastia, decreased libido and fluid retention are not reported in studies using less than 1.25 mg/day for less than 4 weeks.

From our work with using estrogen as an adjunct in the treatment of women with schizophrenia, we hypothesized the estrogen in men would also have a similar effect and conducted a pilot study to test this.

■ Men and estrogen treatment

Results of pilot study

In a pilot study conducted in 1999, 2-mg estradiol valerate was given as an adjunct to 6 men who received antipsychotic drugs and 5 men received oral placebo plus their standard antipsychotic medication. Oral estrogen, rather than transdermal estrogen was used to ensure compliance in acutely psychotic men.

Their psychopathology was measured using the Positive and Negative Symptom Schedule, i.e., PANSS and the Brief Psychiatric Rating Scale (BPRS). Higher scores on both these scales indicate more severe symptoms. Both groups commenced antipsychotic drugs plus estrogen or placebo on day 1 of the trial. However, the dose and type of antipsychotic drug was not standardized in this small pilot study.

Summary of pilot study results

T-test results from the pilot study show that the two groups had no significant difference in psychopathology scores at the start of the study. At day 5, the adjunctive estrogen group had a significantly lower positive PANSS, BPRS score ($P < 0.05$) compared with the placebo adjunct group. The estrogen group had a significantly higher negative PANSS score ($p < 0.05$). There were significant differences in mean hormone levels between the two groups at the start of the study. At day 7, the estrogen group had significantly higher mean estrogen levels, higher LH levels and higher prolactin levels. There was no difference in testosterone levels of FSH at day 7 between the groups.

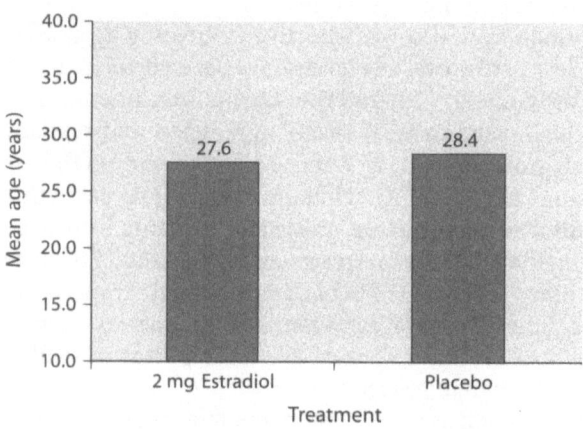

Fig. 8. Mean age of subjects in estrogen and placebo groups.

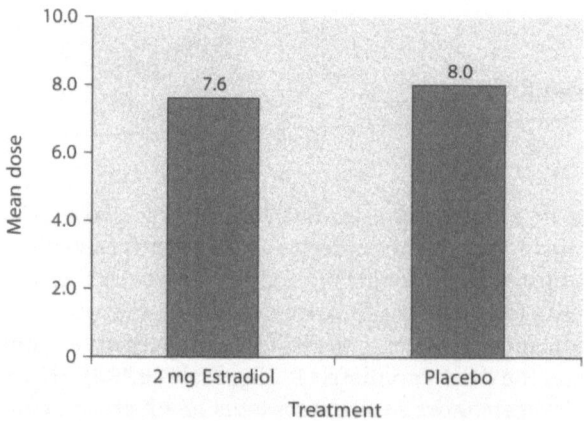

Fig. 9. Mean daily dose of antipsychotics in risperidone equivalents.

Table 2. Mean PANSS change from baseline scores for estrogen and placebo groups

	E2 Group	Placebo Group	P value
PANSS change from baseline to day 14	− 12.38 ± 6.4	−4.38 ± 6.1	0.04
Positive symptom change from 0 – day 14	−3.6 ± 2.6	−2.5 ± 4.4	NS
Negative symptom change. 0 – day 14	−2.3 ± 5.1	−0.75 ± 4.1	NS
General symptom change. 0 – day 14	−6.7 ± 4.3	−1.1 ± 4.1	0.02

Current study

We are currently investigating the effect of adding 2-mg oral estradiol valerate to standardized antipsychotic drug treatment in a group of men with schizophrenia for a 2-week double-blind trial. A target number of 60 patients will be recruited over a 3-year period with equal numbers being allocated to either the adjunctive estradiol or adjunctive placebo group, for 2 weeks.

Results. A total of 16 men with DSM IV schizophrenia have been recruited since May 2001. Eight received adjunctive 2-mg estradiol and 8 received adjunctive placebo. All patients received standardized antipsychotic drugs.

Demographic data revealed no differences between the two groups in terms of age, race, diagnosis, illness duration or antipsychotic drug treatment. The following graphs of the mean age and risperidone equivalent doses show no difference between the two groups.

The estrogen adjunct group was more unwell at the start of the trial as per the PANSS ratings. To compare the two groups' improvement across the 14-day trial, change from baseline measures were calculated. Using this change measures the following results were obtained:

These results show that the estrogen adjunct group made a more significant improvement over the 14-day trial as shown by the decrease in PANSS scores from baseline. In particular the most significant difference was in the PANSS general subscale symptoms (see Figs. 10–13).

Hormone results. There were significant changes between the two groups in terms of the estrogen group had significantly higher day 14 estrogen levels (p = 0.002), and lower testosterone levels (p = 0.04). Change from baseline measures did not show a significant difference across time in LH levels.

This is a study in progress and is also a dose finding study. Patients are closely monitored and no serious adverse effects have been noted.

Conclusions to date

The use of estrogen as a potential treatment in schizophrenia opens up exciting new avenues of preventative and acute treatment for schizophrenia in both men and women. The rapid development of new estrogen compounds, the Selective

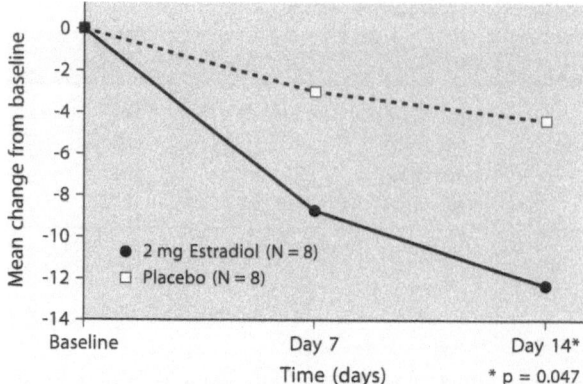

Fig. 10. Mean change from baseline for total PANSS scores for the two groups.

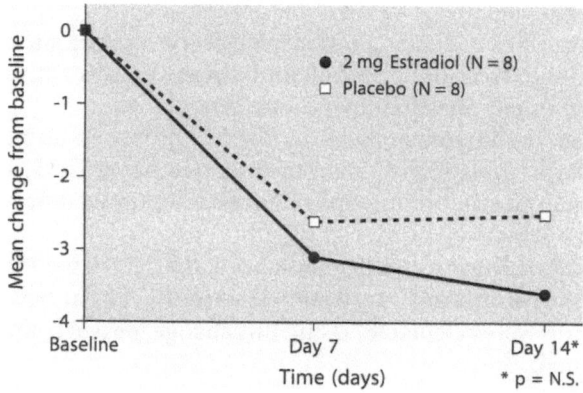

Fig. 11. Mean change from baseline for PANSS positive subscale for the two groups.

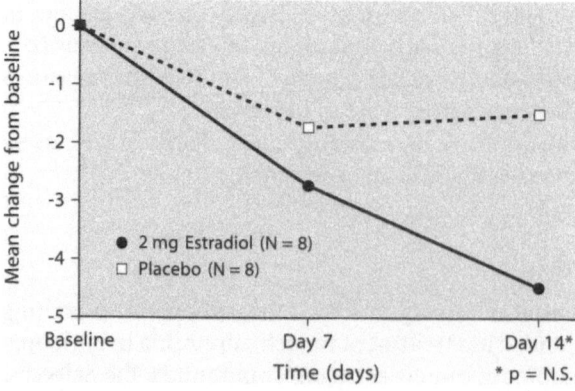

Fig. 12. Mean change from baseline for PANSS negative subscale for the two groups.

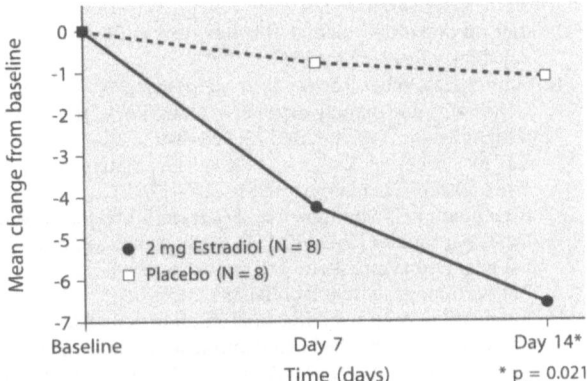

Fig. 13. Mean change from baseline for PANSS general subscale for the two groups.

Estrogen Receptor Modulators – or "brain estrogens" further expands the area of hormone treatments. Studying the mechanisms, by which estrogen potentially provides treatment of psychotic symptoms, may also open up new avenues to understand etiological aspects of schizophrenia, in particular the reasons for why schizophrenia is a post-pubertal disease.

▓ References

1. Arnold SE (1993) Estrogen for refractory aggression after traumatic brain injury. Am J Psychiatry 150: 1564–1565
2. Bedard P, Boucher R, Daigle MM, Di Paolo T (1984) Similar effect of estradiol and haloperidol on experimental tardive dyskinesia in monkeys. Psychoneuroendocrinology 9: 375–379
3. Bell R (1978) Hormone influences on human aggression. Irish J Med Sci 147: 5–9
4. Del Rio G, Velardo A, Zizzo G, Avogaro A, Cipolli C, Della Casa L, Marrama P, MacDonald IA (1994) Effect of estradiol on the normal sympathoadrenal response to mental stress in normal men. J Clin Endocrinology and Metabolism 79: 836–840
5. Di Paolo T, Payet P, Labrie F (1981) Effect of chronic estradiol and haloperidol treatment on striatal dopamine receptors. Eur J Pharmacol 73: 105–106
6. Dupond A, Di Paolo T, Gagne B, Baarden N (1981) Effects of chronic estrogen treatment on dopamine concentrations and turnover in discrete brain nuclei of ovariectomized rats. Neurosci Lett 22: 69–74
7. Ehrenkranz J, Bliss E, Sheard MH (1974) Plasma testosterone: correlation with aggressive behaviour and social dominance in man. Psychosomatic Med 36: 469–475
8. Endo M, Daiguji M, Asano Y, Yamashita I, Takahashi S (1978) Periodic psychoses recurring in association with menstrual cycle. J Clin Psychiatry 39: 456–461
9. Foreman MM, Porter JC (1980) Effects of catechol estrogens and catecholamines on hypothalamicand corpus striatal tyrosine hydroxylase activity. J Neurochem 34: 1175–1183
10. Goldstein JM (1988) Gender differences in the course of schizophrenia. Am J Psychiatry 145: 684–689
11. Goldstein JM, Tsuang MT (1990) Gender and schizophrenia: an introduction and synthesis of findings. Schizophr Bull 16: 179–183
12. Gordon JH, Borison RL, Diamond BI (1980) Modulation of dopamine receptor sensitivity by estrogen. Biol Psychiatry 15: 389–396

13. Hafner H, Behrens S, De Vry J, Gatttaz WF (1991) An animal model for the effects of estradiol on dopamine-mediated behaviour: implications for sex differences in schizophrenia. Psychiatry Res 38: 125–134
14. Hafner H, Riecher Rossler A, an der Heiden W, Maurer K, Fatkenheuer B, Loffler W (1993) Generating and testing a casual explanation of the gender difference in age at first onset of schizophrenia. Psychol med 23: 925–940
15. Kay SR, Fisbein A, Opler LA (1987) The positive and negative syndrome scale (PANSS) for schizophrenia. Schizophr Bull 13: 261–276
16. Kirschbaum C, Schommer N, Federenko I, Gaab J, Neumann O, Oellers M, Rohleder N, Uniedt A, Hanker J Pirke KM (1996) Short term estradiol treatment enhances pituitary-adrenal axis and sympathetic responses to psychological stress in healthy young men. J Clin Endocrinology and Metabolism 81: 3639–3643
17. Koller WC, Weiner WJ, Klawans HL, Nausieda PA (1980) Influence of female sex hormones on neuroleptic-induced behavioural supersensitivity. Neuropharmacology 19: 387–391
18. Kreuz LE, Rose RM (1972) Assessment of aggressive behaviour and plasma testosterone in a young criminal population. Psychosomatic Med 34: 321–332
19. Kulkarni J, de Castella A, Smith D, Taffe J, Keks N, Copolov D (1996) A clinical trial of the effects of estrogen in acutely psychotic women. Schizophr Res 20: 247–252
20. Kulkarni J, de Castella A, Thompson K (1997) Assessment of menstrual cycle phase in women with schizophrenia. The VIth International Congress on Schizophrenia research. Colorado Springs Colorado USA. April 12–16 1997. Abstracts Schizophr Res 24 (1–2) 1-288 Schizophr Res 26 (1) 81-82 erratum
21. Kulkarni J, Riedel A, de Castella A, Fitzgerald PB, Rolfe TJ, Taffe J, Burger H (2001) Estrogen – a potential treatment for schizophrenia. Schizophr Res 48: 137–144
22. Kyomen HH, Nobel KW, Wei JY (1991) The use of estrogen to decrease aggressive physical behaviour in elderly men with dementia. J Am Geriatric Soc 39: 1110–1112
23. Riecher-Rossler A, Hafner H, Dutsch-Strobel A, Oster M, Stumbaum M, van Gulick-Bailer M, Loffler W (1994) Further evidence for a specific role of estradiol in schizophrenia? Biol Psychiatry 36: 492–494
24. Seeman MV (1986) Current outcome in schizophrenia: women vs men. Acta Psychiatr Scand 73: 609–617
25. Seeman MV, Lang M (1990) The role of estrogens in schizophrenia gender differences. Schizophr Bull 16: 185–194
26. Seeman MV (1996) The role of estrogen in schizophrenia. J Psychiatry Neurosci 21: 123–128
27. Sumner BE, Fink G (1998) Testosterone as well as estrogen increases serotonin 2A receptor mRNA and binding site densities in the male rat brain. Brain Res Mol Brain Res 59: 205–214

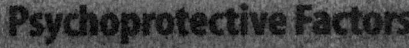

Psychoprotective Factors

Family interventions: empirical evidence of efficacy and open questions

S. Klingberg

Department of Psychiatry and Psychotherapy, University of Tübingen, Germany

▦ Introduction

The development of psychoeducational and behavioral family intervention was inspired by the research of Brown and of Vaughn & Leff [6, 7, 30]. They found a correlation between the so-called "high expressed emotion behavior" in families of schizophrenic patients and the relapse rate of patients after discharge from hospital. Consequently, intervention strategies were developed to address family communication. The underlying assumption of these interventions strategies is that improved communication in the family may lead to a reduced stress level in the patient and therefore helps prevent relapses.

In the meantime the efficacy of family interventions for relapse prevention has been investigated by a considerable number of studies. We will give a summary of the available evidence for the efficacy of family interventions. Today, the efficacy of psychoeducational and behavioral family intervention programs is well established.

However, there are many open questions. We will give an overview over the most import issues that should be addressed in the future. One of the most important issues in the future will be the identification of active ingredients. We do not know exactly how family interventions work in reducing relapse. Most recent studies challenge the assumption that the reduction of high-EE behavior is the most important factor. Therefore we do not know in detail, which components of the various family intervention programs are essential.

Nevertheless, the available evidence is sufficient to demand an improved implementation of family intervention in routine care. The questions of generalizability and implementation will be focused on in the final section of this paper.

▦ Content of family interventions

Gingerich & Bellack [4] described the following aspects as common for family intervention:
- ▦ The family is treated as an ally. This is a very important point and represents a shift in the perception of the relatives. Earlier theories on the causes of schizophrenia stated that the family (especially the mothers' behavior) plays

a crucial role in the pathogenesis of schizophrenia. These theories have not been proven to be valid. Nevertheless, they have resulted in a very distant relationship between therapists and relatives. Today it is important to emphasize that the family is the most important source of support for the patients in most cases.

▪ Treatment session are held on a regular basis ranging from weekly to monthly.
▪ Family treatment programs are long-term interventions, usually at least one year.
▪ Treatment teams are multi-disciplinary. Medication is followed closely. Psychosocial intervention is not designed to be an alternative to medication but to build upon the effects of stable medication. Treatment effects are conceptualized as additional. Today nearly all studies in the field of psychosocial intervention combine pharmacological treatment with psychosocial treatment.

There are different models of family intervention. One aspect of variation is the format of the intervention. Treatment is conducted with:
▪ Individual family units [13]
▪ Individual family plus relatives' groups [27]
▪ Relatives-only groups [20]
▪ Multiple family groups [23]
▪ Parallel patients and family groups [8]

The different formats imply partly different content of the intervention. One of the best-known approaches is the behavioral family intervention as described by Falloon et al. [13]. The format is a single-family intervention. It starts providing information about schizophrenia and treatment. In order to help prevent further relapses, the family is trained to detect and manage early signs of relapse. A training of communication and social problem solving in the family follows. Finally individual problems of the respective family are addressed.

▪ Efficacy of family intervention for relapse prevention: meta-analyses and reviews

Among the variety of psychosocial interventions behavioral and psychoeducational family interventions has been the most extensively researched modality. The available evidence was reviewed several times [19, 22]. Most recently two meta-analyses were published. We will focus in this paper on the results of these meta-analyses.

Pitschel-Walz et al. [25] stated that the "relapse rate can be reduced by 20 percent if relatives are included in the treatment". This statement is based on 25 intervention studies. Moreover, Pitschel-Walz et al. [25] concluded that family intervention has additional positive effects regarding family burden, knowledge about the illness, medication compliance, social adjustment and quality of life.

It should be kept in mind that such analyses combine effects deriving from different formats and types of family interventions as well as effects resulting from the comparison with different control groups. Another limitation is that the original studies usually report results about patients with relatives who are willing to participate and who are in contact with the patient.

Pharoah et al. [24] conducted the Cochrane Review applying meta-analytical methods. They state that family intervention may decrease the frequency of relapse. They report a significant odds ratio of 0.57 (CL 0.4–0.8) with respect to the relapse rate one year after inclusion. Two years after inclusion in the study the odds ratio was 0.52 (CL 0.3–0.8). As Pitschel-Walz et al. [25] they analyzed effects regarding other endpoints. However, Pharoah et al. [24] discussed effects on social adjustment and family outcomes more critically. The authors conclude that the evidence for these endpoints has to be improved.

The available evidence has also led to recommendations in treatment guidelines. The American Psychiatric Association recommended in the treatment guidelines for schizophrenia that the involvement of family members should be ongoing in the stabilization and stable phase [1]. This recommendation has been classified as grade I, indicating substantial clinical confidence.

The Task Force on "Empirically validated treatments" of the American Psychological Association [11] has chosen another approach. This task force has engaged in an on-going endeavor to review the psychological treatment literature in order to identify empirically supported treatments. The most important criterion is that there have to be at least two independent studies demonstrating superiority to a control group. The task force lists "family education programs for schizophrenia" as a well-established treatment. In the field of schizophrenia this is the only treatment in this level of evidence. The two studies that the task force refers to are Hogarty et al. [17] and Falloon et al. [13]. Thus, this evaluation of evidence is based on first-generation studies of family intervention.

In conclusion, it seems to be justified to state that the inclusion of families in the treatment helps improve the course of illness in the patients. However, in order to develop more efficacious treatments it is important to look into the available evidence in more detail.

Meta-analyses and reviews combine several studies that implemented different formats and types of family intervention. It has been investigated whether different approaches show different results. Pitschel-Walz et al. [25] included six studies directly comparing two types of family intervention and found that the more intensive treatments show better results. However, a clear indication for a superiority of a certain type or format did not emerge from these analyses. Pitschel-Walz et al. [25] concluded that different types of *comprehensive* family interventions have similar results. Barbato & D'Avanzo [2] state that it is still unclear to what extent interventions need to be structured according to a particular model.

One consistent finding, however, is that it seems to be necessary to include the patient in the family intervention. Studies on interventions in relatives alone without any psychosocial intervention offered to the patient did not show effect-sizes that are comparable to studies that include patients in the intervention.

In addition, the duration of a family intervention is of importance. There is some evidence that short-term interventions are less efficacious than long-term interventions. Studies evaluating interventions of less than 3-month duration did not find effect-sizes comparable with studies conducting interventions of 9–12 months. That is a conclusion shared by Pitschel-Walz et al. [25] and Barbato & D'Avanzo [2].

The results of studies on efficacy depend to a great extent on the kind of the selected control group. The so-called first generation family intervention studies compared family intervention to untreated controls receiving only a very basic treatment. Presumably this is the reason why this generation of studies showed the strongest effects. Family intervention studies of the last decade reported smaller effect-sizes. On the background of these findings, Dixon [12] concluded that family psychoeducation is likely to show added benefit in terms of relapse reduction in settings with basic, unenriched services. In contrast, enriched individual models or other innovative programs may be as effective as family psychoeducation.

Tarrier et al. [29] reported one of the most striking findings in the field. They found reduced relapses rates even 5 and 8 years after a family intervention. Their study examined the relapse rates of a high-EE family intervention group, a high-EE control condition and a low-EE control condition. It could be shown that the relapse rate of the high-EE intervention group was similar to the low-EE control group, whereas the high-EE control group had significantly more relapses. This result suggests that there is a durable change in the course of illness of persons with schizophrenia due to a comparably short family intervention. Replication of such findings would be very important.

▪ Active ingredients in family intervention

On the basis of meta-analyses, reviews and treatment recommendations the efficacy of family intervention can be qualified as well established.

On the other hand, the knowledge about active ingredients is very limited. Several variables are discussed in the literature as possibly responsible for the efficacy of family interventions. First of all, the reduction of high expressed emotion behavior is assumed to contribute to the effects of family treatment. Moreover, the communication skills of family members are hypothesized to be critical for the success of relapse prevention. The assumption is that improved communication skills might lead to reduced stress for the patient and therefore lead to a reduced risk of relapse. Intervention types that focus on psychoeducation refer to the improved knowledge about the illness and the treatment as the most important ingredient. In addition, burden of care and the resources of the relatives are discussed in the literature.

The research on expressed emotion could clearly establish a correlation between overprotective behavior and criticism on the one hand and the relapse rate on the other hand. This correlation has been shown to be significant in several studies [4, 10]. However, correlations do not say anything about causal relationships.

King [18] addressed this question by assessing expressed emotion in families with the Camberwell Family Interview (CFI) and symptoms of the patients (Brief Psychiatric Rating Scale, BPRS) three times in 18 months. A sophisticated statistical analysis, a path analysis or cross-lagged panel analysis, was conducted in order to investigate the direction of influence between the assessed variables. The result was that negative symptoms predict mothers' emotional overinvolvement and criticism, but no evidence was found that high-EE behavior resulted in symptoms of the patient. Schulze Mönking et al. [28] found similar results. They assessed the CFI at baseline and 20 months later. Patients living in families with high-EE rating at both assessments had more relapses than patients living in families with a maximum of one high-EE rating. As a consequence, the association between expressed emotion and course of illness has to be seen as complex and transactional.

Another consideration refers to the TSS (Treatment Strategies in Schizophrenia) study [27]. In addition to a comparison of three pharmacological treatment strategies this study compared two family intervention conditions. All families took part in psychoeducational workshops and regular multiple family meetings. The intervention type without further treatment was called supportive family treatment. The applied family intervention group took part in an additional communication and problem solving training. The TSS study found no difference between these two conditions. The additional communication and problem solving training did not lead to an additional effect in terms of relapse rates. These findings raised some questions about the relationship of familial communication skills and relapse.

Last year, Bellack et al. [5] published a more detailed analysis of the results of the TSS study concerning this issue. The question was whether applied family management is superior in improving familial communication when compared to supportive family management. The authors used videotaped problem solving tasks to assess familial communications skills. The main result was that there is no group difference between applied and supportive treatment with respect to communication skills. Families of both treatment conditions performed on similar skills levels. In addition, communication skills did not predict time to rehospitalization. These results indicate that familial communication skills were not related to the course of illness in this study.

As a consequence, central assumptions did not find support in most recent studies. High-expressed emotion behavior does not seem to cause symptoms. In addition, communication skills do not seem to be related to enhanced relapse rates. These findings contrasted to earlier results that family interventions were efficacious in reducing expressed emotion. Nevertheless, Pharoah et al. [24] found the evidence as equivocal in this respect. Of course, there is more research needed on this issue. However, a causal relationship between expressed emotion, familial communication and relapse is not supported by these results.

As the research on expressed emotions, the research on the burden of care focuses on the relatives. Nevertheless, relatives are perceived in this context as persons challenged to cope with the illness or their relatives. In the framework of a vulnerability-stress model of schizophrenia the distress of the relatives may be conceptualized as one of many stress factors on the side of the patient.

There are some important findings in this field. Magliano et al. [21] found that the burden of care decreases if the social functioning of the patients could be improved. In addition, an association between burden of care and symptoms could be found. In a study of Provencher & Mueser [26] negative symptom severity was related to objective burden of care. In contrast, positive and negative symptoms correlated with subjective burden. This finding stresses the importance of negative symptoms as perceived by the relatives. Moreover, a very interesting finding of Magliano et al. [21] indicates that intervention may help reduce the relatives' burden. They found that relatives whose coping abilities improved over the time perceived a reduced burden.

As in the research on expressed emotion, a serious limitation in this field is the lack of evidence for a causal relationship between relapse of patients and burden of care of the relatives. In particular, we do not know yet, whether the burden does only vary with the severity of symptoms or whether a reduction of the burden can contribute to the symptom reduction in the patient.

Another approach to the question of active ingredients is to simply ask the relatives what they find helpful in family intervention. Unfortunately, there are only small studies addressing this question. Budd & Hughes [9] asked 20 relatives what they found to be most helpful in family intervention. The relatives' answers included increased knowledge, the feeling of support, the availability of a contact person in case of crisis, the therapeutic alliance and finally an improvement of familial communication. Hence, problems with familial communications do not seem to be first priority.

Barrowclough et al. [3] identified the following factors as main problems of carers of schizophrenic patients: finding support with regard to relapse prevention, lack of information about the illness, negative emotions associated with the illness, psychotic symptoms and antisocial symptoms.

To sum up, the question of active ingredients is still unanswered. Most recent research challenges the assumption that an improvement of familial communication or the reduction of high-expressed emotion behavior in the family is the major active ingredient in family intervention. The relatives report a need for information and support to deal with exacerbations and persistent symptoms. In the field of psychotherapy research, the so-called common factors are well known. Many authors state that these factors are responsible for treatment effects to a great extent. Therefore, we do not know exactly how family intervention works, but it has to be kept in mind that we do know that family therapy is efficacious as mentioned before. More research is needed in this field.

■ Generalizability and implementation

Family intervention studies include only patients who have relatives that are willing to participate in the treatment. As a consequence, it has to be asked whether the generalizability of the results is restricted to this group. Hogarty et al. published a study on a psychosocial intervention program called personal therapy [16, 17]. They conducted two separate studies, one for patients living with their family and another for patients living independent of their family. One important finding of this study was that the effects of personal therapy were different in these two groups of patients. For patients with a family personal therapy contributed to a reduction of the relapse rate. On the other hand patients living alone showed higher relapse rates in the personal therapy group. Presumably the two groups of patients have different needs regarding psychosocial intervention. Such differences also have to be taken into account for the interpretation of studies on family intervention.

The problems of implementation will be the final focus of this paper. The available evidence for the efficacy of family intervention has not led to a wide spread implementation of this kind of treatment, at least in Germany. There are many obstacles including the following: family intervention as a long-term treatment needs an adequate organizational background. It needs time. Therapists need adequate training. Relatives fear being stigmatized if participating in family intervention. In addition, relatives are afraid that professionals misunderstand research on expressed emotion. They fear being held responsible for the disorder. Other relatives do not participate in intervention programs because of feelings of guilt. Moreover, patients suffering from persistent symptoms (e.g., suspiciousness) may not agree with the participation of their relatives.

As a consequence, only a subgroup of relatives takes part in family intervention programs in routine care, even if the treatment is available.

In Tübingen we are currently conducting a randomized clinical trial on a cognitive-behavioral intervention program. The treatment program is implemented in routine care. We make an effort to include all relatives in psychoeducational relatives-only groups. Up to now 63 patients were allocated to the treatment condition. Of these patients, 21 % do not have any relative. The relatives of 30 % of the patients refused to participate or had to be excluded. Relatives were excluded only if they do not have sufficient language skills or if patients refused to give their consent. In conclusion, only 49 % of the patients had relatives participating in the intervention.

These data are comparable with data of an effectiveness trial of Barrowclough et al. [3]. In this study 27 % of carers refused to participate in a family intervention program.

In conclusion, efforts have to be made to assure a maximum degree of generalizability. However, patients living with a family represent only a subgroup of schizophrenic patients. Regarding implementation, there are a variety of factors that prevent the relatives' participation. It remains the responsibility of the respective health care systems to provide optimal care for this group of severely ill patients.

■ Conclusions

It seems justified to state that the efficacy of family psychoeducation and behavioral family intervention is widely acknowledged. There are meta-analyses and reviews clearly indicating that family intervention is efficacious in reducing the relapse rate and therefore improving the course of the illness in schizophrenic patients. However, there are a lot of open questions with respect to the content and the format of the intervention. It seems to be necessary to include the patient in the intervention. The treatments duration should not be less than 9 months. When compared to alternative psychosocial intervention programs, no clear superiority could be found. However, the evidence for the efficacy is convincing, when family intervention is compared to routine care.

The knowledge about active ingredients in family intervention is limited. The hypothesis that improvement of familial communication is a major, active factor has been challenged by most recent findings. In this field much more research is necessary.

We have to be aware that studies on family intervention represent only patients living together with a family. The implementation of family intervention in routine care is restricted to this group. There is evidence that about 20 – 50 % of the patients cannot be included in family intervention programs because they do not have any relative or because their relatives are not willing to participate. For this group of patients other psychosocial interventions may be helpful.

■ References

1. American Psychiatric Association (1997) Practice Guideline for the Treatment of Patients with Schizophrenia. American Journal of Psychiatry 154 (Suppl): 1–63
2. Barbato A, D'Avanzo B (2000) Family interventions in schizophrenia and related disorders: a critical review of clinical trials. Acta Psychiatrica Scandinavica 102: 81–97
3. Barrowclough C, Tarrier N, Lewis S, Sellwood W, Mainwaring J, Quinn J et al. (1999) Randomised controlled effectiveness trial of a needs-based psychosocial intervention service for carers of people with schizophrenia. British Journal of Psychiatry 174: 505–511
4. Bebbington PE, Kuipers L (1994) The predictive utility of expressed emotion in schizophrenia: an aggregate analysis. Psychological Medicine 24: 707–718
5. Bellack AS, Haas GL, Schooler NR, Flory JD (2000) Effects of behavioural family management on family communication and patient outcomes in schizophrenia. British Journal of Psychiatry 177: 434–439
6. Brown GW, Birley JLT, Wing JK (1972) Influence of family life on the course of schizophrenic disorders: a replication. British Journal of Psychiatry 121: 241–258
7. Brown GW, Monck EM, Carstairs EM, Wing JK (1962) Influence of family life on the course of schizophrenic illness. Brit J Prev Soc Med 16: 55–68
8. Buchkremer G, Klingberg S, Holle R, Schulze Mönking H, Hornung WP (1997) Psychoeducational psychotherapy for schizophrenic patients and their key relatives or care-givers: results of a 2-year follow-up. Acta Psychiatrica Scandinavica 96: 483–491
9. Budd RJ, Hughes ICT (1997) What do relatives of people with schizophrenia find helpful about family intervention. Schizophrenia Bulletin 23: 341–347
10. Butzlaff RL, Hooley JM (1998) Expressed emotion and psychiatric relapse. A meta-analysis. Archives of General Psychiatry 55: 547–552
11. Chambless D, Baker M, Baucom DH, Beutler L, Calhoun KS, Crits-Christoph P et al. (1998) Update on empirically validated therapies, II. The Clinical Psychologist 51: 3–16
12. Dixon LB, Adams C, Lucksted A (2000) Update on Family Psychoeducation for Schizophrenia. Schizophrenia Bulletin 26: 5–20
13. Falloon IRH, Boyd JL, McGill CW, Williamson M, Razani J, Moss HB et al. (1985) Familiy management in the prevention of morbidity of schizophrenia. Clincal outcome of a two-year longitudinal study. Archives of General Psychiatry 42: 887–896

14. Gingerich SL, Bellack AS (1995) Research-based family interventions for the treatment of Schizophrenia. The Clinical Psychologist 48: 24–27
15. Hogarty GE, Anderson CM, Reiss DJ, Kornblith SJ, Greenwald DP, Javna CD et al. (1986) Family psychoeducation, social skills training, and maintenance chemotherapy in the aftercare treatment of schizophrenia. I. One-year effects of a controlled study on relapse and expressed emotion. Archives of General Psychiatry 43: 633–642
16. Hogarty GE, Greenwald D, Ulrich RF, Kornblith SJ, DiBarry AL, Cooley S et al. (1997a) Three-year trials of personal therapy among schizophrenic patients living with or independent of family, II: Effects on adjustment of patients. American Journal of Psychiatry 154: 1514–1524
17. Hogarty GE, Kornblith SJ, Greenwald D, DiBarry AL, Cooley S, Ulrich RF et al. (1997b) Three-year trials of personal therapy among schizophrenic patients living with or independent of family, I: Description of study and effects on relapse rates. American Journal of Psychiatry 154: 1504–1513
18. King S (2000) Is expressed emotion cause or effect in the mothers of schizophrenic young adults? Schizophrenia Research 45: 65–78
19. Lam DH (1991) Psychosocial family intervention in schizophrenia: a review of empirical studies. Psychological Medicine 21: 423–441
20. Leff J (1994) Working with the families of schizophrenic patients. British Journal of Psychiatry 164 (suppl 23): 71–76
21. Magliano L, Fadden G, Economou M, Held T, Xavier M, Guarneri M et al. (2000) Family burden and coping strategies in schizophrenia: 1-year follow-up data from the BIOMED I study. Social Psychiatry and Psychiatric Epidemiology 35: 109–115
22. Mari J, Streiner DL (1994) An overview of family interventions and relapse on schizophrenia: meta-analysis of research findings. Psychological Medicine 24: 565–578
23. McFarlane WR, Lukens E, Link B, Dushay R, Deakins SA, Newmark M et al. (1995) Multiple-family groups and psychoeducation in the treatment of schizophrenia. Archives of General Psychiatry 52: 679–687
24. Pharoah FM, Mari JJ, Streiner DL (2001) Family intervention for schizophrenia (Cochrane Review). In: Anonymous Cochrane Library. Oxford: Update Software
25. Pitschel-Walz G, Leucht S, Bäuml J, Kissling W, Engel R (2001) The effect of family interventions on relapse and rehospitalization in schizophrenia – a meta-analysis. Schizophrenia Bulletin 27: 73–92
26. Provencher HL, Mueser KT (1997) Positive and negative symptom behaviors and caregiver burden in the relatives of persons with schizophrenia. Schizophrenia Research 26: 71–80
27. Schooler NR, Keith SJ, Severe JB, Matthews SM, Bellack AS, Glick ID et al. (1997) Relapse and rehospitalization during maintenance treatment of schizophrenia. The effects of dose reduction and family treatment. Archives of General Psychiatry 54: 453–463
28. Schulze Mönking H, Hornung WP, Stricker K, Buchkremer G (1997) Expressed-emotion development and course of schizophrenic illness: considerations based on results of a CFI replication. European Archives of Psychiatry and Clinical Neurosciences 247: 31–34
29. Tarrier N, Barrowclough C, Porceddu K, Fitzpatrick E (1994) The Salford family intervention project: relapse rates of schizophrenia at five and eight years. British Journal of Psychiatry 165: 829–832
30. Vaughn CE, Leff JP (1976) The influence of family and social factors on the course of psychiatric illness: a comparison of schizophrenic and depressed neurotic patients. British Journal of Psychiatry 129: 125–137

Cognitive-behavior therapy in the treatment of schizophrenia

N. TARRIER
Academic Division of Clinical Psychology, School of Psychiatry and Behavioral Sciences, University of Manchester, Wythenshawe Hospital, Manchester, UK

Cognitive-behavior therapy (CBT) was originally developed for the treatment of patients suffering non-psychotic disorders, such as those suffering depression and anxiety disorders [8] but it has recently been used in the treatment of schizophrenic patients both in the acute and chronic phases of the disorder. A review of the literature on the use of psychological treatments for psychosis has recently demonstrated that not all psychological approaches are relevant for people with schizophrenia, though psychotherapies using a cognitive-behavioural approach have shown particular promise [6, 9]. In the CBT approach the individual patient, working collaboratively with a therapist, acquires a range of practical techniques for the better control of their psychotic symptoms. In most studies that have investigated CBT, it has been used as an adjunct to antipsychotic medication. The fact that CBT appears successful in decreasing psychotic symptoms has challenged the conventional psychiatric thinking that psychotic symptoms are not amenable to non-drug therapies. Furthermore, there is evidence that schizophrenic patients can learn to cope with their psychotic experience and to some extent bring their symptoms under voluntary control. There have recently been two meta-analyses of CBT in the treatment of schizophrenia which have indicated moderate to good effect sizes reported from the published studies [4, 13]. The research on evaluation of CBT in the treatment will now be briefly described. The major studies are presented in summary form in Table 1.

In the initial studies, the primary aim of CBT was to reduce medication-resistant positive symptoms in chronic patients. Other aims for CBT were the reduction of negative and affective symptoms, and especially the high levels of distress that resulted from the experience of hallucinations and delusions. More recently CBT has been used with acutely ill patients with the aim to promote faster recovery from the acute episode and buffer against subsequent relapse.

CBT in chronic schizophrenia

Randomised controlled trials (RCTs) are the gold standard by which to evaluate therapeutic interventions. Although case studies and small trials can provide useful information it is the larger methodologically rigorous RCTs that provide the substantial evidence for the efficacy of a therapy. In the UK, three major trials comparing CBT with routine care and/or another form of psychological therapy

Table 1. Randomised controlled trials of CBT with schizophrenia

Study	Treatment condition	Patients	N	Frequency and duration of treatment	Follow-up assessments	Results
Tarrier et al. (1993)	1. CBT + RC 2. S + RC 3. 50% wait list control	Chronic schizophrenic, persistent symptoms	27	10 sessions 2 per week for 5 weeks	Post-treatment 6 months FU	CBT and PS showed significant improvements in positive symptoms compared to wait list
Haddock et al. (1998a)	1. Distraction 2. Focussing	Chronic schizophrenic, persistent auditory hallucinations	33	18–20 sessions weekly treatment of hallucinations only	Post-treatment 24 months FU	Both groups showed a reduction in hallucinations at post-treatment, which was not maintained at FU
London–East Anglia Study, Kuipers et al. (1997), Kuipers et al. (1998)	1. CBT + RC 2. RC	Chronic schizophrenic, persistent symptoms	60 initially 47 at FU	Mean 19 sessions (0–50) over 9 months, initially weekly then fortnightly	Post-treatment 9 months FU	CBT significantly improved on the BPRS rating score, maintained at FU
Manchester Study, Tarrier et a.l (1998a) Tarrier et al. (1999a) Tarrier et al. (2000) Tarrier et a.l (2001)	1. CBT + RC 2. SC + RC 3. RC	Chronic schizophrenic, persistent symptoms	87 initially 70 at 12 months 61 at 24 months	20 sessions over 3 months 2 per week plus 4 monthly boosters	Post-treatment 12 month and 24 month FU	CBT significantly improved on positive and negative symptoms compared to RC and in hallucination compared to SC. At 12 and 18 months FU, CBT and SC significantly improved compared to RC
Sensky et al. (2000)	1. CBT + RC 2. Befriending	Chronic schizophrenic, persistent symptoms	90 at post-treatment and FU	Flexible mean 19 sessions, (2–33) over 9 months	Post-treatment 9 months FU	Improvements in both groups at post-treatment but no group differences at FU. CBT significantly improved compared to befriending

Cont. Table 1.

Study	Treatment condition	Patients	N	Frequency and duration of treatment	Follow-up assessments	Results
Barrowclough et al. (2001)	1. CBT + FI + MI + family support + RC 3. RC + family support	Dual diagnosis (schizophrenia + substance abuse) with close family contact	36	MI – 5 sessions CBT – 24 sessions weekly then fortnightly FI – 10–16 sessions	Post-treatment 12 months FU	Significant improvement in positive symptoms and functioning, reduced relapse and decreased substance abuse in CBT and FI group
Drury et al. (1996a) Drury et al. (1996b)	1. CBT (individual + group + family engagement) + RC 2. Semi-structured recreation and support activities + TAU	Acutely ill hospitalised schizophrenic	40	Flexible 8 hours per week for a maximum of 6 months	Post-treatment 3 months FU	Greater and faster (25–50 %) reduction in symptoms in the CBT group
Haddock et al. (1999)	1. CBT + RC 2. SC + RC	Acutely ill hospitalised schizophrenic with illness detection <5 years	21	Flexible mean 10 sessions over 5 weeks pass-admission + 4 monthly boosters	Post-treatment 24 months FU	Improvement in both groups on group differences at post-treatment, not significantly fewer releases in CBT over FU
SoCRATES Study, Lewis et al. (2001)	1. CBT + RC 2. SC + RC 3. RC	Acutely ill recent onset (80 % first episode, 20 % second episode) hospitalised schizophrenic	309	Flexible up to 20 hours over 5 weeks post-admission, mean = 16 sessions mean duration of session = 40 minutes + 4 booster sessions	Post-treatment 18 months FU	CBT shows significantly faster improvement compared to other groups

BPRS Brief Psychiatric Rating Scale, *CBT* Cognitive behavior therapy, *FI* Family intervention, *FU* Follow-up (follow-up assessments are dated from the post-treatment assessment) *MI* Motivational interviewing, *PS* Problem solving, *SC* Supportive counselling, *RC* Routine Care have been reported: the Manchester trial [19–21], the London and East Anglia trial [10, 11] and the London-Newcastle trial [17]. These trials are sufficiently rigorous in their methodology to provide reliable information concerning the efficacy of CBT in reducing positive symptoms in chronic schizophrenia. All of these trials showed that CBT can be useful as an adjunct in the management of patients with chronic schizophrenia. Immediately after treatment, CBT plus treatment as usual (TAU) was found to be superior to TAU alone in terms of positive symptoms [10, 19], and CBT was superior to supportive care, with regard to hallucinations [20]. At the 9-12 month follow-up, TAU alone was inferior to CBT [11] or supportive counselling [20]. At the 24-month follow-up, TAU was found inferior to both CBT and supportive counselling in terms of positive and negative symptoms and relapse rate [21]. When hallucinations were examined separately patients who received supportive counselling did significantly worse than those who received CBT [22]. In the Newcastle-London study, CBT and befriending (a treatment similar to supportive counselling) produced equivalent, statistically significantly reductions in symptoms immediately after treatment [17]. However, the benefits of CBT were still maintained at the 9-month follow-up, whereas those of befriending were not. There is a different pattern of results between the Manchester and London-Newcastle trials. Both these trials included an active psychotherapy control group, termed supportive counselling in the Manchester trial and befriending in the London-Newcastle trial. In the Manchester trial there is a convergence over time with the difference between CBT and supportive counselling that was present at post-treatment decreasing over the 12 and 24 month follow-up periods. In the London-Newcastle trial, however, there was no difference between CBT and befriending at post-treatment but subsequently there was divergence between these two groups over the follow-up period, in contrast to the convergence reported by Tarrier et al. [21].

■ CBT in acute/recent-onset schizophrenia

CBT has largely been investigated in patients with chronic schizophrenia; though recently, researchers have been investigating CBT in patients with recent-onset and acute psychosis. An increasing body of evidence indicates that the advances made in chronic psychosis can also be applied to acutely ill and recent-onset patients. There have been three main trials in this area. The Birmingham trial compared CBT plus TAU with various recreation and support activities plus TAU in acutely ill hospitalised schizophrenic patients, and found much greater and faster reduction in symptoms in the CBT group [2, 3]. This was a very innovative study in which the magnitude of difference between the two groups was very large. However, in this study the intervention included both individual and group therapy, and a brief psycho-educational intervention with families. There were also some methodological weaknesses with this study. The Manchester pilot trial was designed with two aims in mind. Firstly to see whether treating acutely ill schizophrenic patients with CBT was feasible. Secondly to investigate whether the results reported by Drury and colleagues could be replicated if methodological rigor of the study was improved. This pilot study compared CBT plus TAU with supportive counselling plus TAU; both CBT and supportive counselling improved the symptoms of schizophrenia. At the two year follow-up although the trend was in the predicted direction differences were not significant [7]. This suggested that at least in terms of the magnitude of the treatment effect the results of Drury et al. could be due to bias resulting from poor methodology. To further investigate the efficacy of CBT in acutely ill patients the SOCRATES trial was designed. This was a large multi-centre trial designed to compare CBT plus TAU, with supportive counselling plus TAU and also with TAU alone. Patients were restricted to those experiencing a first episode or a second episode within two years. Treatment was initiated as quickly as possible after admission to an in-patient unit or in a few cases to a day hospital. The trial was analysed over two phases, the acute phase in which symptom improvement over the first 50 days after admission was analysed and the follow-up phase over the subsequent 18 month period. During the acute phase all patients showed a significant improvement in their psychotic symptoms, with a trend of patients in the CBT group showing a faster improvement in symptoms that those in the other groups [12]. When hallucinations were examined separately, patients who received supportive counselling did worse than those who received CBT. This difference was a trend that approached significance. Over the 18 month follow-up period there were no differences in relapses between the three groups, with relapse rates at about just over 50%. However, in terms of symptoms measured at 18 months the patients who received TAU alone had significantly more symptoms than the other two groups. There was also a trend towards significance in which the group who received supportive counselling did significantly worse on hallucinations compared to the CBT group [23].

※ Treatment of dual-diagnosis patients

There is significant comorbidity of schizophrenia and substance abuse [13, 15], and can occur in 30% to 70% of schizophrenic patients. Substance abuse appears to be an indicator of a range of poor outcomes in schizophrenia including self-harm, violence, medication non-compliance and relapse, and re-admission. The only controlled trial of psychological therapy to date in these dual-diagnosis patients investigated the efficacy of CBT and family intervention, and motivational interviewing plus family support, compared with that to TAU plus family support [1]. The experimental treatment consisting of CBT, family intervention and motivational interviewing led to significant improvements in positive symptoms and functioning, fewer relapses and less substance abuse.

Mechanism of action

What is it that makes CBT effective in treating psychotic symptoms? This is very difficult to answer. Most of the trials carried out have been pragmatic trials and there has been little attempt to understand underlying mechanisms [23]. Fur-

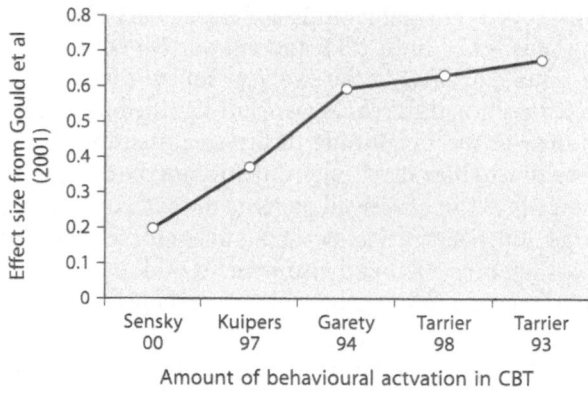

Fig. 1. How much "B" in CBT for psychosis.

thermore, although the CBT approaches of different research groups share many common aspects there are also differences, for example in the emphasis of cognitive or behavioural intervention. To investigate whether this factor was influential in outcome Tarrier & Wykes [23] used the effect sizes of various studies published in Gould et al. [4] and classified these studies in terms of how cognitive or behavioural they were. Studies were ordered along this cognitive-behavioral dimension so as to ascertain whether the effect sizes were related to this order. The relationship between effect sizes and the cognitive-behavioral dimension are presented in Fig. 1. The relationship between cognitive or behavioural elements in the intervention was significantly related to effect size (r = .87) in favour of the more behavioural interventions.

⬛ Conclusion

CBT can be an effect adjunct treatment when used in combination with anti-psychotic medication and optimal psychiatric services. CBT can be used with both chronic and acutely ill patient and with those suffering from co-morbid substance abuse.

⬛ References

1. Barrowclough C, Haddock G, Tarrier N et al. (2000) Randomised controlled trial of motivational interviewing and cognitive behavioural intervention for schizophrenia patients with associated drug or alcohol misuse. American Journal of Psychiatry 158: 1706–1713
2. Drury V, Birchwood M, Cochrane R et al. (1996a) Cognitive therapy and recovery from acute psychosis: a controlled trial I. Impact on psychotic symptoms. Br J Psychiatry 169: 593–601
3. Drury V, Birchwood M, Cochrane R et al. (1996b) Cognitive therapy and recovery from acute psychosis: a controlled trial II. Impact on recovery time. Br J Psychiatry 169: 602–607
4. Gould RA, Robert A, Mueser KT, Bolton E, Mays V, Goff D (2001) Cognitive therapy for psychosis in schizophrenia: an effect size analysis. Schizophrenia Research 48: 335–342
5. Haddock G, Morrison AP, Hopkis R et al. (1998) Individual cognitive-behavioural interventions in early psychosis. Br J Psychiatry 172 (suppl): 101–106

6. Haddock G, Tarrier N, Spaulding W et al. (1998) Individual cognitive-behavioural therapy in the treatment of hallucinations and delusions: a review. Clin Psychol Rev 18: 821–838
7. Haddock G, Tarrier N, Morrison AP et al. (1999) A pilot study evaluating the effectiveness of individual inpatient cognitive-behavioural therapy in early psychosis. Soc Psychiatry Psychiatr Epidemiol 34: 254–258
8. Hawton K, Salkovskis P, Clark DM, Kirk J (1989) Cognitive behaviour therapy for psychiatric problems: a practical guide. Oxford University Press, Oxford
9. Jackson H, McGorry P, Edwards J et al. (1998) Cognitively-oriented psychotherapy for early psychosis (COPE). Preliminary results. Br J Psychiatry 172 (suppl 33): 93–100
10. Kuipers E, Garety P, Fowler D et al. (1997) London-East Anglia randomised controlled trial of cognitive-behavioural therapy for psychosis, I: effects of the treatment phase. Br J Psychiatry 171: 319–327
11. Kuipers E, Fowler D, Garety P et al. (1998) London-East Anglia randomised controlled trial of cognitive-behavioural therapy for psychosis, III: Follow-up and economic evaluation at 18 months. Br J Psychiatry 173: 61–68
12. Lewis SW, Tarrier N, Haddock G et al. (2002) A randomised controlled trial of cognitive behaviour therapy in early schizophrenia: acute phase outcomes in the SOCRATES trial. British Journal of Psychiatry (in press)
13. Pristach CA, Smith CM (1990) Medication compliance and substance abuse among schizophrenic patients. Hosp Community Psychiatry 41: 1345–1348
14. Rector NA, Beck AT (2001) Cognitive behavioral therapy for schizophrenia: an empirical review. Journal of Nervous and Mental Disease 189: 278–287
15. Salloum IM, Moss HB, Daley DC (1991) Substance abuse and schizophrenia: impediments to optimal care. Am J Drug Alcohol Abuse 17: 321–336
16. Soni SD, Brownlee M (1991) Alcohol abuse in chronic schizophrenics: implications for management in the community. Acta Psychiatr Scand 84: 272–276
17. Sensky T, Turkington D, Kingdon D et al. (2000) A randomised controlled trial of cognitive-behavioural therapy for persistent symptoms in schizophreniea resistant to medication. Arch Gen Psychiatry 57: 165–172
18. Tarrier N, Beckett R, Harwood S et al. (1993) A trial of two cognitive-behavioural methods of treating drug resistant residual psychotic symptoms in schizophrenia patients: 1. Outcome. Br J Psychiatry 162: 524–532
19. Tarrier N, Yusopoff L, Kinney C et al. (1998) Randomised controlled trial of intensive cognitive behaviour therapy in patients with schizophrenia. Br Med J 317: 303–307
20. Tarrier N, Wittkowski A, Kinney C et al. (1999) The durability of the effects of cognitive behaviour therapy and supportive counselling in the treatment of chronic schizophrenia: twelve months follow-up. Br J Psychiatr 174: 500–504
21. Tarrier N, Kinney C, McCarthy E et al. (2000) Two year follow-up of cognitive behaviour therapy and supportive counselling in the treatment of persistent positive symptoms in chronic schizophrenia. J Consult Clin Psychol 68: 917–922
22. Tarrier N, Kinney C, McCarthy E et al. (2001) Are some types of psychotic symptoms more responsive to CBT? Behav Cogn Psychother 29: 45–55
23. Tarrier N, Wykes T (2002) Cognitive-behavioural treatments of psychosis: clinical trials and methodological issues in clinical psychology. In: Day S, Green S, Machin D (eds) Textbook of clinical trials. Wiley, Chichester (in press)

Coping and social support as protective factors

K. Maurer, H. Häfner
Schizophrenia Research Unit, Central Institute of Mental Health, Mannheim, Germany

■ Introduction

Research in early detection of schizophrenia is usually concerned with specific risk factors, which are the basis for the evaluation of the actual risk of psychotic transitions in people in an 'at risk mental state'. Research in factors protecting against the risk of developing psychosis is somewhat neglected, although the focus on protective factors allows a more positive view compared to the exclusive view on risk factors. In fact, one can always assume a set of risk and of protective factors acting simultaneously, and the more and especially important protectors are, the more they are able to balance risk factors and to reduce the probability of a psychotic transition. It is possible to distinguish biological and social risk factors, or protective factors. Many risk factors are of a biological nature, like familial load, obstetric and birth complications, delayed and disturbed developmental processes during early childhood, but also some are protective like estrogen in women. There are also social risks like stressful life events, and social protective factors like adequate coping strategies for mental problems, or stable relationships with family members, partners or friends. The following analysis is based on the working hypothesis that social factors like coping, social network and social support are protective factors, reducing the risk of onset, and having some positive impact on the further development and course of schizophrenia.

Coping strategies are not only dependent on the personality, attitudes and abilities of a patient, but also from the people who constitute his/her social network [21]. There is a close interrelationship between coping abilities and social network conditions. The way a patient copes with the (beginning) psychosis is determined by his/her individual resources and by the social support he/she receives and by the social network functioning as a buffer against stress. Hultman et al. [11], who studied general coping style and social support as protecting psycho-social factors, suggest a buffering effect of social factors, as the time between some burdening life event and relapse was extended in patients with close relationships and active support seeking coping strategies. Buchanan [4] presented an interactive model with social support as a protective factor that facilitates coping and social competence. As Salokangas [18, 19] demonstrated in a 5 year prospective study, patients living with a spouse or partner had superior values on different course indicators (like neuroleptic dosage, days in hospital) compared to patients living with their parents or living alone. Therefore, the clinical and functional outcome is influenced also by the living situation and the social network. In a qualitative analysis, McNally & Goldberg [17] studied natural cognitive strategies in 10 drug-resistant patients. They identified 55 coping strategies and as a major category a cognitive strategy which they called 'self talk', which itself was composed of nine lower-level categories, used by schizophrenic patients to manage their psychotic symptoms. Lalonde et al. [13] identified four main problem areas schizophrenic patients are confronted with – symptoms, coping strategies, organization of daily activities and interpersonal contacts – and two basic coping strategies: confrontation and emotional coping.

Especially for patients with treatment resistant positive symptoms, mainly with auditory hallucinations, cognitive behavior therapy (CBT) was applied as a technique to learn how to cope with these symptoms [12, 14, 26, 27, etc.]. Braun-Scharm [3] reports for the initial phase that adolescents with schizophrenia developed considerably fewer active coping strategies compared to adolescents with some other disorder. Especially for positive symptoms active coping is least prominent. Boschi et al. [2] also analyzed coping with positive symptoms after the first hospitalization and the relation to psychosocial functioning. Most frequently cognitive strategies were applied, while the most helpful strategies were behavioral, as the patients who described the use of active coping strategies as most helpful demonstrated better psychosocial functioning at the 2 year follow-up. Sayer et al. [20] studied the relationship of coping with positive symptoms and attributional styles. There were clear correlations of a resistive coping style and the attribution of malevolence to voices on the one hand and an emerging coping style and benevolent attribution on the other. In a recent study by Andrews et al. [1] the effects of a coping-oriented group therapy for schizophrenic and schizoaffective patients was compared to a supportive group therapy. The best predictor of the one year outcome was an active and problem-focused coping strategy. As in the ABC study, coping and social network/support were assessed at the time of first admission; it seemed to be worthwhile to present some descriptive data and to show how these protective factors are related to several indicators of the early course.

■ Sample and assessment instruments

The statistical analysis is based on the first episode sample of the Mannheim ABC Schizophrenia Study. This sample has been described in detail in several publications [7, 8, 15]: it consists in 232 first illness episodes admitted with an ICD-9 diagnosis 295, 296, 297.3 and .4, and an inclusion age between 12 and 59 years. A total of 108 (46.6%) of the sample are men; 124 (53.4%) are women. The mean age at first admission is 28.2 years for men and 32.2 years for women (p < 0.001). To assess social development, pathways to care, the development of symptoms and signs of a beginning mental disorder, the "Interview for the Retrospective Assessment of the Onset of Schizophrenia" (IRAOS, [5, 6, 10]) was used, which was applied retrospectively during the first hospital stay. First admission dates back to the years 1987 to 1989. Meanwhile, a 12 year follow-up of the ABC sample has been completed.

Social network and social support were assessed by use of a revised version of the "Mannheimer Interview zur Sozialen Unterstützung (MISU)" [25], which is subdivided in three parts: the first for structural variables, the second for interaction variables and the assessment of the quality of social interactions. In the third part functional variables are assessed, which means the availability of help in critical situations. Further details of the MISU follow in the Results below.

The "Interview zur Krankheitsbewältigung (IKB)" [22, 24] was used to assess coping with the disease. Due to the limited interview time in the ABC study, only three of a total of eleven subsections were applied [16, 23]. In the first section coping with positive symptoms (thought disorders, hallucinations, delusions) is assessed, in the next one coping with non-specific symptoms (non-specific, depressive and negative symptoms) here called 'subjective complaints'. Finally, questions about everyday situations – which may lead to irritability and worsening of symptoms – are presented in the last section. More details about the IKB are presented in the Results below.

■ Results

The Results are subdivided in three sections. Part I describes social network and social support at the time of first hospitalization. Part II is concerned with disease-related coping behavior at the same point in time, and part III describes the relationship of measures of the early course (like duration of the prodrome and the duration of the psychotic pre-phase, symptom accumulation during the early course, age at symptom onset) and global measures of social support and coping strategies. The analyses were conducted by SPSS version 10 for PC.

Social support and social network at the time of first admission (part I)

The MISU is subdivided in three parts: the first one considers structural variables, the second variables on interaction and the quality of close relationships, the third considers functional variables, which relate on the availability of help in specified hypothetical situations. In the following sections, the results from the three MISU subsections are presented.

Structural variables: network density. Structural variables relate to the number of people who constitute the patient's social network. For eight patients of the ABC first-episode sample, the MISU interview could not be conducted. Therefore the sample size for the analysis of social support/network variables is reduced to 224 patients. The maximum number of people, defining network density is 32 for one patient. As a minimum one patient mentioned only one other person defining his social network. The mean number of persons constituting the overall social network is 12.8, and 50% of the patients mentioned at least 12 people.

The overall social network is subdivided into specific sub-nets concerning the family, friends and acquaintances, neighbors, clubs, groups and organizations, colleagues at work, school or studies, and finally people who offer professional assistance like doctors, therapists, but also lawyers or clergymen. Of the patients, 35.7% had a partner, and more than half of the patients had contacts to at least 3 (mean: 3.21) core family members (parents, siblings, children). The maximum number of core family persons was ten, but ten (4.3%) patients had no contact to the core family, and in relation to the whole family (including the core family), 6 (2.6%) patients had no contacts to any family member. The maximum number of family members is 15, the mean is 5.37, and the median is 5.

Two further important aspects in relation to the density of the social network are contacts outside the family, like contacts with friends, colleagues and neighbors, but also contacts with people who offer professional help (like doctors, therapists, priests, lawyers, etc.), and others who fulfill some important function for the patient. Fifteen patients (6.5% of the sample) had no friends and another 20 (8.6%) only one close friend or colleague. A mean number of 6.10 friends (median: 5) were mentioned, and the maximum was 21. In relation to people who offer professional help, more then 50% of the sample did not mention anybody (mean: 0.93). A total of 61 (27.2%) patients named exactly one person, 44 (19.6%)

Table 1. Index for the evaluation of an intact social network

Familial social network			Non-familial social network			Total social network		
	n	%		n	%	N	%	N	%
						0		5	2.2
1	15	6.7	1	50	22.3	1		40	17.9
2	137	61.2	2	87	38.8	2		69	30.8
3	72	32.1	3	87	38.8	3		76	33.9
						4		34	15.2
total	224	100.0	total	224	100.0	total		224	100.0

Familial network:
1 = not sufficient: no partner & (core family < 2 or total family < 4)
2 = sufficient: (partner & (core family < 2 or total family < 4)) or (no partner & (core family ≥ 2 or total family ≥ 4))
3 = highly sufficient: (partner & (core family ≥ 2 or total family ≥ 4))
Non-familial network:
1 = not sufficient: ≤ 2 friends
2 = sufficient: ≥ 3 friends and no professional help
3 = highly sufficient: ≥ 3 friends and professional help
Total social network:
0 = family = 1 & friends = 1
1 = (family = 2 & friends = 1) or (family = 1 & friends = 2)
2 = (family = 2 & friends = 2) or (family = 3 & friends = 1) or (family = 1 & friends = 3)
3 = (family = 2 & friends = 3) or (family = 3 & friends = 2)
4 = family = 3 & friends = 3

between 2 and 5 persons, and only 4 (1.8%) patients more than five (maximum: 9) persons offering professional help.

Which relationships and connections must be present as a minimum to allow the assumption of a sufficiently established social network? What are the conditions to define such a network as moderately good? When are obvious weaknesses in the network and, finally, when must it be considered insufficient? An index, based on the evaluation of familial relationships and relationships outside the family, is suggested. First, for the family network three conditions (excellent, intermediate, poor) were defined, as well as for non-familial relations (Table 1). Then, both indices are combined into one overall index of completeness of the social network which differentiates five levels: 4 = both conditions excellent; 3 = one condition excellent, the other one intermediate; 2 = both conditions intermediate or one excellent, the other one poor; 1 = one condition intermediate, the other one poor, and finally 0: both conditions poor. If a patient had a partnership and a sufficient number of familial relationships, and additionally several friends and at least one professional help offering contact, this was taken as a most sufficient and established social network. On the other extreme, if there was no partner, and no or only one member of the core family or a maximum of 3 family members in total, combined with a maximum of one friend only and missing professional assistance, this indicated a mostly insufficient social network. In 72 (32.1%) of the patients, the family network was excellent, and in most cases (n = 137; 61.2%) it was sufficient. Only in a small group of 15 (6.7%) patients was the familial network very poor. Concerning the network outside the family, it seems to be excellent in 87 (38.8%) of the patients and for the same number of cases (n = 87; 38.8%) at least acceptable. There remains a subgroup of 50 (22.3%) patients without an adequate network outside the family.

Combining both sub-networks – inside and outside the family – 110 (49.1%) patients had an at least sufficiently good social network, and 114 (50.8%) a restricted or insufficient one.

Interaction and quality of interaction with key persons. The patients were asked to name the five most important people, who are especially important and close to them, whom they prefer to talk with and whose company they like mostly. Only 84 (36.2%) patients were able to name 5 people with those characteristics, but 94.4% (n = 219) of the patients mentioned at least one close person. Most often, important key persons are either the partners or somebody belonging to the core family. Friends also play an important role, whereas colleagues, neighbors, teachers, doctors and other professional authorities, at this early time do not play a significant role.

The mean age of the key persons in the most important position was 41.4 years, and age was reduced over the 5 positions reaching a mean age of 34.9 years at position 5. This is due to the growing importance of siblings and especially of friends on these lower ranks. The duration of the relationship is on average 19.1 years for position 1, and declines over the positions to an mean duration of 14.9 years for position 5. Overall, the mean age of these most important persons as well as the long duration of the relationships show that patients have trustful, long-lasting and stable relations mostly, with some older and life-experienced person.

Concerning the availability of key persons, 44.2 % of the most important persons are living in the same household, and about 1/3 of the second and 1/4 of the third key persons. There are enough possibilities for frequent contacts: for the first three key persons, either daily or at least weekly contacts are usual for more than 70 % of the patients. 75 % of the most important key persons and between 63 % (for the second important person) and 54 % (for the fifth important person) are emotionally available at any time, and they most often are also living in the same town or village, and to a high percentage in the same house or flat or in the neighborhood of the patient.

Functional variables for help seeking situations. In the MISU, functional variables relate to hypothetical situations arranged in a 4-fold scheme: there are two aspects in relation to the sort of help (instrumental vs. psychological) and another two concerning the type of the situation (everyday vs. crisis). If the situation relates to instrumental help, it is further differentiated into real practical assistance or into supply of relevant information. If it relates to psychic help, emotional assistance versus active help in the stabilization of the self-esteem are considered.

For all these situations (Table 2), more than 50 % of the patients named at least two people, who will offer some help or assistance. For the first two situations – where some instrumental help in everyday situations is sought – even an average of 4 and 3 people are named. The percentage of patients who indicate that no help is possible is between 5 % and 10 % for five situations and above 10 % (with the maximum of 13 %) in 4 situations.

Finally, an indicator of good, intermediate and poor help resources was determined. About half of the sample (52.5 %) had very good resources, as they mentioned at least one person they could ask for help in 9 or 10 of the everyday and crisis situations. Another 28.4 % knew somebody to ask for help in at least half of the situations, and only 11 (5.0 %) of the patients could ask for help in less than half of the situations. There was only one patient in the sample, who answered for each of the ten questions, that there is nobody he could ask for help.

Finally, the patients were asked, if the five most important key persons offer help in specific situations. The most important person offers help in 52 % (C1: financial problems) up to 73 % (B2: advice in everyday situations). Those percentages are reduced gradually over the five different key persons for every of the ten situations, reaching percentages between 20.5 % (C1) and 55.4 % (B1: ask for some favor) for the fifth person mentioned.

MISU variables as dependent variables. In part III the relationship of indicators of the early course and variables of social support and coping is reported. For this analysis, the MISU offers some global measures, like structural variables on network density (the overall number of people defining the network, the number of family members, the number of friends, the number of persons representing help agencies). But to use also some data on the quality of the social network and its

Table 2. Functional variables: 10 difficult situations and numbers of people in the social network who will be asked for help

Situations	Everyday situation/ crisis situation	Instrumental/ psychic	If instrumental: practical/ Information	If psychic: emotional/ active	Min/ Max	Mean/ (Std. Dev.)	Median	Patient wants more possibilities n (%)	No help at all n (%)
B1	Everyday	Instrumental	Practical	–	0 / 22	5.0 (4.6)	4	40 (18.5)	6 (2.8)
B2	Everyday	Instrumental	Information	–	0 / 25	4.6 (5.2)	3	23 (20.5)	9 (7.9)
B3	Everyday	Psychic	–	Emotional	0 / 24	3.4 (4.0)	2	39 (19.3)	25 (12.1)
C1	Crisis	Instrumental	Practical	–	0 / 15	2.2 (2.1)	2	50 (23.9)	28 (13.0)
C2	Crisis	Instrumental	Practical	–	0 / 15	2.7 (2.2)	2	46 (21.4)	11 (5.0)
C3	Crisis	Instrumental	Information	–	0 / 22	2.4 (2.4)	2	48 (22.2)	18 (8.3)
C4	Crisis	Psychic	–	Emotional	0 / 22	2.7 (2.8)	2	54 (25.7)	17 (8.0)
D1	Crisis	Psychic	–	Emotional	0 / 17	3.2 (3.1)	2	57 (27.4)	14 (6.6)
D2	Crisis	Psychic	–	Emotional	0 / 24	2.6 (2.7)	2	53 (25.5)	25 (11.7)
D3	Crisis	Psychic	–	Active	0 / 14	2.5 (2.1)	2	68 (32.9)	26 (12.1)

Situation B1 Whom could you ask for some favor (like help in preparing a party, help when moving etc.).

Situation B2 Whom could you ask for advice in everyday problems and decisions (where to spent holidays, which new furniture to buy).

Situation B3 Where to get advice in everyday problems (what to dress; which present to buy for a friend).

Situation C1 Financial problems.

Situation C2 Severely ill.

Situation C3 Severe loss (of home, work, financial resources).

Situation C4 Severe decision with long lasting consequences (change of work, to become highly indebted).

Situation D1 Loss of a close friend or a family member.

Situation D2 Severe personal failure.

Situation D3 Desperate mood, down, discouraged; who helps to regain self-confidence?

ability to offer help in difficult situations, the variables introduced to define the degree of completeness of the network as well as the number of critical situations in which the patients have some person offering help also are used as dependent variables.

Coping strategies at the time of first admission (part II)

The "Interview zur Krankheitsbewältigung" (IKB, [22]) was used to assess coping with the disease. The presentation of the results follows the three sections remaining in the shortened interview version: first, coping with psychotic symptoms; second, coping with non-psychotic symptoms (here called 'subjective complaints'); and, finally, coping with everyday situations, which might increase the relapse risk or the risk for disease aggravation in vulnerable people.

Coping with positive symptoms. In the first section for three groups of positive symptoms (thought disorders, hallucinations, delusions), the patient answers how distracting these symptoms were during the month before the interview, and if he/she thinks that he/she is able to do something against them. Finally he/she was asked to select from a list of 13 coping reactions those he/she uses to cope with positive symptoms.

In relation to thought disorders and hallucinations, the most frequent answer about subjective burden and the patient's estimation, if he or she can do something against the symptom, was "I don't know". The main reason for this is that 73 (31.5%) of the first episode sample did not experience any hallucinations and 89 (38.4%) had no thought disorders yet. For others the psychotic symptoms probably have been experienced in such a way that they had no idea how to manage them. Actually, 53% of the patients did not know if thought disorders are burdening, and 47% gave this answer in relation to hallucinations. Of the sample, 31% experienced thought disorders as stressful in a strong or even very strong degree, and only 9% said those symptoms were not stressful or only stressful to some mild degree. Twenty-seven percent experienced hallucinations as strongly or very strongly burdening, and 14% rated them as only slightly stressful or not stressful at all. As delusional experiences had occurred in a high number of patients (95.7%), the "I don't know" answers are reduced but still occur in 18.5%. Of the sample, 61% had (very) stressful delusional experiences, and in only 11% of the patients were they not stressful or only stressful to some minor degree.

Of the sample, 27% had the opinion, they could do something to regulate thought disorders, 22% gave this answer in relation to hallucinations and 20% reported that regulation of delusional experience is possible. Those patients were asked which coping reaction they use in relation to thought disorders, hallucinations and delusions. A set of 13 possible coping reactions (see Table 4) was presented, and the patients answered by yes or no to indicate which one they use as coping strategy for the respective symptom. The coping strategies for the different positive symptoms are quite similar: for all three symptom groups, the most frequently used strategy was "I think what I could do about the

Table 3. Non-specific symptoms (subjective complaints)

Subjective complaints	Percentages			
	Complaints present		The most burdening	
	n	%	n	%
1. Reduced interest in activities	127	58.5	29	15.4
2. Reduced intensity of emotions	94	43.9	17	9.0
3. Tthinking and speaking more difficult	119	54.8	25	13.3
4. More difficult to concentrate	140	64.8	43	22.9
5. Reduced enjoyment in hobbies and activities	106	49.5	5	2.7
6. Difficulties in everyday activities like self care	84	38.5	16	8.5
7. lifficulties to remember	105	47.7	19	10.1
8. Increase of sadness and depression	105	48.2	34	18.1

total n (item nr.)
complaints present: n (1,3) = 217; n (2,5) =214; n (4) = 216; n (6,8) = 218; n (7) = 220 ;
most burdening: n = 189

Table 4. Coping reactions for the most burdening non-specific symptoms (= complaints) and for the most burdening everyday situation

Coping reactions	Non-specific symptom			Everyday situation		
	n	%	Val. %	n	%	Val. %
1. I avoid certain people and situations	51	22.0	29.3	91	39.2	45.5
2. I speak out my mind		35.8	48.0	104	44.8	52.8
3. I distract myself (by sports, reading, music, work, driving my car, etc.)	84	36.2	48.3	91	39.2	46.0
4. I wait until the situation changes	61	26.3	35.5	56	24.1	28.3
5. I try to change the situation in an active way	89	38.4	52.0	110	47.4	55.0
6. I think about the problem and evaluate the situation	73	31.5	42.7	87	37.5	44.2
7. I allow myself something enjoyable	72	31.0	46.6	72	31.0	36.5
8. I encourage myself	93	40.1	53.4	98	42.2	49.0
9. I say to myself that there are more important things in my life	51	22.0	29.7	65	28.0	33.0
10. I go to the doctor and take the medication (which he or she prescribes)	65	28.0	38.0	44	19.0	22.3
11. I think what I could do against the problem	88	37.9	50.9	117	50.4	58.8
12. I'm seeking for a rest inside by praying, meditation, exercises to relax	70	30.2	40.2	66	28.4	33.2
13. I try to make the best out of my situation	86	37.1	49.1	111	47.8	55.8

Missing data = I-don't-know answers

problem", and the less frequent one was "I say that there are more important things in life".

Coping with non-specific symptoms. In addition to the three positive symptoms, the IKB is concerned with coping behavior in the context of non-specific symptoms (Table 3). Aggravation during the last four weeks was assessed for eight representative and important negative and depressive symptoms. High percentages of the sample – between 38.5% for "difficulties in everyday activities like self-care" and 65% for "reduced ability to concentrate" – suffered from increasing severity of these symptoms during the last month. The patients were asked which of the eight symptoms was experienced as the most burdening. Most frequently (in 23% of cases) this was the "reduced ability to concentrate". This symptom did not only occur most often, but it was also the most burdening. Increasing "sadness and depression" was most burdening in 18% and "reduction of activities" in 15% of the sample. On the other hand, "loss of interest in hobbies" and "reduced abilities to fulfill everyday tasks like self-care" are only mentioned as the most burdening symptoms in less than 10% of the patients.

For the most burdening subjective complaint (i.e., non-specific symptom), all patients had to tell which of the 13 coping reactions they use to cope with. All coping reactions were mentioned by a considerable number of patients: between 22% (avoidance of certain people and situations) and 40% (encouraging oneself) of the sample said they apply these different coping reactions (Table 4). If patients with "I don't know" answers are excluded, positive answers to the coping reactions are between 29% and 53%.

Coping with everyday situations. The final part of the IKB presents eleven probably burdening everyday situations, leading to irritability and which also might have a worsening effect on psychiatric symptoms (Table 5).

The most burdening situation was "to be alone too much", indicated as such by 24% of the patients. Another four situations, all of them indicating problems in the relationship with other people like "criticism or rejection", "arguments or conflicts", "ambiguous situations", and "being patronized by others", were for 10% to 14% of the sample the most burdening situations. The minimum effect on symptom aggravation is expected for the "situation to talk while others are talking", but still 27% do expect this. The maximum expected symptom aggravation effect is 67% for "being on your own too much", which had already been mentioned as the most burdening situation. But more than half of the sample (58%) answered yes, when they were asked if they are able to do something against the most burdening situation. The coping reaction used most often is "I think what I could do against the problem", and the one with the minimum frequency is "to go to the doctor and take the medication". It is easy to understand that this answer is seldom for everyday situations, as the consultation of the doctor or the intake of medication seems – from the view of the patients – not to be an adequate measure against the problems mentioned. There is a lack of information that psychological or psychotherapeutic intervention is also probably available for these problems.

Table 5. Burdening everyday situations leading to irritability and symptom aggravation

Burdening everyday situations	Percentages			
	Symptom aggravation		The most burdening	
	n	%	n	%
1. Criticism or rejection	100	55.6	24	11.6
2. Arguments or conflicts	115	62.8	28	13.5
3. Intense emotions	67	45.9	16	7.7
4. Ambiguous situations	90	38.8	21	10.1
5. Exciting or upsetting topics	64	44.4	7	3.4
6. Being patronized by others	100	55.9	29	14.0
7. To talk while others are talking	35	26.9	6	2.9
8. To concentrate while others are busy and noisy	57	39.3	5	2.4
9. To work under pressure of time	93	62.4	15	7.2
10. Sudden change in daily routine	57	43.8	7	3.4
11. Being on your own too much	103	66.5	49	23.7

total n for answering the question about
symptom aggravation: n (1) = 180; n (2) = 183; n (3) = 146; n (4) = 181; n (5) = 144 ; n (6) 179;
                                     n (7) = 130; n (8) = 145; n (9) = 149; n (10) = 130; n (11) = 155;
n for the question about the most burdening situation: n = 207

IKB variables as dependent variables. The coping reactions presented in the IKB and offered to the patients as a representative list are quite different in nature: some seem to be rather passive, possibly aiming at relaxation and stress reduction, others are concerned with active behavior, which is not directly disease related. Some coping reactions are active and indicate a direct initiative against symptoms or problems. In a first attempt the 13 coping reactions were grouped on a passivity and activity dimension by the interviewers of our team. This attempt was in accordance with the result of a factor analysis with a forced 2-factor solution. But without restriction of the factor number and applying the Eigenwert criterion >1, three factors have been extracted [16]: one passivity factor and two activity factors, one for "non-directed activities", the other for "directed activities".

In the following analysis (in part III), a score is used to indicate the total number of coping reactions summed up over the five different situations: coping with thought disorders, hallucinations, delusions, distracting situations (non-specific symptoms) and burdening everyday situations. But in addition to this global score, sub-scores based on the result of the 3-factor solution are used: a sub-score for non-direct active, direct active and passive coping strategies was determined, and finally, a differences score of active and passive coping styles was computed and used as an additional dependent variable.

The relationship of variables of the early course and social support/coping at first admission (part III)

To study the relationship of variables characterizing the early course of the disease (e.g., age at onset, duration of the prodrome and duration of the psychotic phase, duration of the total early course from symptom onset until first admission) with indicators of coping and social support at the time of first admission, Product Moment Correlations (Pearson Correlations) were determined. To study the influence of the early course on the coping behavior and social network at the time of first admission, a regression analysis was conducted.

Correlations of variables of the early course and coping. The indicators of coping behavior did not correlate with the duration of the early course, but with the number of symptoms, irrespective of which indicator of coping behavior was used, the total number of coping reactions, active and directed reactions, active

Table 6. Variables of the early course and coping at first admission

a Pearson correlations (* p < 0.05; ** p < 0.01; ***p < 0.001)

Variables of the early course	Total coping repertory	Direct active coping	Non-direct active coping	Passive coping	Difference active – passive
Number of thought disorders	0.28 ***	0.24 ***	0.25 ***	0.25 ***	–
Number of hallucinations	0.29 ***	0.27 ***	0.25 ***	0.24 ***	–
Number of delusions	0.29 ***	0.25 ***	0.27 ***	0.24 ***	–
Number of non-specific symptoms	0.29 ***	0.30 ***	0.24 ***	0.25 ***	–
Number of negative symptoms	0.30 ***	0.31 ***	0.25 ***	0.24 ***	0.14 *
Number of positive symptoms	0.38 ***	0.34 ***	0.35 ***	0.33 ***	–
Number of social disabilities	0.31 ***	0.30 ***	0.28 ***	0.22 ***	0.14 *
Total number of symptoms	0.43 ***	0.42 ***	0.38 ***	0.35 ***	0.16 *

Duration of the prodrome; duration of the psychotic pre-phase; duration of the early course; age at symptom onset; age at psychotic onset; gender: no significant correlations

b Multiple regression analysis: beta weights (* p < 0.05; ** p < 0.01; ***p < 0.001)

Variables of the early course	Total coping repertory	Direct active coping	Non-direct active coping	Passive coping	Difference active – passive
Duration of the early course	–	-0.14 *	–	-0.15 *	–
Number of hallucinations	–	0.15 *	–	–	–
Number of non-specific symptoms	–0.27 *	–	–0.27 *	–	–
Total number of symptoms	0.64 ***	0.37 ***	0.59 ***	0.37 ***	0.17 *

Dduration of the prodrome; duration of the psychotic pre-phase; number of thought disorders; number of delusions; number of negative symptoms; number of positive symptoms; number of social disabilities; age at symptom onset; age at psychotic onset; gender: no significant beta weights indirect reactions or passive reactions – the Pearson Correlations were between 0.24 and 0.29 for the number of thought disorders, hallucinations and delusions, all significantly different from zero ($p < 0.001$). They are even somewhat higher for the total number of symptoms in the early course, the number of non-specific symptoms, the number of positive and negative symptoms and the number of social disabilities (Table 6). Only for the difference score of active and passive coping strategies were the correlations either not significant or somewhat reduced, compared to the other coping indices. The number of coping reactions does not correlate with age at onset, irrespective of the definition of onset, and it also is not influenced by gender. The maximum correlations resulted for the total number of symptoms with the total repertory of coping reactions ($r = 0.43$) and with actively directed coping reactions ($r = 0.42$). These results demonstrate that coping reactions are only influenced by symptom load and not by symptom duration or age at symptom onset. Coping strategies seem to be activated only when it is necessary due to the accumulation of symptoms.

Table 7. Variables of the early course and social network at first admission

a Pearson correlations (* $p < 0.05$; ** $p < 0.01$; ***$p < 0.001$)

Variables of the early course	Intact family net	Intact net outside the family	Intact total network	Number of help giving people	Total network density
Number of delusions	−0.16*	–	−0.13*	–	–
Number of positive symptoms	−0.18**	–	−0.14*	–	–
Age at symptom onset	0.24***	–	0.17**	–	–
Age at psychotic onset	0.31***	–	0.21***	–	–
Gender	0.18**	0.22***	0.26***	0.19**	0.25***

Duration of the prodrome; duration of the psychotic pre-phase; duration of the early course; number of thought disorders; number of hallucinations; number of non-specific symptoms; number of negative symptoms; number of social disabilities; total number of symptoms: no significant Pearson correlations

b Multiple regression analysis: beta weights (* $p<.05$; ** $p<.01$; ***$p<.001$)

Variables of the early course	Intact family net	Intact net outside the family	Intact total network	Number of help giving people	Total network density
Number of delusions	–	–	−0.14*	–	–
Number of positive symptoms	−0.30***	–	–	–	–
Total number of symptoms	0.23*	–	–	–	–
Age at symptom onset	–	–	–	−0.14*	–
Age at psychotic onset	0.32***	–	0.14*	–	–
Gender	–	0.21**	0.23**	0.20**	0.25**

Duration of the prodrome; duration of the psychotic pre-phase; duration of the early course; number of thought disorders; number of hallucinations; number of non-specific symptoms; number of negative symptoms; number of social disabilities: no significant beta weights

Correlations of variables of the early course and the social network. If a social network has some protective function, patients with an intact and functioning social network should come to treatment earlier, as assistance in a developing mental disorder should be of such a kind that some relative or friend should reinforce the help-seeking behavior of the risk person. But generally, there are no significant correlations of overall network density and duration of the sub-phases or the total early course. Only for an adequate family network – but not for the network outside the family – a low but negative correlation with the total number of positive symptoms ($r = -0.18$; $p < 0.01$) did result. As the intactness of the total social network depends from an intact network inside and outside the family, the correlation for the total network is reduced, but it still remains significant ($r = -0.14$ ($p < 0.05$). The correlations of age at onset and age at psychotic onset show that with growing age the network density is normally increased, and the positive correlations of network indicators and gender simply demonstrate the larger social networks of women (Table 7).

The correlations of the variables of the early course and densities of sub-networks make it clear that only for the partner do we find a negative correlation with delusions and total number of positive symptoms, whereas for the number of persons in the core family and total family are positive (Table 8).

Table 8. Variables of the early course and social sub-network at first admission

a Pearson correlations (* $p < 0.05$; ** $p < 0.01$; *** $p < 0.001$)

Variables of the early course	Partner	Core Family	Total family	Friends	Functional relations
Number of delusions	−0.14 *	0.14 *	–	–	–
Number of positive symptoms	−0.15 *	–	–	–	–
Age at symptom onset	0.25 ***	0.14 *	0.16 *	–	–
Age at psychotic onset	0.31 ***	0.18 **	0.17 **	–	–
Gender	0.22 ***	–	0.13 *	0.20 **	0.16 *

Duration of the prodrome; duration of the psychotic pre-phase; duration of the early course; number of thought disorders; number of hallucinations; number of non-specific symptoms; number of negative symptoms; number of social disabilities; total number of symptoms: no significant Pearson correlations

b Multiple regression analysis: beta weights (* $p<.05$; ** $p<.01$; *** $p<.001$)

Variables of the early course	Partner	Core Family	Total family	Friends	Functional relations
Number of delusions	−0.13 *	0.15 *	–	–	–
Psychotic onset	0.27 ***	0.20 ***	0.17 **	–	–
Gender	0.17 *	–	–	0.20 **	0.16 *

Duration of the prodrome; duration of the psychotic pre-phase; duration of the early course; number of thought disorders; number of hallucinations; number of non-specific symptoms; number of negative symptoms; number of positive symptoms; number of social disabilities; total number of symptoms; age at symptom onset: no significant beta weights

Multiple regression of the variables of the early course on coping at first admission. After the presentation of bivariate correlation coefficients, a regression analysis was conducted with indicators of age at onset, symptom severity and symptom duration in the early course as independent variables – which are at least to some degree redundant predictor variables – and indicators of coping strategies and social network variables as criteria (see Table 6b). The method of entering the predictors in the models was stepwise. The total number of symptoms in the early course was identified as a significant predictor for the different coping variables used in the analysis. For the total coping repertoire and for the number of indirect active strategies, the number of non-specific symptoms also are significant predictors, but with negative signs of the beta weights. This is an interesting result which shows that after controlling for the positive relationship of overall symptom load, the relation of non-specific symptoms indicates that people with more coping strategies have a lower number of non-specific symptoms. Also for the number of problem-oriented direct coping strategies and for the number of passive coping mechanism the duration of the early course is a significant predictor with negative beta weights. The active problem directed strategy is also determined by the number of hallucinations in the early course.

Multiple regression of the variables of the early course on social network and social support at first admission. Turning to the prediction of social network variables, we find in general that the number of family members and especially the presence of a partner are related to significant predictors in the early course (see Tables 7b and 8b), whereas for relationships outside the family, no such predictors are found. Gender did not play a role in the prediction of the coping strategies, but it is important for the density of the social network. In the regression analysis for the prediction of the network density, measures of the early course are related to the family network, but not to the network of friends and other persons outside the family. For mostly the same variables with significant correlations and significant beta weights with identical signs are found. Therefore, the interpretation of the results is generally the same. The intact network outside the family is only influenced by the patient's gender, as females usually have larger social networks, and woman are older at symptom onset and the social networks also grow with age.

■ Discussion and summary

In the ABC study, coping strategies and social network variables as possible protective factors were assessed for the first time at first admission. Unfortunately, there are no indicators of coping and social support at onset of the prodrome or at psychotic onset available in our data, and therefore it is not possible to demonstrate if and how coping style and social support will influence the early course, and if coping behavior and social network variables themselves will change as a consequence of the beginning psychosis. In the ABC first episode sample, all patients were psychotic. Therefore, it is not possible to study the influence of coping or social network variables on the risk for schizophrenia, and to study these variables as predictors of the duration of the untreated psychosis (DUP) or the duration of the untreated illness (DUI). It only is possible to test if certain coping styles and social network conditions at first admission are associated with several aspects of the prodromal or psychotic pre-phase.

Based on the analysis of variables of social interaction and the quality and availability of key persons, we concluded that most of the patients were able to mention several close persons, whom they can trust and where they find help and understanding. Most key persons belong to the core family, and the relationships are of a long duration and of a high stability. The key persons are available either always or most often, they are in reach, and most of them living in the same town. Personal contacts take place very often, either daily or at least once a week. Therefore, for the time of first admission, the social network of the patients – at least as one relates to very close key persons – seems to be rather intact. On the other hand, we have no data to compare patients and normal controls to demonstrate, whether social networks in beginning schizophrenia are comparable to networks in healthy people of the same age and gender and with a comparable socio-economic background, or if there are already some negative influences of the developing disease already demonstrable in first admitted schizophrenic patients. Häfner et al. [8, 9] demonstrated that the proportion of patients with work or own income, and with a partner are comparable to a control sample from the healthy population when patients experienced their symptom onset, but there was a growing disadvantage of the schizophrenic group over time and during the early course, with a stagnation in the younger age groups and a remarkable decline of the social status in the older subgroup of the ABC sample, in comparison to the further positive social development in the control sample. Similar processes in the early course are plausible in relation to the social network variables, the presence of people who offer help in difficult situations and probably in the repertory of active and passive strategies to cope with difficult situations.

■ References

1. Andrews K, Pfanmatter M, Garst F, Teschner C, Brenner HD (2000) Effects of a coping-oriented group therapy for schizophrenia and schizoaffective patients: a pilot study. Acta Psychiatrica Scandinavica 101: 318–322
2. Boschi J, Adams RE, Bromet EJ, Lavelle JE, Everett E, Galambos N (2000) Coping with psychotic symptoms in the early phase of schizophrenia. American Journal of Orthopsychiatry 70: 242–252
3. Braun-Scharm H (2001) Coping bei schizophrenen Jugendlichen. Praxis der Kinderpsychologie und Kinderpsychiatrie 50: 104–118
4. Buchanan J (1995) Social support and schizophrenia: a review of the literature. Archives of Psychiatric Nursing 9: 68–76
5. Häfner H, Riecher A, Meissner S, Maurer K (1992a) Interview zur retrospektiven Einschätzung des Erkrankungsbeginns (IRAOS). Selbstverlag, Mannheim
6. Häfner H, Riecher-Rössler A, Fätkenheuer B, Maurer K, Meissner S, Löffler W (1992b) Interview for the retrospective assessment of the onset of schizophrenia (IRAOS). Translation: G. Patton, Selbstverlag, Mannheim

7. Häfner H, Maurer K, Löffler W, Riecher-Rössler A (1993) The influence of age and sex on the onset and early course of schizophrenia. British Journal of Psychiatry 162: 80–86

8. Häfner H, Maurer K, Löffler W, Bustamante S, an der Heiden W, Riecher-Rössler A, Nowotny B (1995) Onset and early course of schizophrenia. In: Häfner H, Gattaz WF (eds) Search for the Causes of Schizophrenia. Vol. III. Springer, Berlin Heidelberg New York, pp 41–66

9. Häfner H, Nowotny B, Löffler W, an der Heiden W, Maurer K (1995) When and how does schizophrenia produce social deficits? European Archives of Psychiatry and Clinical Neuroscience 246: 17–28

10. Häfner H, Löffler W, Maurer K, Riecher-Rössler A, Stein A (1999) IRAOS. Interview für die retrospektive Erfassung des Erkrankungsbeginns und -verlaufs bei Schizophrenie und anderen Psychosen. Verlag Hans Huber, Bern Göttingen Toronto Seattle

11. Hultman CM, Wieselgren IM, Ohman A (1997) Relationships between social support, social coping and life events in the relapse of schizophrenic patients. Scandinavian Journal of Psychology 38: 3–13

12. Jenner JA, van de Willige G, Wiersma D (1998) Effectiveness of cognitive therapy with coping training for persistent auditory hallucinations: a retrospective study of attenders of a psychiatrist out-patient department. Acta Psychiatrica Scandinavica 98: 384–389

13. Lalonde P, Lesage A, Comtois G, Morin C, Likavcanova W, L'Ecuyer G (1996) Strategies de coping la schizophrenie. L'Encephale 22: 240–246

14. Leclerc C, Lesage AD, Ricard N, Lecompte T, Cyr M (2000) Assessment of a new rehabilitative coping skills module for persons with schizophrenia. American Journal of Orthopsychiatry 70: 380–388

15. Maurer K, Häfner H (1995) Methodological aspects of onset assessment in schizophrenia. Schizophrenia Research 15: 265–276

16. Maurer K, Häfner H (1998) The impact of coping abilities on the development of schizophrenia. In: Lopez-Ibor JJ, Lieh-Mak F, Visotsky HM, Maj M (eds) One World, One Language – Paving the Way to Better Perspectives for Mental Health. Proceedings of the X World Congress of Psychiatry. Hogrefe & Huber Publishers, pp 228–239

17. McNally SE, Goldberg JO (1997) Natural cognitive coping strategies in schizophrenia. British Journal of Medical Psychology 70: 159–167

18. Salokangas RKR (1996) Living situation and social network in schizophrenia. A prospective 5-year follow-up study. Nordic Journal of Psychiatry 50: 35–42

19. Salokangas RKR (1997) Living situation, social network and outcome in schizophrenia: a five-year prospective follow-up study. Acta Psychiatrica Scandinavica 96: 459–468

20. Sayer J, Ritter S, Gournay K (2000) Beliefs about voices and their effects on coping strategies. Journal of Advanced Nursing 31: 1199–1205

21. Stark FM, Stolle R (1994) Schizophrenie: Subjektive Krankheitstheorien. Eine explorative Studie. Teil I: Patienten. Psychiatrische Praxis 21: 74–78

22. Thurm I, Häfner H (1987) Perceived vulnerability, relapse risk and coping in schizophrenia. An explorative study. European Archives of Psychiatry and Neurological Science 237: 46–53

23. Thurm-Mussgay I, Galle K, Rey E-R (1987) Interview zur Krankheitsbewältigung (IKB). Unveröffentlichte Version

24. Thurm-Mussgay I, Galle K, Häfner H (1991) Krankheitsbewältigung Sxchizophrener: Ein theoretisches Konzept zur Erfassung und erste Erfahrungen mit einem neuen Messinstrument. Verhaltenstherapie 1: 293–300

25. Veiel HOF (1990) The Mannheim Interview on Social Support. Reliability and validity data from three samples. Social Psychiatry and Psychiatric Epidemiology 25: 250-259

26. Wiersma D, Jenner JA, van den Willige G, Spakman M, Nienhuis FJ (2001) Cognitive behaviour therapy with coping training for persistent auditory hallucinations in schizophrenia: a naturalistic follow-up study of the durability of effects. Acta Psychiatrica Scandinavica 103: 393–399

27. Wykes T, Parr AM, Landau S (1999) Group treatment of auditory hallucinations. Exploratory study of effectiveness. British Journal of Psychiatry 175: 180–185

Discussion: protective interventions in schizophrenia

F. Resch
Dept. of Child and Adolescent Psychiatry, University of Heidelberg, Germany

It is indeed a great honor and pleasure to discuss these three outstanding papers on psychotherapeutic aspects of schizophrenia within the framework of early prevention.

According to Dr. Tarrier's notion cognitive behavior therapy has a high impact on positive symptoms in acute and chronic conditions of schizophrenia and especially in patients with persistent symptomatology after a drug therapy trial. But in the long run, cognitive behavior therapy seems to be equally effective with supportive counseling compared to standard procedures of routine care. Could this mean, that a positive *interpersonal relationship* constitutes the most striking working factor in psychotherapy of schizophrenia – and psychoeducative elements may exert specific additional influences upon particular psychological features? Noteworthy, this question is part of an ongoing "psychotherapy debate" [7]. Taking relationship aspects for serious, one could argue about psychodynamic approaches to psychotherapy of psychoses anew: at this point an activity of the International Society for Psychological Approaches to Therapy of Schizophrenia (ISPS) may be announced. ISPS is promoting a task force under the leading authorship of Tor Larsen (Stavanger) concerning the evidence that relationship-focused therapies do have clinical effects.

Could it be proposed that a therapeutic relationship could also be performed by other members of the therapeutic team than medical doctors or psychologists giving way to nurses or social workers – if they are trained enough? This fact could have high impact on therapeutic management in the future!

In the family therapy approaches we notice different formats of intervention. Dr. Klingberg does not only focus on the individual family unit, but also includes other relatives' groups, multiple family groups and parallel patients and family groups. In fact, various family interventions do seem to have a positive impact on the course of schizophrenia. We notice a development of pathogenetic concepts from blaming the parents for dysfunctional behavior causing patients' behavior – like Bateson's [1] concept of double-bind communication or the early expressed emotion-concepts of Vaughn and Leff [6] – to a more sophisticated view of recognizing parents and their emotional reactions as mirrors of the patient!

Modern views of pervasive developmental disorders like autism and schizophrenia do not blame the parents any more – on the contrary – people are concerned with the heavy burden mothers and fathers of schizophrenics carry with them in caring for their inflicted children! Expressed-emotions patterns of critical and over-involved attitudes may be the expression of special concern and care for the patient more reflecting the deteriorating state of health than an independent atmospheric factor of relapse. Expressed-emotions patterns of critique and over-involvement seem to be reactive, secondary communicative structures and provide information about parents' response tendencies and symptoms of the patients. While emotional over-involvement of mothers seems to be associated with increased risk of relapse, its the critical component of fathers that may be part of the relapse pattern in the families, like King [3] pointed out recently. These new vistas have a revolutionary impact on work with the families in cases of schizophrenia – because they force us to look quite thoroughly upon differential aspects of verbal and nonverbal communication. In one of our pilot studies [4], expressed emotion in adolescent schizophrenics and key relative interactions were addressed considering emotional aspects of verbal behavior and head positions. Fifteen adolescent patients with schizophrenia or schizoaffective psychosis in an age range from 14 to 21 years (9 males, 6 females) were examined during a 10-minute dialogue with a key relative. Healthy adolescents matched for age and sex served as controls in a dialogue with their relative. Expressed emotion was assessed with a 5-minute speech sample. In addition, nonverbal interaction was assessed with the Berne System for assessment of nonverbal interaction according to Frey [2]. The expressed emotion level of key relatives indicates indifferent nonverbal behaviors between schizophrenic and nonschizophrenic adolescents. Schizophrenic patients with highly emotionally expressure parents present a very prominent pattern of refusal behavior by turning their head away, negating open communication. Whereas normal adolescents do not spend more time in looking away from their parents, even if they are high-EE compared to low-EE. So dysfunctional nonverbal behavior as a form of drawback from face-to-face communication seems to be increased in schizophrenic adolescents with high-EE parents.

The actual psychosocial context of the schizophrenic person remains important. There is an ongoing vulnerability that has to be addressed. As Dr. Maurer points out clearly, we know that cognitive and neurobehavioral variables interact with social environmental factors in the development of prodromal phase symptomatology. Concluding from the information of the three papers, we may propose an integrative model of the psychotic transition process: three domains of schizophrenic vulnerability may be described: a cognitive deficit consisting of impairments in associative thinking, deficits of working memory and several other disturbances of thought and language go together with disorders of attention and deficits of complex memory function. Another basic deficit can be detected in affective regulatory processes. Abnormal affectedness and hyperarousal may have a negative impact on cognitive processes by inducing mental states of negative emotions. Last but not least, a deficit in communication can be described. Schizophrenics do show problems with reading affective signals and seem to have a tendency to misinterpret social contexts. They lack and avoid social contact and present with difficulties in the establishment of social relationships [5]. These cognitive emotional and communicative deficits constitute a vicious circle of schizophrenic pathogenesis. Basic deficits of appraisal

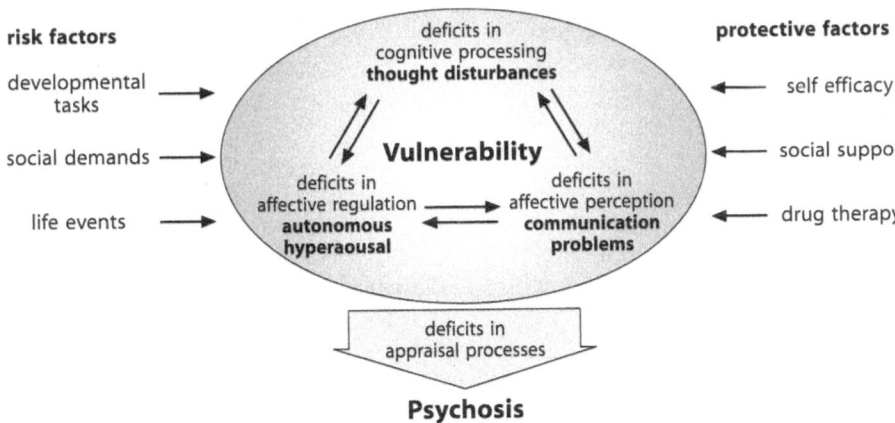

Fig. 1. The vulnerability hypothesis

processes concerning the establishment of meaning in a world of uncertainty characterize the psychotic process (see Fig. 1).

We cannot hinder the world from inflicting our patients: developmental tasks, social demands and life events will take their toll. But what we have learned from todays' presentations is that psychosocial therapies may exert protective influences on the patient, in the domains of self-regulation and communication. These two domains seem to represent the basic targets of psychopreventive strategies.

The following questions have to be raised:

■ What kind of therapy do we need?
■ How specific should therapy be?
■ How can therapy be applied in relation to the psychotic process?
■ When to perform the right therapy in the right context?

■ References

1. Bateson G (1981) Oekologie des Geistes. Anthropologische, psychologische, biologische und epistemologische Perspektiven. Frankfurt: Suhrkamp
2. Frey S, Hirsbrunner HP, Pod J, Daw W (1981) Das Berner-System zur Untersuchung nonverbaler Interaktion: Die Erhebung des Rohdatenprotokolls. In: Winkler P (ed) Methoden der Analyse von face-to-face-Situationen. Stuttgart: Metzler-Verlag, pp 203–236
3. King S (2000) Is expressed emotion cause or effect in the mothers of schizophrenic young adults? Schizophrenia Research 45 (1-2): 65–78
4. Ramsauer B (2001) Expressed Emotion (EE) in Interaktion jugendlicher schizophrener Patienten mit Angehörigen unter Berücksichtigung emotionaler Aspekte des Verbal- und Kopfpositionierungsverhaltens. Aachen: Shaker
5. Resch F, Parzer P, Brunner R, Koch E (2002) Early detection of Psychosis and preventive Strategies in Adolescence. In: Brenner HD, Strik WK, Genner R (eds) Preventive Intervention in Schizophrenia. Bern: Hogrefe und Huber (in press)
6. Vaughn CE, Leff JP (1976) The measurement of expressed emotion in the families of psychiatric patients. British Journal of Psychiatry 121: 241–258
7. Wampold BE (2001) The Great Psychotherapy debate. Models, Methods and Findings. London, New Jersey: Lawrence L. Baum Associates

Developments and Perspectives

Risk and protective factors in schizophrenia. Towards a conceptual model of the disease process

P. B. Jones
Department of Psychiatry, University of Cambridge, Addenbrooke's Hospital, Cambridge, U.K.

With 20 papers presented, and 7 discussants leading lively debate and exchange of views, the conference achieved much, despite not agreeing on a new or satisfactory model of schizophrenia. However, much was learned about the design of such a model of the disease process. It must incorporate dynamic mechanisms operating over the lifecourse, it must be realistically complex, and it must be based upon interactions between genetics, environment, neurobiology and behavior. Understanding and acknowledging what we do not yet know is as important as synthesising islands of certainty, and not understanding the determinants of normal variation remains an important lacuna.

In the final session, we discussed interpretations of words and phrases in the conference title and the task that it set. All had been used in a number of ways, reflecting the diversity of approaches and the enormous task of considering an explanatory model. Risk factors, for instance, were originally conceived as pointers towards causal factors, with a variety of frameworks being developed to aid the process of inferential judgement regarding causation [1, 6]. However, the field of prediction and prevention uses risk factor in a different way, as something pointing towards an outcome rather than backwards towards a cause. Several causal models have been assumed in the presentations, where individual characteristics act as indicators of outcome or true modifiers of risk. Other models had been predicated upon notions of necessary versus sufficient causes, with no such models being found to be applicable to schizophrenia. Stress-vulnerability models had been debated, particularly by Verdoux, van Os, and Parnas, in which predisposing, precipitating and perpetuating causes supported the longitudinal view of the disease process that is current, and that was generally supported by the conference. The important, German contributions on the early manifestations, prodromal features and course are the clinical aspect to this formulation.

The important, but often neglected fact that the strength or importance of a causal factor may depend upon its prevalence became apparent in the presentations from Harrison and Mortenson when considering possible environmental factors. When these factors are common, then other factors may determine disease outcome or be rate-limiting, necessary factors, for example Rose's [4] point. His illustration was lung cancer: if everybody smoked, then bronchial tumors would appear to be a genetic disorder determined on the basis of vulnerability genes. Finally, many presenters and discussants, including those above, emphasised the importance of longitudinal models where causal constellations [5] build up over time.

The characteristics of protective factors were an exciting aspect of the conference. Moreover, these protective factors were not considered merely in terms of absence of risk, but as true, additional and malleable characteristics, both physiological and psychological, that are amenable to manipulation. The links to the important concept of psychological resilience were made by Done, and the possible role of protective genes and pleiotropy covered by Weiser.

Thus, the conference took care to consider models in a conceptual sense, but, rather perversely, did not take the opportunity to debate the nature of schizophrenia. Perhaps this was just a step too far, or maybe we felt we needed to turn our backs on that nosological swamp and keep to firmer ground. There was consensus that a longitudinal view of disease processes means that schizophrenia can be considered as an outcome, or perhaps as a transitory expression of an underlying process. The debate was far from the phenomenological views of schizophrenia that characterised the initial descriptions of the disease. However, we were reminded of the cognitive psychological approach taken by Kraepelin and Bleuler and its reflection in current views of a cognitive endophenotype for the disorder. This begged the question of the cognitive basis of normal behaviour and a recurring theme for the conference that much more needed to be known concerning the broad church of normality before the determinants of abnormality could be fully understood.

In the light of this general discussion, how did conceptual models change? There was consensus about the importance of *dynamic* models that evolve over time; the whole concept of a risk factor is a longitudinal one involving prior action. However, rather than only the one-to-one relationship between cause and outcome, the phenotype was considered as a punctuation or definition of a life-course trajectory. This is important because it implies the same abnormal or vulnerable underlying processes acting before and after disease expression. This allows for considerable dynamism for many years before schizophrenia is manifest, and models involving both abnormal trajectories and transitions between trajectories. Thus, there are many changes to be understood, and that may be amenable to intervention.

The idea as to how complex a useful model of schizophrenia will most likely be was raised by a comment from Harrison, who noted that epidemiological and social approaches had been put at the beginning of the conference programme. Discussion included the fact that a useful and realistically complex model of the disorder has to account for all, or at least a large proportion of, characteristics. There is no room for hierarchical approaches in terms of social models being trumped by physiological or psychological models. An adequate model needs to explain why schizophrenia is more common in migrant groups (see Harrison, this volume) and why it is more common in urban settings (Mortenson, this volume), just as much as it needs to explain why ectopic pre-alpha cells occur in the parahippocampal gyrus (Falkai, this volume).

The conference acknowledged that *complete* understanding must explain all aspects of the disorder. Even if this is not a realistic expectation now, it is a necessary aim. Whilst any one area may produce a step-change or paradigm shift in understanding, no single area can be primary in terms of *complete* understanding. In our current, intermediate situation, the conference acknowledged that clear statements of what is not understood are, perhaps, more important than aiming for naïve and overarching models that may result in new ideas being stifled rather than fostered.

Aspects of this complexity were captured in several areas of the conference. Interactions between different types of risk factor were the subject of several different presentations. Verdoux, Parnas, van Os, Falkai, and Tienari all ranged over the various combinations of interactions between genes, environment, family and behavioural factors that mould the normal mind. Harrison reminded us of the importance of the longitudinal view, where changes in behaviour can alter the immediate environment of an individual, leading to further deviation through a variety of mechanisms; something referred to previously as a self-perpetuating cascade [3]. A variety of seemingly trivial events may trigger the transitions referred to earlier, and define outcome in a distant part of the lifecourse; a new, chaotic view that was addressed in structural terms by Schröder. These are all examples of the realistic complexity that we must build into new conceptual models of schizophrenia.

There were two important contributions concerning genetics, important because they pointed us away from the original ideas of psychiatric disorders being due to single gene effects. Maier reviewed the area and pointed out that the evidence is heavily against schizophrenia as a single gene disorder, rather, the evidence suggests, multiple genes of small effect. This model leads us away from the idea of "bad genes". Rather, different combinations of genes have different effects, and, again, may interact with events, environmental or behavioural, that are themselves trivial but, in combination with the particular genetic diathesis, lead towards bad outcomes. An analogy might be genes as individual playing cards being dealt as a hand. None of the cards is, *per se*, good or bad, but their combination leads to a good or bad hand. Interactive effects, such as calling one suit of cards as a trump, can radically change the importance of individual cards, suits or combinations. The contribution from Jones suggested that different sets of cognitive strategies that develop to subsume particular tasks (on which there may be evolutionary pressure) may be understood as continuous risk factors for schizophrenia in the same way

The second contribution introducing new models of genetic effects came from Peter Falkai, who not only introduced new developments within neuropathology, but also the new technologies of functional genomics and proteomics. Thus, we are now able to go beyond thinking of the presence or absence of a gene, or whether it is abnormal in probabilistic terms. We can now assess the expression of genes in terms of messenger RNA, and their protein products, including the myriad of post-translational changes.

This "new, new genetics" will lead to a mushrooming of facts and findings, much as resulted from the new technologies in imaging that we have seen over the last 30 years. We will, therefore, have a new vocabulary to add to models of schizophrenia. However, along with these new facts and findings we need a conceptual model as to how the formation of proteins can lead to schizophrenia. We have realised for some time that genes code for proteins, not for delusions and hallucinations [2], bur incorporating this truism into a model is not straightforward.

These developments lead to two aspects that we may wish to incorporate into our models of the disease process in schizophrenia. First, genes do not recognise the neck in terms of the powerful and malign influence that this anatomical structure has on medical thought; physical disease and mental disorder have long been foreign lands to each other. However, all cells, other than gametes and the vagaries of mitochondrial DNA, contain all genes. An abnormality in gene expression, protein folding, or other post-translational change may be manifest in the brain and elsewhere in the body. Thus, the phenotypes for which we search may involve mental and physical manifestations. The presentation by Weiser on the Israeli conscript study, showing that diabetes and asthma could be associated with psychological traits (intelligence) and with mental disorder may demonstrate this, assuming a genetic mechanism is involved.

The second consequence of the new, new genetics is that we may find unexpected, cross-cutting mechanisms that link some risk factors to disease. Gattaz demonstrated a strong association between early-life exposure to meningitis and subsequent schizophrenia in adult life. This hypothesis-led investigation, along with other work concerning early-life risk factors, suggests a mechanism concerning oxidative stress. It may be that vulnerability to oxidative stress could be a mechanism linking this risk factor with the schizophrenia phenotype.

Such an idea leads to thoughts of new interventions, and the conference enjoyed a range of presentations concerning the possibility that these may include neuro-protective agents (see Siren and Behl). Already becoming established in other disease areas, their efficacy in schizophrenia would lead to important advances in therapy alongside fundamental changes in the way that we would understand this disorder (see Kulkani). The section on psycho-protective factors (see contributions by Klingberg, Tarrier and Maurer) further stressed the importance of complexity in a complete conceptual model of schizophrenia. It must encompass processes operating after the first signs of psychosis that affect recovery and outcome, rather than those beforehand that are seen in terms of risk of onset. My own view is that we should look for continuity of these processes and that there may be more parsimony present than is obvious from the way that different approaches claim different areas. The conference was fortunate having two sections on protection, one biological and the second largely psychosocial to remind participants that both approaches are be required for a broad understanding.

In conclusion, we know much more at the end of our conference than at the beginning about the specifications of new models of schizophrenia. We know that we have far to go in understanding normal variation and its determinants before we can interpret the causes and mechanisms for a disease state such as schizophrenia. We know that the determinants of schizophrenia will not only be many and various, but that they will interact with each other. Sometimes, perhaps rarely, this will result in psychosis, and sometimes, perhaps more commonly, in other probably unexpected phenotypes; some of these will be within the range of normal variation, others will not. Longitudinal processes are important, and these combinations and interactions may evolve over long periods of time, perhaps with schizophrenia but one, age-dependant outcome or manifestation of endophenotypes. In this complex situation we are unlikely soon to have a complete model of schizophrenia. Serendipity will play a part in our progress, but working at the interface between our traditional approaches and listening to others working in distant fields will most likely result in new understanding and hypotheses.

▓ References

1. Hill AB (1965) The environment and disease: association or causation? Procedings of the Royal Society of Medicine 58: 295–300
2. Jones P, Murray RM (1991) The genetics of schizophrenia is the genetics of neurodevelopment. British Journal of Psychiatry 158: 615–623
3. Jones PB, Rodgers B, Murray RM, Marmot MG (1994) Child developmental risk factors for adult schizophrenia in the British 1946 birth cohort. Lancet 344: 1398–1402
4. Rose G (1992) The Strategy of Preventive Medicine. Oxford: Oxford University Press
5. Rothman KJ (1976) Causes. American Journal of Epidemiology 104: 587–592
6. Susser MW (1991) What is a cause and how do we know one? American Journal of Epidemiology 133: 635–648